A CULTURAL HISTORY
OF MEDICINE

VOLUME 5

A Cultural History of Medicine
General Editor: Roger Cooter

A CULTURAL HISTORY
OF MEDICINE

IN THE AGE
OF EMPIRE

Edited by Jonathan Reinarz

BLOOMSBURY ACADEMIC

LONDON • NEW YORK • OXFORD • NEW DELHI • SYDNEY

BLOOMSBURY ACADEMIC
Bloomsbury Publishing Plc
50 Bedford Square, London, WC1B 3DP, UK
1385 Broadway, New York, NY 10018, USA
29 Earlsfort Terrace, Dublin 2, Ireland

BLOOMSBURY, BLOOMSBURY ACADEMIC and the Diana logo are trademarks
of Bloomsbury Publishing Plc

First published in Great Britain 2021
This paperback edition first published 2024

A catalogue record for this book is available from the British Library.

Library of Congress Cataloging-in-Publication Data
Names: Cooter, Roger, editor.
Title: A cultural history of medicine / general editor, Roger Cooter.
Description: London ; New York : Bloomsbury Academic, 2021. |
Series: The cultural histories series | Includes bibliographical references and index. |
Identifiers: LCCN 2020051490 | ISBN 9781472569936 (hardback)
Subjects: LCSH: Medicine–History.
Classification: LCC R131 .C78 2021 | DDC 610.9—dc23
LC record available at https://lccn.loc.gov/2020051490

ISBN: HB: 978-1-4725-6989-9
         Set: 978-1-4725-6987-5
         PB: 978-1-3504-5161-2
         Set: 978-1-3504-5164-3

Series: The Cultural Histories Series

Typeset by RefineCatch Limited, Bungay, Suffolk
Printed and bound in Great Britain

To find out more about our authors and books visit www.bloomsbury.com
and sign up for our newsletters.

CONTENTS

ILLUSTRATIONS

CHAPTER 2

CHAPTER 3

CHAPTER 4

CHAPTER 5

CHAPTER 8

GENERAL EDITOR'S PREFACE

ROGER COOTER

The cultural history of medicine is all embracing. Virtually nothing can be excluded from it – the body in all its literary and other representations over time, ideas of civilization and humankind, and the sociology, anthropology and epistemology of health and welfare, not to mention the existential experiences of pain, disease, suffering and death and the way professionals have endeavoured to deal with them. To contain much of this vastness, the volumes in this series focus on eight categories, all of contemporary relevance: Environment, Food, Disease, Animals, Objects, Experience, Mind/Brain and Authority. From the ancient through to the postmodern world these themes are pursued with critical breadth, depth and novelty by dedicated experts. Transnational perspectives are widely entertained. Above all, these volumes attend to and illuminate what exactly is a *cultural* history of medicine, a category of investigation and an epistemological concept that has its emergence in the 1980s.

Introduction: Culturing Medicine in the Age of Empire

JONATHAN REINARZ

On 10 June 1883, as New York was in the midst of a new diphtheria epidemic, the disease claimed another young victim in what now averaged an annual death toll of 1,000, a mortality rate of 48.6 per thousand deaths. An upper-respiratory tract infection most fatal among children under the age of five, diphtheria appeared to spread indiscriminately through the 40-square-mile island of Manhattan and its toll would not abate for several more years. On this particular Sunday, seven-year-old Ernst Jacobi and his younger sister, Mary, who had repeatedly been stricken with diphtheria, were again confined to their beds. The first of his father's seven children to live past the seventh birthday, Ernst was expected to recover as he had already survived the most vulnerable years of infancy. But infections like diphtheria were unpredictable and continued to carry off children from rich and poor households alike, whether in urban or rural districts. Yet this conceptualization of the disease was about to alter as dramatically as the Jacobi family. In 1883, and following Dr Robert Koch's postulates, the four criteria designed to establish a causative relationship between a microbe and a disease, the German-Swiss pathologist Edwin Klebs had fulfilled two of these key suppositions in an emerging field of biomedical research by isolating and growing the club-shaped bacterium responsible for the disease. Koch had performed a similar test in 1877 when he isolated the bacillus that causes anthrax; soon after, he identified the mycobacterium causing tuberculosis (TB) and, as

Klebs toiled away in his lab, and Ernst died in bed in Manhattan, Koch was en route to investigate an outbreak of cholera in Egypt. In the case of diphtheria, the third postulate, which Klebs found so difficult to verify, was eventually confirmed by Koch's student, Friedrich Loeffler, who publicized his ability to communicate the disease to animals (in this case, guinea pigs, rabbits and small birds) the following year. However, unable to locate the bacillus outside the immediate injection site, Loeffler put forth his own 'postulate', namely that death in the case of diphtheria was likely caused by some other substance, possibly a toxin. His hypothesis was eventually confirmed in 1888 in another laboratory, in Paris, where Louis Pasteur's colleagues – Emile Roux, who also investigated cholera in Egypt, and one of Pasteur's pupils, Alexandre Yersin, who had visited Koch's Institute in Berlin – demonstrated that the bacillus was accompanied by especially potent toxins. Antitoxin trials, validated by quantitative measurements, followed in 1894 and the bacteriological explanation for diphtheria, not to mention some dozen other infectious diseases, including anthrax, TB, cholera and plague, rapidly began to transform established narratives of medicine, let alone infectious disease, in the closing years of the nineteenth century.

It is now recognized that the work undertaken in Berlin, Paris and other research centres, dependent on laboratory inquiry and clinical examination, and not least a new coded language of disease investigation, paved the way for modern bacteriology. Unfortunately, these findings came too late to save Ernst, or any of the 43,000 other fatalities in New York attributed to diphtheria between 1866 and 1890 (Cone 1979: 109). Instead, Ernst was laid to rest in a plot situated in 478 acres of gently rolling ground in Brooklyn's Green-Wood Cemetery alongside two of his father's previous wives and five other children. A further memorial to Ernst was erected by his parents on the shores of Lake George on Hiawatha Island in Tioga County, New York, which Ernst's father visited on each subsequent anniversary of his son's death (Bittel 2009: 171). Ernst's passing had a tremendous impact on his father; his mourning was 'profound and lengthy' (171), despite his evident familiarity with death. Not only were fatalities, such as Ernst's, ubiquitous in the nineteenth century, but similar stories of morbidity and mortality are regularly recounted in the opening pages of countless histories of medicine, with such emotional illness narratives often being related by scholars determined to reconstruct the patient's, rather than the practitioner's, perspective of illness. However, Ernst, as any parent might claim about their progeny, was no ordinary child. To begin with, his long-grieving father was Abraham Jacobi (1830–1919), regarded by many to be the 'father' of American paediatrics. His mother was also a physician, the scientist and reformer Mary Putnam Jacobi (1834–1906), the first woman to graduate from Paris's École de Médecine and one of the earliest American women to qualify in medicine. As such, Ernst's case sheds light on more than just the experience of illness in 1880s New York; his story has the unique potential to open an alternative perspective on medicine's past, one encapsulating the culture that came to define an epoch spanning more than a century and described here as the 'age of empire'.

Like other medical moments, aspects of which have been explored by at least three generations of medical historians, it appears ripe for reinterpretation.[1] The diverse accounts spawned by this tragic episode, emerging from documents produced by medical practitioners, journalists and Ernst's parents, and republished in newspapers, periodicals and scholarly studies, comprise a rich collection of cultural symbols or signs, both written and visual, that signify the ideology of a world we have lost, but regularly revisit and repeatedly reconstruct from our own contemporary perspectives. Each time scholars have done so, they have highlighted new elements of the tale or left out others, for medicine's stories, like those composed by historians generally, are now recognized to be culturally-contingent constructions and therefore rich in meaning when carefully examined. The world into which Ernst Jacobi was born, for example, understood diphtheria in terms of 'fever nests' and 'miasma', yet the early twentieth century one in which his parents died, imagined it as one of 'germs' and 'carriers'.[2] One might even argue that the emotionally charged stories of sickness and suffering are especially suited to such detailed 'thick description', a technique regularly employed by cultural historians and most often associated with the anthropologist Clifford Geertz. Over many decades, Geertz and other anthropologists in particular have tutored scholars in the ways such singular or seemingly unusual events might be employed to access more generalizable patterns of historical circumstance. In Geertz's own research, the specific ritual of the Balinese cock fight was employed to illustrate the workings of an entire culture.[3] Through an analysis of the symbolic dimensions comprising the Jacobi's lives, one might similarly plunge into the ideologies, mentalities and science that characterized a particular age in its most fully emotionalized form (Geertz 1973: 30). Historians of medicine will recognize the wider meanings of Ernst's story, despite it being in no sense 'typical'. Its value comes from being a mutually intelligible network of signs, the various components of which can be methodically unpacked in order to explore the changing cultural framework of a nineteenth-century mindset, let alone its medical practices.

My decision to place diphtheria centre stage, on the other hand, may seem unusual, for this infection is not usually described as the quintessential nineteenth-century disease, as plague had been for the fourteenth – that crown has been bestowed on cholera (Rosenberg 1962: 1) – but it could be. By the end of the nineteenth century, an army of microbiologists and public health experts successfully applied the principles of germ theory to its diagnosis, treatment and prevention, thereby heralding a new bacteriological approach to disease. The lessons of this endeavour were then successively and successfully applied to 'fight' (and historians use such military expressions intentionally) other diseases. While diphtheria had undoubtedly claimed lives since antiquity and was responsible for numerous previous epidemics, such as the 'malady of bladders in the windpipe' described by American minister Cotton Mather in the early 1700s, it was the French doctor and founder of the medical school at Tours, Pierre Bretonneau (1778–1862), who employed the methods of the Paris school to distinguish the disease from scarlet fever in 1826 and gave it a new name. Bretonneau had examined the disease outside Tours' hospital clinic (1818–21), describing its initial appearance in military barracks and subsequent rampage through neighbouring quarters of the city. Although cholera has become a far more familiar character in historical studies in recent years – thanks to the work of some of the field's most respected practitioners,[4] who have described its far more class-specific impact on populations in even more densely packed cities from Europe to Japan, and its defiance of national borders thanks to improved and more rapid networks of trade and communication – diphtheria might equally be employed as a disease that defined the long nineteenth century. Certainly from the 1850s, when the child had entered its modern sentimental significance and diphtheria took greater hold on French and British populations, it exercised a particularly tight grip on the throats of children, who were frequently suffocated by the disease's characteristic pseudo-membrane that formed in victims' larynx. Although its local pathology continued to confuse investigators, many regarded the disease to be equally dependent on local insanitary conditions, whether characterized by manure-filled streets, or ditches in which pestilential run-off accumulated, and elicited fear among the public akin to that inspired by the Boston strangler, let alone a water-borne infection like cholera (Hardy 1993: 81). But, ultimately, diphtheria epitomized the emergence of modern medicine, or at least a type of medicine that represented all that was modern at the close of the nineteenth century. Its conceptualization from the time it was renamed by Bretonneau until the moment its causative organism was isolated in a laboratory was radically different from its previous image. Or, to paraphrase Charles Rosenberg (on cholera), between diphtheria's forceful emergence in the 1850s and its reconceptualization by scientists in the 1890s, medical thought 'had passed seemingly through centuries rather than decades' (Rosenberg 1962: 226) (see Figure 0.1).

By the end of the period covered by this volume, new ideas, assumptions and habits of thought appeared to supplant those of the mid-nineteenth century. Additionally, these changes are clearly palatable in the lives and careers of the Jacobis. More than the disease that claimed the life of Ernst Jacobi, diphtheria was the subject of his parents' research, a regular part of their practice and even came to define their medical careers. Coincidentally, even cruelly, Abraham Jacobi was the first practitioner on America's Atlantic coast to write about diphtheria in 1860, and published the first book-length study of the disease in 1880. Given that Mary Putnam Jacobi also wrote an article on 'Croup and Diphtheria' in 1877, it might be said that their story is intimately linked to transformations in medicine during these years. This is underscored by the

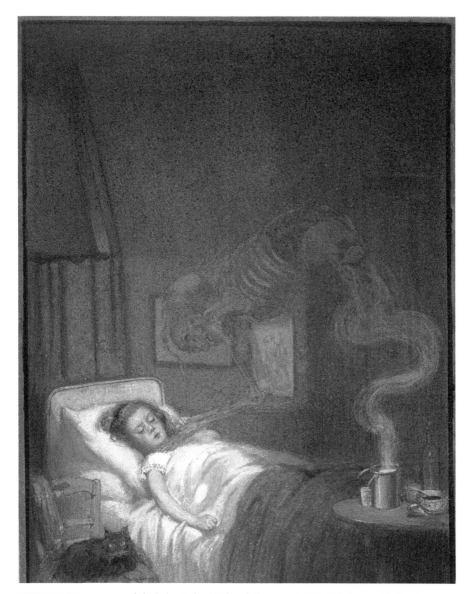

FIGURE 0.1: Image of diphtheria by Richard Cooper, 1912. Wellcome Collection.

contemporaneous rise of medical specialties, such as paediatrics, the field to which both arguably belonged, as well as other defining innovations of this period, including the routine use of statistics in medicine, the admission of women into medical schools, and laboratory investigation more generally. While this introduction indeed touches on the principal topics that structure subsequent chapters, it does not do so equally. Instead, its composite sections strive to highlight some of the key concepts and approaches that have come to define the cultural history of medicine over recent decades. For example, the first section acknowledges the work of Foucault and the birth of the clinic, or Paris medicine, and examines how a new medical gaze, or way of seeing, altered the practice of governance in Western medical culture. The second part explores the rise of new intellectual cultures, primarily through medical specialization and the emergence of paediatrics in particular. Subsequent sections examine the entrance of practitioners to the laboratory and women to medical schools, in order to acknowledge the gendered culture of medicine, as well as the material and spatial turns taken by historians more recently. As such, vignettes from the Jacobis' lives, together with a final section which attempts to merge the main tenets of this account, should adequately prepare the ground for an entire volume that seeks to situate the most significant cultural currents and shifts that came to define medicine in the age of empire.

ACCOUNTING FOR HEALTH

Although it was perhaps unfathomable to the Jacobis that their son would become just another mortality statistic in the story of diphtheria, the quantification of medicine became a science in its own right during the years that frame this book. The rational quantification of infant mortality practised in England and France in the eighteenth century has been described as the first serious measure of public health (Jorland et al. 2005: 6). With the introduction of mandatory national censuses in many European countries during that century, numbers gradually became part of the ordinary discourse of life and death, let alone medicine, in the early nineteenth century (Higgs 1991). So much had counting become an obsession that a steady stream of numbers quickly developed into a torrent by mid-century (Crook and O'Hara 2011: 1); early advocates of the numerate method might have preferred the metaphor of a rich harvest, as captured in the official symbol of the Statistical Society of London (a wheatsheaf), given numbers' scientific and political uses (Schweber 2006: 101). Either way, one could describe this epoch as the statistical century. In a story which has grown familiar, Sweden led the way, introducing bookkeeping to modern governance in 1748. A year later, set apart from earlier methods of political arithmetic through the process of naming, the term 'statistics' was first employed by Gottfried Achenwall (Rosen 1942: 95). In 1791, the French national assembly established its statistical office led by scientist Antoine Lavoisier. England arguably started counting on 10 March 1801, its politicians apparently more interested in agricultural employment, trade and manufacture than in the names and addresses of 10.9 million citizens. If this exercise was tied to issues of health and illness, it was through challenging prevailing pessimistic views that revealed growing, not shrinking, populations when repeated every ten years (Huzel 2006: 116–17). For example, although New York comprised 30,000 inhabitants in 1800, the city doubled in size with each passing decade, bringing all of the challenges associated with such rapid growth. By the 1870s, its population, 80% of which comprised immigrants, including Abraham Jacobi, surpassed a million. Like England, France subjected its citizens to the statistical gaze in 1801, its organizers claiming a greater commitment to 'science', and quickly channelled their numerical interests into various health surveys to improve the country's self-knowledge (Schweber 2006: 171). Armed with expanding datasets that would make their respective 'societies of strangers' legible in new ways (Vernon 2007: 18), experts claimed to see how populations were changing and determined more authoritatively how each should best be governed.

At this time, a new variety of hospital-based medicine was being practised in Paris, one that was based on the careful study of bodies, reliant on clinical observation, pathological anatomy, new methods of diagnosis, but also a discernible *numerical method* (Ackerknecht 1967: 11). This last characteristic is epitomized by the work of the hygienist Louis-René Villermé, whose previous studies of soldiers, labourers and prisoners were inspired by Lavoisier and his fellow savants in the 1780s before this statistical gaze settled onto Europe's urban poor more generally (Bynum 1994: 25–54). Being numbered, however, did not mean that all these lives counted equally in the eyes of rulers. Like his countryman A. J. P. Parent-Duchâtelet, who concerned himself primarily with the distribution of sewage, prostitutes and dead horses, Villermé quickly learned to manipulate his numbers to support a dubious moral vision, thereby making him a worthy candidate for the title of first 'spin doctor'. While inspiring the work of Edwin Chadwick, Christopher Hamlin has argued that Chadwick equally adopted Villermé's and Parent-Duchâtelet's derogatory narrative strategies, thereby transforming the occupants of urban slums into sinister lower animals, whilst simultaneously elevating the status and authority of his social peers (Hamlin 1998: 167). The vital statistics collected by newly-appointed medical officers of health and the offices of registrars general were never value free. Early detective work usually led sanitarians into noted pestiferous zones in regional centres, nearby rural districts and more distant colonies, and to the usual suspects. Michael Brown has convincingly argued that the physician Thomas Southwood-Smith's commitment to sanitary reform was grounded in spiritual belief, the minister-reformer having envisaged a direct cosmological link between sin and filth and the punishment of pestilence in the English communities he studied (Brown 2008). A similar set of rhetorical strategies was employed by his contemporaries who enumerated the overseas empires that European imperialists acquired at this time. Interestingly, these territories were usually too vast and complex to classify accurately and, therefore, remained less legible than European populations throughout this era.

In their edited collection *Constructing Paris Medicine*, La Berge and Hannaway reiterate just how dependent the main components of Paris medicine were on numbers (Hannaway and La Berge 1998: 4). This singular transformation in hospital practice resulted in doctors no longer seeing sick individuals and symptoms, but rather a vast collection of disease statistics, from which averages and anomalies could more easily be deduced, even if one had not set out to identify such norms. As greater numbers of students from Europe and North America flocked to the French capital, its hospital wards became theatres in which physicians, often the most vocal and flamboyant, became the 'lead actors'. Given the heightened emphasis on observing, treating and dissecting cases, many others, not least students themselves, gained unrivalled opportunities to enter the performance and practice medicine. One of the many renowned stars of this show was Pierre Louis, described as the 'inventor' of medicine's numerical method, and whose analysis of disease and treatment through statistics started with the ubiquitous nineteenth-century practice of phlebotomy, which he revealed to be less successful than originally thought (La Berge 2005: 90). Bloodletting, like counting, had a long history in medicine, but had been reintroduced to medicine by the flamboyant liberal revolutionary Francois-Joseph-Victor Broussais in a way that appeared very modern. Relaunched as a means of effectively treating illnesses caused by overstimulation, bloodletting was quickly made to appear useless through statistical means. Not the first to use statistics, Louis is recognized as the first to make them the basis of medicine, regarding medical facts to be without value unless enumerated (Ackerknecht 1967: 9–10). Combined with the institutional structure of Paris medicine, statistics had wide applicability, potentially perfecting physicians' observations, especially when drawing on the city's largest hospital wards, which were simultaneously being reorganized into specialist institutions in which practitioners more easily located their patients and organs of preference. Plunging themselves into overcrowded wards granted students and practitioners many lessons, but medical authority also demanded accuracy, and the judgements of physicians who counted badly could not be relied on in the eyes of the public. Though appearing uncontroversial, this ultimately pitted a numerically-literate school against those who defended an earlier medical art, based on judgements made by practitioners after years of experience on the grounds that they homogenized individual differences between their patients; among the non-numerate, this generated fears that their skills accumulated after decades of private practice were being displaced by mechanical procedures and a small group of hospital-based experts, whose critics claimed erroneously to seek certainly, where none was to be found (Jorland 2005: 7, 13). In another early and influential study of the practice of lithotomy, French doctor J. Civale gathered data from surgeons to demonstrate that cutting for the stone was eight times more likely than lithotrity to end fatally; through his study, Civale reframed a tried and tested method of calculus surgery as a dangerous procedure through the application of the 'calculus of probability' (La Berge 2005: 91). From this period onwards, statistics would frighten surgeons as much as their scalpels and lancets had previously terrified their patients.

Numbers also had the potential to reframe diseases, including diphtheria. Before the Klebs–Loeffler bacillus was identified and accepted, several theories aiming to explain the cause and transmission of diphtheria were in circulation. The miasmatic theory linking filth and diphtheria, held by England's Registrar-General in 1858, was particularly popular among sanitarians and the public. However, diphtheria, which had become a global pandemic by the 1850s, was still regarded by many to be a disease of the countryside, whose inhabitants had long suffered from typhoid, TB and cholera and merely returned the compliment of urban disease by exporting diphtheria to the cities. This view circulated into the 1890s, when beliefs that diphtheria originated in unhygienic urban environments enjoyed a resurgence, with some experts speculating that it might even be disseminated through horse manure (Hardy 1993: 80–109). This was bolstered by data which suggested that between 100,000 and 200,000 horses were walking the streets of Manhattan at any time in these years. While being kicked or run over by one of these unpredictable, living machines remained a very real danger throughout the 1800s, by century's close concerns had shifted, because estimates (they really were counting everything by this time) suggested that each horse dropped around 24 pounds of manure on the city's thoroughfares daily (McShane and Tarr 2007: 26–7). Many were worked to death during careers that rarely extended beyond three years, the corpses of lowly carthorses literally littering New York's streets in 1880. While similar equine casualties were noted in other financial centres, concerns often varied from one epidemic street to the next. In England, for example, public health experts suggested that diphtheria was associated with meteorological conditions and geology (Hardy 1993: 89–90). Bacteriology-denier and disease historian Charles Creighton even constructed a table demonstrating diphtheria's inverse proportion to density of population (Hardy 1993: 93). By the end of the decade, therefore, diphtheria's alarming rise in cities led the malady, like cholera, to be reframed as an urban hazard and eventually a disease of the poor. More importantly perhaps, diphtheria became a notifiable disease in London and New York in the late 1880s, leading to cases being more likely to be included in government statistics. Once excluded from metropolitan hospitals, diphtheria began to account for nearly a third of admissions in the late 1890s (Hardy 1993: 95–6). Needless to say, therapy was less likely to include blood-letting and counter stimulants than antiseptic gargles, mercury injections and, eventually, antitoxin, and the success or failure of these new methods would similarly be determined by statistical analysis. Diphtheria's victims were also more likely to experience surgical interventions, primarily tracheotomy and intubation, to prevent suffocation should false membranes have formed in patients' throats (Hardy 1992). In turn, surgeons began to colonize hospitals, their cases accounting for far greater proportions of hospital inpatients in the second half of the nineteenth century as a result of the twin practices of anaesthesia and antisepsis. Surgeons' operations would continue to fluctuate with fashions, rising and falling, not unlike empires, well into the twentieth century.

SPECIALIZATION IN INFANCY

Although nineteenth-century hospital records normally distinguished consultants as either physicians or surgeons, the division of labour in medicine discernibly increased in the second half of the period (Weisz 2005: xix). Previously, specialization was perceived to be the hallmark of charlatans, whether well-remunerated tooth-drawer, bone-setter, surgeon-oculist or venereal doctor (Cooter 1993). However, practitioners working in fields previously populated by unlicensed 'quacks' were gaining considerable knowledge and institutional legitimacy by establishing orthopaedic, eye and skin hospitals, for example, as long as they openly declared their commitment to general medicine. The process usually began in large urban centres, where cases accumulated in numbers sufficient to fill specialist wards. Specialization reputedly first emerged in Paris during the 1830s, before changing medical cultures a decade later in Vienna and spreading to other European centres in the 1850s and 1860s. Paris medicine, however, retained its emphasis, and gaze, on specialization after mid-century, leading many to suggest that the formation of branches in medicine was a French peculiarity (Warner 2003: 293). Although many practitioners remained suspicious of such narrowness in training, if not openly critical of the apparent multiplication of oculists or venereal and belly doctors in these years, the time spent in specialist institutions was recognized to increase one's knowledge of specific maladies vastly and simultaneously raised the esteem of orthodox practitioners. The fact that the proliferation of specialists coincided with periods when the profit margin of private practice began to diminish did not go unnoticed either (Malpas 2004: 151).

Combined with a thorough general education, short periods of specialist training in a growing number of medical fields was recognized as an appropriate professional model for medicine in France, Britain and the United States by the last decades of the nineteenth century. Interestingly, specialties were dynamic and changed in ways that allowed practitioners subsequently to recast their interests at key historical moments. The field of ophthalmology, for example, was initially preoccupied with eye diseases which potentially incapacitated legions of European soldiers in colonial contexts, and practitioners who initially populated this field would strategically refocus their attention on a range of conditions thereafter that would lend the field certain and useful degrees of urgency. Ophthalmologists have also historically relied on the elevated status of sight over the other senses since first justifying the existence of their field (Davidson 1996: 332), but many other early specialists were equally adept at framing the 'natural' importance of their particular specialty, depending on prevailing economic and social priorities. Careful not to mimic the promotional methods pioneered by an earlier generation of quacks too closely, these new, more acceptable, specialists regularly used their privileged positions as editors and authors to engage in indirect forms of advertising that furthered their own professional and commercial interests (Malpas 2004: 157). Although the committee of the New York State Medical Society, as represented by Abraham Jacobi in 1875, declared that specialization tended 'to degrade the general practitioner in the estimation of the public' (Rosen 1942: 349), a number of specialist branches were already recognized as both natural and inevitable subdivisions of medicine by the last quarter of the century. This tendency would lead members of the American Medical Association as early as 1869 to declare 'that this Association recognizes specialties as proper and legitimate fields of practice' (Rosen 1942: 352).

Nevertheless, there were still fewer than fifty declared child specialists in the United States in 1880, and none practised on a full-time basis. A specific term to define this emerging field was also still being coined, the majority, like Abraham Jacobi, calling themselves pediatrists (Halpern 1988: 1). As important as naming is to specialty's formation, a defined therapeutic regime that addressed the unique challenges of infancy was already evident in the medical literature on children, which had increased tenfold after 1850 and was now being employed to justify the public institutionalization of this young discipline (Jacobi 1905: 5), starting in 1855 with the foundation of a children's hospital in Philadelphia. By the 1920s, more than 10% of physicians were full-time specialists, and departments of paediatrics existed in many medical schools, both in North America and Europe. While scientific progress is routinely identified as the principle motivator of specialization, the rise of a child care profession appears to have been driven by its own distinct ideological culture. A variant of professionalization, specialization serves as a form of collective advancement, just as paediatricians, in turn, sought the advancement of a wider, and younger, collective. As such, paediatrics is recognized as a field whose evolution has been strongly influenced by intellectual currents and social reform movements outside the medical profession. Originally argued by George Rosen to have been less dependent on technology than other specialist fields, paediatrics has also been described as 'soft and unrigorous' (Halpern 1988: 9–11). While the earliest exponents of the field joked that they were essentially assuming the traditional roles of neighbours and grandmothers, many others tellingly regarded paediatrics as particularly suited to women. Changing notions of childhood and child welfare both shaped its evolution over the next decades and are mirrored in the field's conceptualization. Intrusions into the family grew with the expansion of state powers, as new ways of regulating childhood were introduced to schools, legal systems and private life. Social movements larger than the medical profession therefore remained central to its development, just as they were to Abraham Jacobi's own life and career trajectory.

In an obituary written by F. H. Garrison in August 1919, Abraham Jacobi was already regarded to be the 'father and founder of American pediatrics' (Garrison 1919: 102). Having settled in New York in 1854, along with some 250,000 other German immigrants in this period, Jacobi began to lecture in paediatrics at New York's College of Physicians and Surgeons by 1857, at a time when Lewis Smith was the country's only other recognized representative of the field. By 1860, Jacobi assumed the chair in paediatrics at New York Medical College, in whose building he established a specialist clinic two years later. By this time, there were already children's hospitals in many European capitals, including Vienna (1843), Prague (1842), Moscow (1842) and Berlin (1843), where Jacobi had been arrested as a political agitator less than a decade after the latter institution's foundation. He had escaped political persecution in 1853 by boarding a ship from Hamburg to London, where, incidentally, a children's hospital had been established a year previously; before the end of the 1860s, London supported five children's hospitals (Lomax 1996: 15). Once settled in New York, Jacobi founded his own dispensary in 1856, complete with a department for the diseases of children (Wells 2001: 168). That said, he argued that children had a better chance of survival in the poorest homes than in these early institutions. Although recognized as a specialist, Jacobi, like many of his professional colleagues, publically opposed this tendency in nineteenth-century medicine. Equally, Jacobi's early years were characterized by modest earnings, and he reputedly lacked the 'business manner of the *arriviste*', characteristics that made him a 'respectable' practitioner, let alone a 'rebel' (Haggerty 1997).

It is worth noting that Mary Putnam Jacobi, like other women to enter this field, is rarely recognized as a paediatrician or pioneer, let alone a founding mother. Her obituary in the *British Medical Journal* indeed recalls her professorship at New York Postgraduate Medical School (1868), but fails to note that this appointment involved delivering lectures on children's diseases (Anon. 1906). Although a prolific author and contributing to her husband's work, Mary's output was overshadowed by Abraham Jacobi's collected writings, which filled eight volumes and totalled 4,000 pages, many of which were devoted to children's health care. In terms of his lasting contribution to paediatrics, his 1877 book on diphtheria was recognized by Garrison, and others, as a definitive text. While this alone appeared to justify his 'father of paediatrics' title, he was also throughout his career the quintessential social reformer, remembered by many as a victim of the unsuccessful revolution of 1848 in Prussia, a period which equally awakened pathologist Rudolph Virchow's political conscience. Though nearly achieving the success and renown of his mentor, at career's end, Jacobi was no longer a victim, but recognized as a hero by his peers. Interestingly, he was, to an extent, involved in making his reputation, as well as the history of his speciality, contributing 'authoritative' histories of paediatrics in 1902 and 1913, and one on paediatrics in New York (1917), where he had taught the subject for fifty years. If there were any remaining 'victims' besides the sick children that filled wards named in Jacobi's honour, it was the medical women, who, as was common in early histories, were excluded from these historical narratives.

GHASTLY KITCHENS AND SEEING FURTHER

Well before Jacobi's demise, the celebrated era of Paris medicine came to an end in the middle of the nineteenth century. In place of the hospital clinic, its defining feature, arose a new hallmark of modern medicine, namely the laboratory, fully stocked with its associated fragile, material culture, including glass tubes, flasks, rubber hoses and stoppers, and its key signifier, the microscope, which has more often survived through the generations. Biomedicine's new foundation stone appeared to be laid in the previously undesignated basement rooms adjacent to, but often below, lecture halls and museums, in places where human physiology would be worked out in minute detail, starting with the nervous and sensory systems of lower animals, and described utilizing the relevant industrial and technological metaphors of the day. Less a student of the French clinics and their statistical work, Abraham Jacobi was an early pupil of the Germanic laboratory. While these investigative spaces might not have appeared modern, with an accumulating stock of apparatus resembling modified kitchen utensils, their methods were certainly novel, so much so that the absence of a designated laboratory became shorthand for 'pre-modern' or a substandard hospital or medical school by the end of the era covered by this volume. That said, the first laboratories must occasionally have looked distinctly 'antiquated', with their earliest advocates relying on pre-modern trades, like that of the glass-blower, to craft the swan-necked flasks and other necessary and contrived equipment that were not yet mass-produced. The earliest lab-based researchers, like Johannes Müller (1801–58), had no choice but to improvise wherever space permitted, and practised methods in environments that grew ever more cluttered (Otis 2007: xi). Müller's students formed an evolutionary tree, as described by Darwin a year after Müller's death, which connected their melancholy mentor to Koch; it is through Rudolf Virchow, who convinced physicians to think about disease at the cellular level, that one is able to connect Müller and Abraham Jacobi. Resembling early modern alchemists, these obsessive lab-based toilers also shared working methods with cooks, or even farmers, as Latour famously remarked with reference to Pasteur's research on anthrax (Latour 1983: 146). Many became chemists, whose status noticeably lagged behind that of physicians and surgeons, or even served as anatomists at medical schools. Later compared to bear baiters, or other early modern brutes (Turner 1980: 79–92), many laboratory-based practitioners appeared to be seeking new scientific truths by torturing animals, eventually heralding a new age of bacteriology by attenuating or exalting microbes by passing them through rabbits, guinea pigs and mice. The introduction of anaesthesia may have ameliorated the concerns of some critics, but these practices eventually led authorities to restrict such experiments to licensed individuals, who were required to conduct their work in recognized centres of learning, such as a medical school. Despite some vocal protests, usually following experiments involving 'noble' animals, including dogs, many replicated German practices by appointing full-time professors of physiology, pathology and, eventually, histology and bacteriology (Sturdy 2007: 762). Generally, this involved introducing the exact methods of physics and chemistry to improve medicine, a process interpreted by its exponents as heralding the dawn of a more just and rational society, rather than its downfall (see Figure 0.2).

Abraham Jacobi belonged to that cohort which believed that science was part of utopian public life, and promised to emancipate society. It is therefore curious that, if there was a member of the Jacobi family who remained cautious about laboratory medicine, it was Abraham. Although a product of the German universities, his training ended decades before the onset of the age of bacteriology. Rather than a champion of these methods, he better represents the tension that existed between the laboratory and clinical practice (Sturdy 2011: 739). While not hostile to the new science, he openly declared a desire to keep it 'in its place' (Lawrence 1985: 503–20). Unlike her husband, Mary Putnam Jacobi immersed herself fully in the new experimental method from her admission to New York's College of Pharmacy, where she obtained her first degree and acquired a taste for science in 1863 (Putnam 1925: 59). Throughout her career, she entered the 'black box of the laboratory' and, unlike some of its most renowned theorists, found many extraordinary things in these 'scientific' temples (Latour 1983: 141). Unlike Marie Françoise, Claude Bernard's wife, who divorced 'the prince of vivisectors' after witnessing his callousness towards animals, Mary encouraged her spouse to take a greater interest in laboratory investigation. In fact, rather than being relegated to a supporting role on this occasion, as so many scientifically inclined women were in the late nineteenth and twentieth centuries (Twohig 2005: 6), Mary Putnam Jacobi actively disseminated her scientific knowledge throughout her career by regularly presenting at various medical societies. Thus in the Jacobi family, laboratory life was not a 'family affair' (Twohig 2005: 8). Mary's scientific approach to the

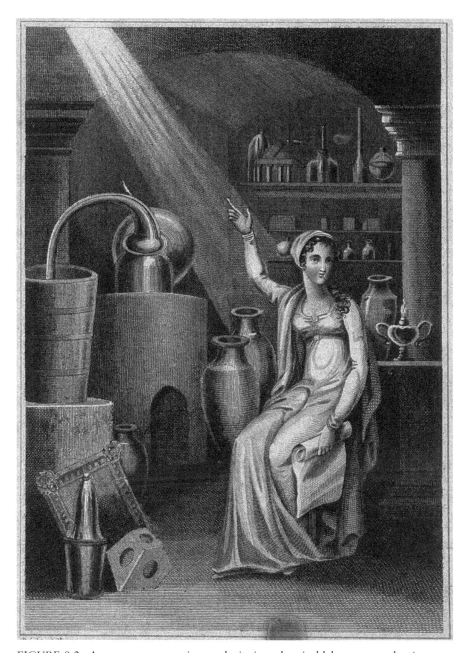

FIGURE 0.2: A woman representing truth sits in a chemical laboratory and points at the source of a ray of light, representing philosophy. Engraving by Crabb, 1817, after G. M. Brighty. Wellcome Collection.

world even grew more complete as a result of her formal rejection of religion (Putnam 1925: 58), though many would have likened her adherence to germ theory to a religious conversion (Tomes 1998: 27).

Just as Pasteur managed to convert various people, from farmers to brewers, to believe in his laboratory experiments (Latour 1988: 143), Mary Putnam Jacobi communicated her passion for the laboratory doctrine to uninitiated colleagues, mainly through her presentations and writings. However, she also popularized a scientific approach to medicine at a time when the language of the laboratory and its emerging methods was still 'micro' in scale. For example, she persuaded mothers to seek out doctors who could advise them on how to 'scientifically' feed and care for their children. While some industrialists had rapidly incorporated the laboratory into production (Latour 1988: 33), Mary explained its relation to infant feeding. Seeking to comfort those who feared the displacement of existing habits, she, like many other laboratory champions, suggested that the incorporation of new ideas into feeding was merely the next logical stage of its evolution (Sturdy 2011: 746). The later part of her career witnessed the merging of bench and bedside in a marriage that was more harmonious than her own matrimonial union. More radically, through her writings she helped displace notions that the refined gentleman was the unquestioned pinnacle of medical learning. While scientists traditionally sought to establish themselves as modern, rational and professional, and simultaneously associate women and other so-called non-scientific social groups as 'passionate', and thereby relegate them to a pre-modern worldview, Putnam challenged such thinking and situated women firmly in this space. Instead, she actively employed science as a means to resist discriminatory institutions and policies and support a case for equal rights. According to Skinner, she asserted a science-driven model of political change in which laboratory findings led directly to an expanded political and social role for women (Skinner 2016: 254). She regularly used science as a weapon to confront bureaucratic structures of domination (Skinner 2016: 258). Employing the latest technical language in her writings and lectures, she seized on the prestige and elite status that came with a mastery of these new ideas, and augmented her own, and women's, authority in the profession (Skinner 2016: 256–7). Furthermore, by employing science in this way, she ultimately made her case for social reform appear both natural and less controversial.

Other practitioners similarly seized upon the potential of laboratory science to leverage their status. Public health workers, for example, became recognized authorities in the diagnosis of infectious diseases when New York established its first diagnosis programme for diphtheria in 1893. As outlined at the outset of this introduction, Klebs and Loeffler, among others, clarified the relationship of bacteria to diphtheria after a series of experiments conducted from 1873. Just as cholera stained red, diphtheria was shown to stain purple using methylene blue, which revealed its characteristic club-like appearance. The Greek term for club, *korynee*, was subsequently incorporated into the name of its causative organism, *Corynebacterium diphtheria*, with which Loeffler inoculated animals. Interestingly, Mary Putnam Jacobi communicated Loeffler's findings at a meeting of the New York Postgraduate Medical School in 1884, and Abraham Jacobi's negative comments in 1885 indicate that scepticism continued to exist (Hammonds 1999: 51). Nevertheless, systematic bacteriological work on diphtheria eventually began in America in 1887 and concentrated in New York, where a diagnostic laboratory was established. A final piece in the diphtheria puzzle fell into place when the role of carriers finally explained the apparently unrelated appearances of the disease. American epidemiologist William Hallock Park established the concept of the carrier in diphtheria, stressing the importance of the dangers posed by both convalescent carriers and symptomless carriers of the disease, whose numbers comprised 1–2% of the childhood population in New York alone (Hammonds 1999: 13). These mild cases were described by Jacobi as the 'pistol bullet', as opposed to 'magic bullets', a term soon after coined by Paul Ehrlich, and from which there was no escape for children, like Ernst, as long as cases went unreported or continued to be concealed (Hammonds 1999: 31). In 1893, doctors in New York were provided with 'culture kits', which provided physicians access to bacteriological diagnosis, transformed the culture of general practice and provided a new and more accurate picture of diphtheria's distribution (Hammonds 1999: 12). Plotting every reported case on maps, the city's health department encouraged new ways of visualizing diseases, and no longer inevitably led investigators to the usual suspects, such as the 'diphtheria nests' of the Lower East Side. As the 'lessons of the laboratory' became part of the fabric of everyday life, fear of microbes was 'exploited' by a variety of entrepreneurs and manufacturers to sell ordinary consumers a wealth of goods and services (Tomes 1998: 11–13).

In 1894, diphtheria became the first infectious disease since smallpox to acquire a specific, or remedy, when the new bacteriology introduced antitoxic serum for the treatment of patients. The treatment was developed and announced in December 1890 by Emil von Behring, who, unlike Koch, was never involved with tropical medicine in the age of empire, but collaborated with a foreign scientist, Shibasaburo Kitasato, in publishing the first account of the essential production of immunity to disease. Though early trials proved disappointing, the rumour that antitoxin was first used on a comatose child in a Berlin clinic on 25 December 1891 instantly lent the drug a certain mythic quality, linking it with the healing traditions of Christianity by suggesting its inventor performed a Christmas miracle (Linton 2005: 9). More extensive and successful trials commenced at the children's hospital in Paris in 1894, which eventually led to the antitoxin's introduction to hospitals across Europe and

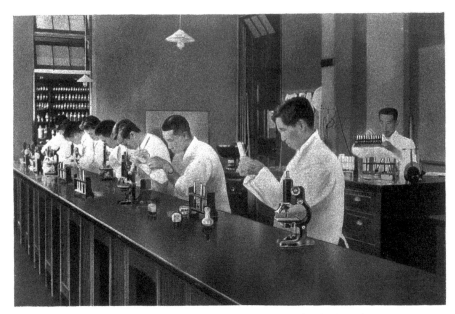

FIGURE 0.3: Students attacking a laboratory problem, School of Medicine, Tsinan, China. From Harold Balme, *China and Modern Medicine: A Study in Medical Missionary Development*, 1921. Reproduced with permission of the Wellcome Trust.

North America the following year. By this time, increased workloads were reported in all diagnostic laboratories, where a new generation of bacteriologists aimed to identify the causative organisms of dozens of infectious diseases, including typhoid, tetanus and plague. As laboratories and tests multiplied, their equipment began to be mass-produced and marketed to a wider range of potential users, filling rooms in hospital basements, public health offices, factories and even classrooms. Equally, laboratories before the end of the age of empire transformed from rooms into buildings, and more disciplined, standardized and complex entities befitting modern industrial society (James 1989: 2). It is at this time that medicine reputedly made its historic power grab that 'transformed doctors from lowly tradesmen to lofty professionals', who subsequently commanded greater respect from patients and the public (Sturdy 2011: 740). While occasionally seized, authority was more often negotiated, as well as dependent and respectful of the new disciplinary boundaries that had emerged over previous decades. Nevertheless, the dominance science bestowed on individuals in the health profession is especially evident in the case of diphtheria, where one of its experts was recognized for his work and invited to join an aristocracy for the modern age; in 1901, Behring was awarded the first Nobel Prize in Medicine for his research that led to the development of antitoxin, a decision which simultaneously linked medicine's cutting edge with an honorific system that, from its very ceremony, appeared a relic of the past. Surprisingly, the prize's first celebrity was a woman, the Polish chemist and physicist Marie Curie. Like competition for medicine's highest honour, laboratory science seemed a global pursuit, its methods and findings appearing universal in nature, reproduced in generic spaces that did not easily betray the regional cultures that shaped the scientific endeavours of its practitioners (Livingstone 2011). With as many as 1,200 Japanese medical students travelling to Germany between 1868 and 1914, for example, one could no longer easily differentiate between German, Japanese or even Western medicine for that matter (Kim 2014: 5). While the diseases they studied were already recognized as international phenomena, medical researchers and practitioners more regularly travelled, as would their ideas (Löwy 2007:466).

THE CIRCULATION OF PEOPLE AND KNOWLEDGE

Although Elizabeth Blackwell had gained international fame even sooner than Curie when she entered the Geneva Medical School in rural New York, that first door to medical qualification for women was quickly slammed shut by the school's dean, who declared her admission to have been an experiment, not a precedent (Bonner 1995: 6). Many other women, however, including Mary Putnam, were inspired by Blackwell's success, some facing even greater obstacles to qualification. In the worst cases of discrimination, women applied to dozens of colleges and travelled to the ends of the earth, before being permitted to commence their studies, while others were hindered beyond admission by a masculine culture sustained by students, as well as staff, concerned with the 'difficulties' potentially caused by admitting members of 'the weaker sex' into schools. As one might expect from the daughter of a publisher, Putnam was a prolific writer throughout her career and some of her correspondence captures the various obstacles she, and others, had to endure, and occasionally avoid, in her quest for medical qualification.

Like so many of the first women to train in medicine, Putnam came from a middle-class family and enjoyed the support of a father who, despite regarding medicine a 'repulsive pursuit' (Putnam 1925: 67), held progressive views about women's education. From childhood, Mary's morning instructions had included French, which later facilitated the decision to study medicine in France, while knowledge of Latin set her apart from the majority of female students, whose ignorance of the classical language was regularly noted (Putnam 1925: 24, 34). Despite gaining admission to medical lectures, complete equality was not yet achieved, for Mary Putnam was required to enter lecture theatres through a side door and sit separately, near the professor's lectern (Bonner 1995: 1). With the help of a network of French physicians who knew and respected her predecessor, Elizabeth Blackwell, Mary eventually gained access to seven of the French capital's renowned teaching hospitals. Finally, in 1868, she became the first woman to graduate from Paris's school of medicine. Her efforts were further rewarded when faculty granted her a bronze medal, one of only three similar prizes awarded to a woman in the first two decades of women's study in the French capital. Interestingly, Putnam specifically chose a topic that was not immediately recognizable as 'feminine', namely the fatty degeneration of the liver. In this way, she initially set herself apart from many of her contemporaries, whose research concentrated on supposedly 'female' complaints, such as migraines, obstetrics or the diseases of children.

Although compared most often to their male peers, female students differed greatly from each other, according to recent research on nineteenth-century medical women. For example, in her research, Susan Wells was unable to identify a single 'unitary, distinctly feminine voice' in this period (Wells 2001: 12). Instead, she unearthed a variety of narrative styles in the writings of female practitioners, who developed diverse strategies for working in a hostile profession. Unpacking the rhetoric of science, Wells suggests that women, like Elizabeth Blackwell, indeed claimed that gender gave them 'a special understanding of some neglected aspect of medicine' (Wells 2001: 5), often describing themselves as less interventionist and more empathetic than their male peers. Others, including Mary Putnam, employed alternative strategies, often resembling masquerade, adopting personas deemed appropriate to particular stages of their careers. Unlike the famed Irish military surgeon, James Miranda Barry, who literally disguised herself as male during a successful career in the British Army, members of the first, openly female generation of women doctors regularly engaged in more subtle, yet equally convincing, 'performance[s] of subversion dressed as compliance' (Wells 2001: 6).

Mary Putnam Jacobi's various performances are particularly interesting, not simply because her multiple identifications constitute gender in ways described by philosopher Judith Butler, but her numerous styles collectively replicate the diverse strategies employed by other woman doctors active in these years. Near the outset of her career, for example, she chose to deflect attention from her sex by publishing her work anonymously. Most famously, in her winning essay submitted for the Boylston Prize for Medical Writing, she employed an overtly 'scientific' argument to refute Harvard Professor Edward Clarke's dire warnings against educating women and challenge his views alleging women's intellectual inferiority (Putnam 1925: 46). Pressed to counter Clarke's view that menstruation incapacitated women for higher education, Putnam amassed statistics claiming that 1.5 million American women already undertook paid employment in industry with no discernible impact on productivity. Additional statistical evidence on French women suggested that the majority reported only very slight pain during menstruation (Harvey 1990: 112). She augmented her statistics with qualitative evidence from a survey, collecting 268 replies from women, a third claiming no discomfort or pain. Anonymized in order to ensure all entries were judged fairly, the panel had no choice but to judge the entry on its merits, rather than the sex of the author.

While Putnam sometimes revealed her gender, at other times she masked it, as when she chose to advertise as 'Dr Putnam' on the sign posted outside her practice (Putnam 1925: 76). Her devotion to her sick siblings, who she nursed early in her career, appears out of place in a career that otherwise challenged the existence of 'natural' gender traits. For example, her autobiography describes a very masculine form of medical initiation, starting with a childhood desire to dissect a rat in order to see its beating heart, an urge that was extinguished by her mother, who repeatedly challenged Putnam, in a more recognizable display of gendered behaviour. Historian Ludmilla Jordanova has argued that the need to unveil the body through dissection was a particularly masculine activity, not unlike the penchant of the flâneur to walk the city streets unchaperoned, as Putnam regularly did whilst a student in Paris. Although clearly driven by a need to please her father, who requested her to make greater efforts to 'be a lady' and 'an attractive and agreeable [doctor]' (Putnam 1925: 68), Mary Putnam appeared to seize every opportunity after qualification to engage in behaviour otherwise deemed unladylike. Likewise, she refuted the generally held view that women should not be surgeons (Wells 2001: 168), despite the fact that idealized surgery in these years was said to require a 'Lady's Hand' (Brock 2017: 16). Unlike Barry, Jacobi was openly identifiable as female at professional meetings, and, as already argued, embraced the latest 'masculine' methods of scientific investigation in an act akin to self-preservation. The condescension she directed at her peers at the Women's Medical College of Pennsylvania in 1860s, whom she described as 'illiterate', therefore appears somewhat unusual behaviour, normally suited to the most vociferous male critics of women's education, who, evidently more concerned with breeding, than reading abilities, regularly described their female colleagues as unsexed.

In collaborations with her spouse, Mary Putnam Jacobi continued to blur gender distinctions, challenging readers to guess which sections of their jointly-authored book, *Infant Diet* (1874), were penned by her and which by Abraham. Given her wide experience writing for the popular press – she wrote 170 pages of medical journalism during her five years in Paris – Putnam was invited by her husband to popularize his nutritional research. Originally presented by Abraham to the New York Public Health Association, the text was doubled in size by Mary while on their honeymoon. Rather than allow scientific feeding to remain the preserve of male practitioners, she disseminated its techniques by incorporating them into common medical discourse (Skinner 2016: 256–7). Whether she was successful is uncertain, given the information on feeding that overwhelmed nineteenth-century publics. In their text, for example, the Jacobis ridiculed the heresy of 'the top milk gospel' whereby families, especially the wealthiest, reserved the top quarter of the milk, in which the cream was concentrated, for infants. Not only did they regard this as too fatty for children, but they urged carers to boil milk. While older folk ideas also continued to circulate, including families' preference for brunette over blonde wet nurses, mathematical formulas had gradually entered feeding debates. Leading attempts to reframe milk diets and remove feeding from the hands of 'charlatans' and parents was Dr Thomas Morgan Rotch, Harvard's professor of paediatrics since 1893. Rotch promoted the 'percentage method' of infant feeding, which called for a highly complex method of dilution, carefully calculated ratios of fat, carbohydrate, cream and sugar, with changes often called for on a day-to-day basis depending on both the condition of the child and the supplier of milk. A glance at his 'simplified' charts should clarify why such recipes began to be referred to as 'formulas' at this time. In particular, Rotch's calculations provoked Abraham Jacobi, who reputedly exclaimed that 'you cannot feed babies with mathematics; you must feed them with brains' (Halpern 1988: 64). Only after 1898 would paediatricians and health workers begin to discuss infant feeding in terms of caloric requirements, and almost as quickly, Rotch's theories were displaced by new and even more simplified narratives (see Figure 0.4).

Despite not championing every scientific approach to infant health care, Mary Putnam Jacobi found herself singled out from the crowd more often than eccentric thinkers like Rotch. In contemporary publications she was regularly described as a 'female writer of insistently masculine medicine' or 'the girl in the horde' (Wells 2001: 172), which highlighted her exceptional abilities but simultaneously reinforced ideas of women's inferiority. In response, she encouraged women to endure attacks when struggling for equality, claiming that their own 'infusion of masculine strength' would come when knocked down in their battles against masculine opposition (Harvey 1990: 114). So completely did she identify with the scientist, however, that she frequently set herself apart from other women doctors, such as Elizabeth Blackwell, who called for a 'feminine' approach to medical practice, which embraced aspects central to the suffrage campaign, including anti-vivisection and temperance. Not only did Putnam recognize a place for animal experimentation and alcohol in medicine, but, having tested the drug atropine on a woman in good health, Jacobi was labelled a human vivisectionist in the last decades of the nineteenth century (Lederer 1997: 75). In her defence, Jacobi claimed the anti-vivisection movement only hurt the women's rights cause 'by reifying women's alliance with sentimentalism' (Bittel 2009: 200). She made her preference for the rational over the emotional evident in most of her writing, and her apparent stoicism in the immediate aftermath of her son Ernst's death must be considered along these lines. Displays of passion, Mary Putnam Jacobi claimed, only

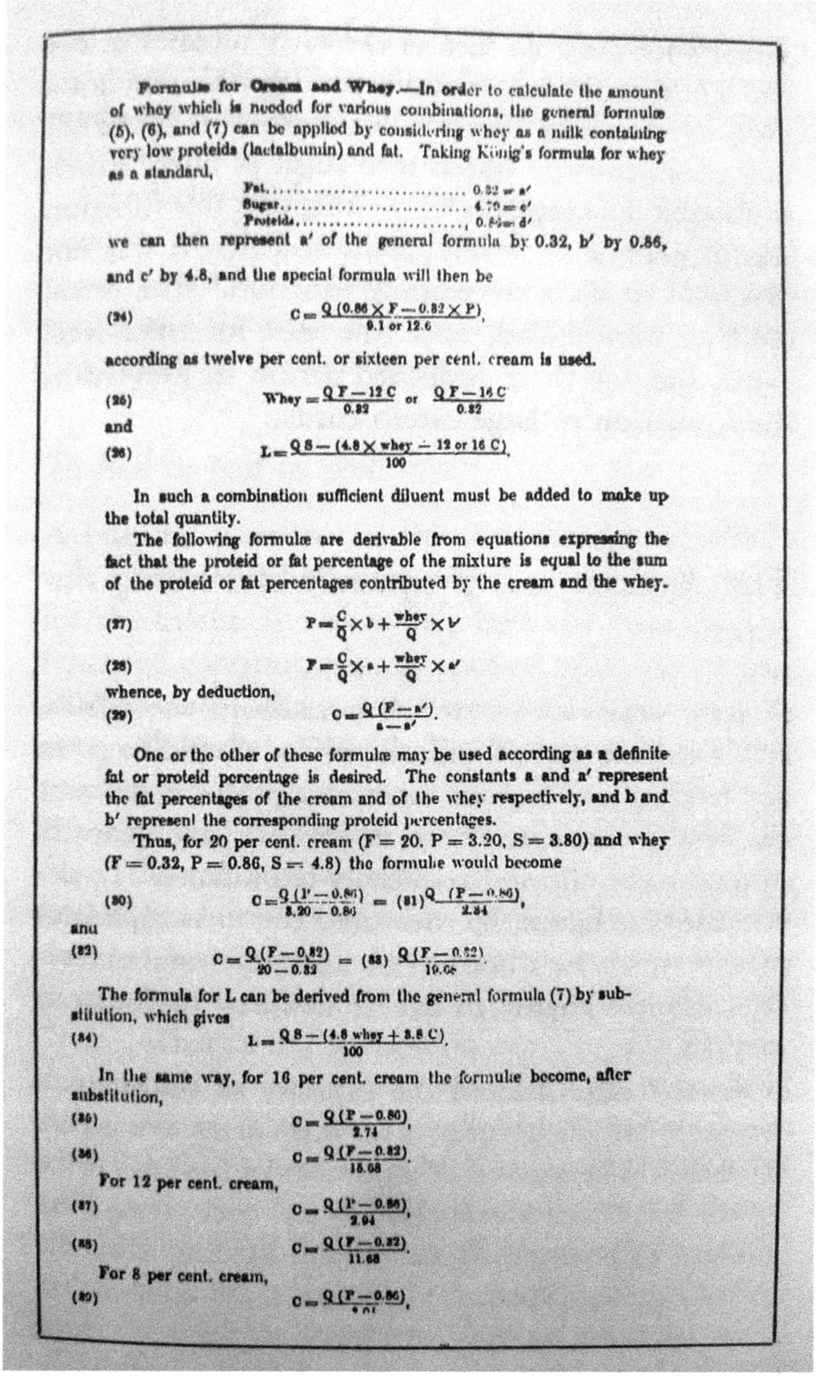

Formulæ for Cream and Whey.—In order to calculate the amount of whey which is needed for various combinations, the general formulæ (5), (6), and (7) can be applied by considering whey as a milk containing very low proteids (lactalbumin) and fat. Taking König's formula for whey as a standard,

$$\text{Fat} \dots \dots \dots \dots \dots 0.32 = a'$$
$$\text{Sugar} \dots \dots \dots \dots \dots 4.79 = c'$$
$$\text{Proteids} \dots \dots \dots \dots \dots 0.86 = d'$$

we can then represent a' of the general formula by 0.32, b' by 0.86, and c' by 4.8, and the special formula will then be

(24) $$C = \frac{Q(0.86 \times F - 0.32 \times P)}{9.1 \text{ or } 12.6},$$

according as twelve per cent. or sixteen per cent. cream is used.

(25) $$\text{Whey} = \frac{Q F - 12 C}{0.32} \text{ or } \frac{Q F - 16 C}{0.32}$$

and

(26) $$L = \frac{Q S - (4.8 \times \text{whey} \div 12 \text{ or } 16 C)}{100}$$

In such a combination sufficient diluent must be added to make up the total quantity.

The following formulæ are derivable from equations expressing the fact that the proteid or fat percentage of the mixture is equal to the sum of the proteid or fat percentages contributed by the cream and the whey.

(27) $$P = \frac{C}{Q} \times b + \frac{\text{whey}}{Q} \times b'$$

(28) $$F = \frac{C}{Q} \times a + \frac{\text{whey}}{Q} \times a'$$

whence, by deduction,

(29) $$C = \frac{Q(F - a')}{a - a'}.$$

One or the other of these formulæ may be used according as a definite fat or proteid percentage is desired. The constants a and a' represent the fat percentages of the cream and of the whey respectively, and b and b' represent the corresponding proteid percentages.

Thus, for 20 per cent. cream (F = 20, P = 3.20, S = 3.80) and whey (F = 0.32, P = 0.86, S = 4.8) the formulæ would become

(30) $$C = \frac{Q(P - 0.86)}{3.20 - 0.86} = (31) \frac{Q(P - 0.86)}{2.34},$$

and

(32) $$C = \frac{Q(F - 0.32)}{20 - 0.32} = (33) \frac{Q(F - 0.32)}{19.68}.$$

The formula for L can be derived from the general formula (7) by substitution, which gives

(34) $$L = \frac{Q S - (4.8 \text{ whey} + 3.8 C)}{100}$$

In the same way, for 16 per cent. cream the formulæ become, after substitution,

(35) $$C = \frac{Q(P - 0.86)}{2.74},$$

(36) $$C = \frac{Q(F - 0.32)}{15.68}.$$

For 12 per cent. cream,

(37) $$C = \frac{Q(P - 0.86)}{2.94},$$

(38) $$C = \frac{Q(F - 0.32)}{11.68}.$$

For 8 per cent. cream,

(39) $$C = \frac{Q(P - 0.86)}{?.??},$$

FIGURE 0.4: A Formula for the Modification of Cow's Milk, from Thomas Morgan Rotch, *Pediatrics*, 4th edition (1903), p. 238.

confirmed doubts about women's intellectual capacity and their ability to participate rationally in public life (Skinner 2016: 262).

While Putnam famously seized the rhetoric of science to reconceptualize gender, scientific language was being employed publically in far more insidious forms, not least as evidence for intellectual difference between races. Science at this time was famously being employed to reshape ideas of race and class specifically to marginalize groups in society. The most common example, which has attracted considerable attention from historians, was the misuse of Darwin's theory of evolution as an ideological weapon to divide society into 'normal' and 'deviant' groups. This is often associated with the work of Italian physician Cesare Lombroso, who, like those who preached women's intellectual inferiority, used statistics, or an 'avalanche of numbers', to lend his racist theories legitimacy. His particular Darwinist arguments honed in on certain features of inherited backwardness reputedly present on the eve of Italian nationhood in order to underscore the threat that atavism posed to that society (Pick 1989: 114–15). Lombroso saw degeneration throughout the newly unified country and not only among the criminal and dangerous classes, but in the paralysed and atrophied upper classes and among its rebels and revolutionaries (Pick 1989: 141–2). Lombroso and his followers of course wished to play a critical role in the construction of the nascent Italian nation, while Putnam had her own fish to fry. Although desiring the improvement of women's lot, Putnam frequently articulated an essentialist view of woman's nature in writings that were not entirely free from the concept of degeneration that infected her generation. She, too, focused on the disorders of an emergent mass society based in the expanding cities, doubting, for example, the fitness of labouring men for participation in elective politics (Skinner 2016: 259).

Responses to Darwinism, like those to women doctors, of course varied with geography, as became evident when the naturalist's ideas spread from England to more remote outposts of British civilization and specific local cultures. Survival of the fittest, for example, could mean very different things in underpopulated parts of the globe. Even in a large and rapidly growing city like New York, the so-called degenerate 'types' identified by Lombroso formed a substantial percentage of the tired, poor and huddled masses arriving in the city in droves during the second half of the nineteenth century. While the perception of difference is even evident in some physical descriptions of Jacobi, he was generally spared the anti-Semitism that was more readily apparent during the late nineteenth century, when large numbers of Jewish immigrants arrived on America's shores. Obituaries of Jacobi indeed addressed his physical appearance, but not the rhetoric surrounding the Jewish body identified by Sander Gilman (1991). In fact, while the German scientific community used physiological references to underline Jewish difference and seed doubts that they could ever become fully German, let alone American, descriptions of Jacobi emphasized his uniqueness, but also his unequalled intellectual capacity. Acclaimed medical historian and Principal Assistant Librarian of the Army Medical Library, Fielding Garrison, indeed drew attention to his 'large, splendid head', which was variously described as 'leonine' and 'magisterial'. To Garrison and others, Jacobi was 'the living embodiment of some great high-priest of knowledge of old'. Earlier portraits of the paediatrician 'betoken extraordinary vigor of mind and body', the lines on his face without a doubt the result of a penchant for 'curious thought' (Garrison 1919: 103–4). According to physician, scientist and professor of experimental pathology Simon Flexner, Jacobi's face was 'lighted by brilliant, searching eyes and moulded by a play of expressions responding to emotions and thoughts the most diverse' (Flexner 1925: 628). While Garrison's obituary addressed Jacobi's Jewish heritage, he was described as 'Hebrew by race, but not clannish, not a sectarian', belonging more to the 'ante-bellum generation that produced figures such as Lincoln', yet retaining some of his otherworldliness. Although European, he evidently belonged to 'the wretched refuse of [that continent's] teaming shore' that was 'yearning to breathe free'.

If his allegiance to America was ever in doubt, Jacobi repeatedly emphasized his rootedness in American soil, the country he claimed was already his 'ideal' when a young man, a belief he demonstrated by turning down in the 1890s a professorship in paediatrics in Berlin. During the First World War, Jacobi again felt compelled to reiterate where his allegiances lay, vocally opposing Germany and declaring the Prussian regime to be anti-democratic. In this way, he shaped his biography in a manner that would shield him from further accusations, even from historians who unanimously appear to regard him to have been patriotic 'in a very fine sense' (Gardner 1959: 286). Although potentially suspect to those familiar with Jacobi's socialist past, including his links to Friedrich Engels and Karl Marx, both of whom he visited while in England in 1853, biographies written soon after the second red scare of the McCarthy era would emphasize that the Revolution of 1848, of which Jacobi was both product and participant, followed the intellectual traditions of the American Revolution (Gardner 1959: 282). Although recognized as a 'revolutionary', Jacobi was also importantly remembered as a 'respectable' rebel (Haggerty 1997), and, after his death, children's wards bearing his name were established in hospitals across America. Similarly, Mary Putnam's connections to French political activities during the time of the Commune were with the Reclus family, whose members supported women's rights and state socialism and were described as leading French 'gentle' anarchists (Harvey 1990: 107, 112). In her own correspondence, Putnam referred to them as 'radical republicans and socialists' (Putnam 1925: 171). During his lifetime, Jacobi was appointed President of the American Medical Association (1912), an honour not normally awarded to a foreign-born practitioner, let alone one with a Jewish background, and on his seventieth birthday was the recipient of the first international festschrift ever organized for a professor. One biographer claimed his 'spirit' belongs to 'the coming generations' (Haggerty 1997: 466). When his home burned in his eighty-eighth year, destroying many of his private papers and the first four chapters of his autobiography, it only ensured that future biographers would have a freer hand when attempting to rewrite and revise his life's story.

Interestingly, recent biographies have addressed Jacobi's physical appearance in very different ways, paediatricians of the later twentieth century frequently commenting on his small stature and his 'sickly' childhood, one in an act of retrospective diagnosis suggesting that he 'probably had rickets' (Haggerty 1997: 462). These features, which were absent from all of Jacobi's obituaries, were later listed in a manner which was to convey Jacobi's suitability and sensitivity to the challenges that faced most immigrant families whose children he treated in New York throughout the second half of the nineteenth century. In this case, signs which were employed to denigrate the intellectual capacity of many other immigrants underscored Jacoby's capacity as a first-generation paediatrician. As David Livingstone has demonstrated in terms of scientific knowledge, time, as well as place, evidently conditions the generation and uptake of ideas (Livingstone 2003).

WELFARE AND WARFARE

While ideas about degeneration varied with geography, the bacteriological diagnosis of diseases such as diphtheria universally created new roles for public health departments and expanded the role of the state in citizens' lives. There are, in fact, countless ways in which the state harnessed medical expertise in the last decades of the age of empire, but the clearest and most sustained use lies in the state's use of expert knowledge around the figure of the child, which became the focus of increasing social anxieties, all seemingly requiring interventions in the late nineteenth century (Cooter 1992). Never one to focus on germs alone, Abraham Jacobi had always regarded the childhood illnesses he encountered in the poorest homes to be the result of faulty diet and, therefore, preventable. Pathologies, it followed, could in future be minimized by simply encouraging mothers to breastfeed children, for example, while other challenges required more aggressive interventions. In an early history of paediatrics penned at the end of his career, Jacobi, sounding a little like Lombroso, argued that 'Human society and the state have to protect themselves by looking out for a healthy, uncontaminated progeny' (Jacobi 1905: 21). The condition of children, he claimed, will determine whether the world will be more 'Cossack' or more 'Republican' (33), in a style more characteristic of a former revolutionary. Following the lines of his most admired predecessors, Jacobi claimed that it was not enough for doctors to 'work at the individual bedside and in a hospital' (33). Merely building hospitals in order to safeguard national health, as was common in the early nineteenth century, was to tackle the problem from the wrong end. The simultaneous establishment of children's law courts, rather than milk depots, only convinced him that America was still some way from the 'promised land'. Only when the nation's desire to avenge brutality was controlled, or asylums replaced state prisons, 'then we shall be a human, become humane, society' (33). He therefore urged physicians to seek out and assume influential roles in school boards, health departments and legislatures. The doctor, and not the politician, in his eyes, was the legitimate advisor to the judge, physicians owing communities their services as an obligation of citizenship. Jacobi even advocated the establishment of a health department led by a person of cabinet status, as became reality in Britain in 1919. Lombroso may have suggested that there was 'no room in politics for an honest man', but he rarely spoke on behalf of his profession, as Jacobi did for most of his later career (34). Lombroso's views openly clashed with those of Jacobi when the latter declared that 'it is time for the physician to participate in politics'. Only a life spent in service to mankind, in Jacobi's opinion, was a life well spent. He advised his medical brethren to '[n]ever stop working', always seek out 'new problems' (34), guidance that, albeit well meaning, might to some extent be responsible for the epidemic of medicalization, which, already evident in the nineteenth century, would run rampant in the next.

All too often regarded as a disjuncture from all that came before, the onset of war in 1914, on this occasion, seems more like continuity. If nothing else, it arguably fuelled the greater involvement of the state in health care, among other sectors. Much recent work on the First World War also reiterates the main themes covered in this introduction, not to mention the subsequent chapters in this volume. For example, the bureaucracy of wartime rapidly turned soldiers, like their peacetime, industrial equivalents, into numbers and statistics. Subjected to the same forces that transformed industrial society over the previous century, the armed forces became increasingly rationalized, professionalized and specialized (Harrison 1999: 2–3). Moreover, the war encouraged the entrance of women into the workforce, many, like Mary Putnam Jacobi, assuming positions formerly regarded as the preserve of male workers. Indeed, admitted to many more medical schools, women entered medicine in numbers that allowed them to dominate the civilian medical workforce in these years, especially as men enlisted. It is estimated that between 45% and 80% of doctors joined the forces in Britain and France (van Bergen 2009: 24–5). As a result, injured or sick soldiers sent home encountered female expertise and authority in ways unfamiliar to previous generations. As hospitals filled with the damaged and fragile bodies of male soldiers, these contrasts only intensified. The military medical environment, as Ana Carden-Coyne has shown, 'destabilised femininity and masculinity' on a larger scale than seen during the Jacobis' lifetimes (Carden-Coyne 2014: 251). Wounded male bodies suddenly appeared weak, many robust recruits from industry having been reduced to what many regarded to be women's natural state. Writings from the period similarly reveal a more complex picture of hospital therapy, with passive and wounded male bodies subjected to the rigours of a 'muscular' rehabilitation regime implemented by women. Previously regarded as vulnerable, female nurses and therapists routinely inflicted pain on injured men rendered 'functionally impotent' by their battle injuries (Carden-Coyne 2008: 143–4). Whereas female neurotic patients were treated with delicacy and sympathy in the nineteenth century, male patients with similar conditions were treated with a firm hand by nurses who more often resembled drill sergeants. Considered alongside other studies, it has become clearer why soldiers quickly became 'discontented with hospital life' (Carden-Coyne 2014: 318). Faced with anxieties produced by mass organized death on the front lines, soldiers often regressed into child-like states (Roper 2009: 1, 8), if their subordinate positions in the military bureaucracy had not already reduced them to 'passive and helpless waifs' (van Bergen 2009: 5). Like the careers of Abraham and Mary Jacobi, the cultural history of the war reveals the complexity of gender dynamics at the close of our period. The Great War indeed continues to appear revolutionary in turning aspects of Western society upside down (Carden-Coyne 2014a: 14).

While most members of contemporary society can only imagine the trauma endured by the Jacobis upon losing their son, Ernst, nearly all Europeans at the conclusion of the First World War were in a position to comprehend the family's loss. Despite a steady decline in mortality from infectious diseases in the twentieth century, families would continue to lose loved ones, often sons, many in youth, only now as the result of war. Twenty million men alone are estimated to have passed through the German and British armies between 1914 and 1918 (Watson 2008: 8), and it is believed that as many people were wounded during a conflict that saw the implementation of new and efficient forms of 'industrial killing' (van Bergen 2009: 11). It was the first conflict to harness industrial technology, allowing the deployment of machine-guns, tanks, gas, aircraft and flame throwers, among other lethal tools of warfare. While fatalities on the German side were counted in millions, British deaths numbered in the hundreds of thousands, and French casualties surpassed British ones. In sum, the war claimed many millions of victims (van Bergen 2009: 16). After the war's end, the lives of the many fallen were commemorated in countless memorials erected in communities globally. It is no surprise that the conflict was said to be responsible for 'the crucifixion of the youth of the world' (Powell 2009: 20).

Like those remembered in war memorials, Ernst Jacobi was laid to rest in a collective grave, marked 'The Babies'. Located in Brooklyn, the cemetery physically tied his final resting place to a location of serenity, rather than the 'battlefields' of urban Manhattan. Ernst's empty tomb on the shore of Lake

George was even more symbolically removed from the squalid urban environment with which his death and those of countless other children were associated in this era. Like those who would commemorate the slaughter of the First World War each Armistice Day after the conflict's end, Abraham Jacobi would undertake an annual pilgrimage to the Lake George site, which became an antidote to the trauma he had suffered (Winter 2014: 233). While the mortality of babies unusually halted its rise during the war, modern war memorials listed every soldier's name and thereby captured the devastation reaped by such conflict. According to Leo van Bergen, not only did death discard its scythe and become a 'machine operator' in the First World War, but he reminds us that, in contrast to the days of hand-to-hand combat, soldiers now usually came under attack from a distance. Unknown soldiers' lives were taken by unknown combatants firing bullets, shells or dropping bombs and, as a result, death became impersonal. Many were reduced to fragments and buried in unmarked graves, with only four in ten of the dead actually identified (van Bergen 2009: 483). In some respects, their plight resembles that of the patient, or sick man, in accounts of medicine throughout this period. The wounded and dead in war, like patients subjected to uniform tests, were often reduced to statistics during the conflict. The way their dismembered bodies were treated may equally remind scholars of the way in which medical students a generation earlier occasionally treated cadavers, even if this, in the case of war, was only the result of expediency (van Bergen 2009: 48). The incalculable losses sustained on all sides during the conflict, let alone its worst atrocities, left a generation traumatized and searching for a suitable language with which to describe the unparalleled loss and devastation they had experienced. Not surprisingly, martial terminology gradually seeped into medicine in the years that followed, while the heroic language of the military was adopted by members of the public who desperately sought a discourse appropriate to their collective bereavement (Winter 2014: 5, 53, 224). Heroic narratives have naturally endured in annual remembrance ceremonies, but they have also found their way into the accounts of military historians. Perhaps unsurprisingly, these reappeared in the publications of medical historians who first attempted to describe the sweeping transformations in medicine during the age of empire. And just as post-war society struggled to make sense of the Great War, medical historians, too, have more regularly searched for meaning in medicine's past.

NOTES

The author is grateful to Roger Cooter, Lisa Smith and Rebecca Wynter for reading and commenting on earlier drafts of this introduction.
1. Historical studies of the Jacobis include Truax 1952; Gardner 1959; Haggerty 1997; Bittel 2009; and Wells 2012.

2. For the best description of these transformations between the mid-nineteenth century and the pre-Second World War period, see Hammond 1999.

3. Chapter 15 in C. Geertz's *The Interpretation of Cultures* (412–53) provides a detailed account of the way in which the rituals of the Balinese cock fight gradually became apparent to Geertz and his wife, who arrived in Bali in 1958 to begin their fieldwork.

4. These include Briggs 1961; Rosenberg 1962; Morris 1976; Arnold 1986; Evans 198; and Hamlin 2009.

CHAPTER ONE

Environment

MATTHEW NEWSOM KERR

Medicine and environment intersect repeatedly and thoroughly. In fact there is hardly any other more well-established notion in any medical tradition than the one assuming that health and disease are invariably an expression in some way of natural and human landscapes. It has only been a little more recently, however, that this notion has been both delved into and critiqued as a question of substance for cultural history. The nineteenth century was a period of tremendous change for ancient notions of 'airs, waters and places'. Thus it is unsurprising that scholars have looked to unpack some of the ways that certain of these configurations were reconfigured by the age of empire.

For historians, medicine's connection to the environment is at once well established and at the same time now also ever more flexible and unstable. One way to approach this paradox is by reference to critical theories of space. We are a few decades into the spatial turn in the humanities and the 'new' cultural geography no longer seems all that new. We have long been advised to take *space* seriously and also to question how a sense of *place* is constructed and contingent. 'Space implies, contains, and dissimulates social relations,' Henri Lefebvre memorably instructed. 'Space lays down the law because it implies a certain order – and hence a certain disorder ... Space commands bodies' (Lefebvre 1992: 83–4, 142–3). These ideas were taken up first by urban social historians, who proposed that spatial contexts could no longer be relegated to mere backgrounds of historical events. This aligned with the arguments of critical geographers, looking to destabilize location and placedness itself as fixed coordinates and thus to challenge assumptions about the neutrality or naturalness of space. The lesson was that space was at once the product of social life and also the constricting medium giving shape to society. This critical

attitude shared many of the same concerns as the wave of cultural histories of
the body appearing in the 1980s. The main instigator here was undoubtedly
Michel Foucault, who propelled a radically historicist project aimed at
questioning how modernity invests bodies as sites and vessels of governance – a
development, not incidentally, in which he credited medicine in a key role.
Foucault's geographies of power reflect how critical theory had already moved
from production of space as central to the historical ordering of societies
(which had served to legitimate history's contribution as a social science) and
more toward this spatial production being part and parcel of the messy and
contradictory process of organizing meaning.

More broadly, as far as science studies is concerned, the spatial turn has
helped to refashion what had been discussed as the social construction of
knowledge into what was to become the cultural destabilization of knowledge.
The body and its architectural enclosure was one of the first targets of this
spatial disassemblement. It was followed eventually by a critical deciphering of
environments, terrains, landscapes, geographies, milieus and territories. These
could all be examined as *effects* of representation. They were not the stage
underneath, but rather part of the staging of identity, imagination, narrative,
memory and aesthetics. They were found, elicited and expressed through
language and text. In this light, 'the natural environment' (which had emerged
as a major analytical category and political concern in the 1960s and 1970s)
started to look not quite so natural. The environment, it turned out, was also
something that historically was *naturalized* by discourse. All of this goes some
way toward explaining the still-active fault lines between critical cultural history
and environmental history. The latter grew out of left-leaning social history
scholarship which viewed itself as a challenge to Western technoscientific
development. Most environmental historians have seemed wary of reducing the
environment to text, discourse and representation. Meanwhile, a smaller
segment of the environmental humanities (known sometimes as ecocriticism)
had arisen alongside feminist science studies and its interest in the cultural
production of nature (Heise, Christensen and Niemann 2017). It was critical
cultural studies that displayed openness to displacing the environment as a
natural given and to considering it a product of cultural discourse. These
inclinations played their own part in the academic culture wars of the 1990s
and featured in debates over whether medicine, science and reality itself are
reducible to systems of signification.

The aim of this chapter is far more modest. It traces some of the ways that
health and disease were spatialized – put into place, displaced and relocated as
a matter of culture – during the age of empire. Although discourses pertaining
to natural and human landscapes had always been central to medical
understanding, it is important to acknowledge that 'the environment' as we talk
about it today is not exactly the same as the geographic and topographical

imagination that proved so fertile for nineteenth-century medical thought. That being said, the methods and concerns of cultural history can help greatly in elucidating how the general understanding of 'the environment' was at once the product of medicine and also the constricting medium giving shape to medicine. Medical thought and practice 'took place' within and in relation to particular locations and idealized milieus. For this reason we are perhaps best served by considering the multiple, divergent as well as intersecting *environments* wherein Western medical thought and practice was constructed, as well as the environments which by means of this construction were themselves also transformed by medicine. Finally, this chapter also wants to suggest that cultural histories of medicine have already performed an important role in resituating the environment as a category of critical inquiry and have raised vital new questions about the cultural production of health and illness. The move to radically historicize medicine intersects in some important ways with the project of historicizing the environment both as a cultural resource and also as a product of culture. As it turns out, much of work completed in this field tends to attach to practices and discourses surrounding the rise of public hygiene and sanitation. Perhaps this has to do with the evident spatiality of these topics. In any case, for this chapter I have decided to focus on examples in relation to cholera, tuberculosis and malaria. I start with a general outline of the places and meanings of medical topography and conclude with some more specific arguments about the locations and uses of tropical medicine.

MEDICAL TOPOGRAPHIES

Johann Peter Frank's monumental *A System of Complete Medical Police* (published in nine volumes from 1779 to 1827) signifies the shifting importance of medical topography in modern systems of governance. The German professor of physiology and hygiene stressed that every publicly employed doctor should 'supply the medical description of his region as accurately as possible, and compare every change in weather, every phenomenon concerning the healthiness of a place, with his site so that the science of the influence of human dwellings and the climate of each country becomes better known' (Frank 1976: 180). On the one hand, Frank's treatise is clearly a continuation of ancient advice regarding health and environment, which stressed the medical significance of certain natural landscapes, airs, waters, elevations and climates. On the other hand, his work also shows how the medical understanding of environments was becoming incorporated as a political and economic problem of great importance and increasingly situated at the very jurisdictional core of *raison d'état*. The health of the people, previously really only emerging as a matter of concern during extraordinary crises like plague epidemics and involving only the negative suppression of threats, was newly conceived as a technical and epistemological project and was starting to reach beyond the 'political topographies' urged by mercantilist theorists since the sixteenth century as a means of cataloging the resources at the disposal of the ruler. Statistics – knowledge of the state – had emerged as an indispensible tool of effective governance, if simply because it was a representation of the power to know the governed terrain. It encompassed the 'political arithmetic' compiled and arranged by medical police and featured in the absolutist arsenal of surveillance and control (Rosen 1958: 84–6, 109–20). This understanding of the environment, however, also came to represent knowledge critical to representative and limited governance; it made possible a *positive* politics of health (or 'biopower' as described by Foucault) and a mode of government corresponding to liberal techniques for indirectly managing realms like scarcity, mortality and so on – milieus that have their own natural regularities and dispositions that cannot be completely controlled but may be guided to result in more favorable outcomes (Foucault 2007).

The task of ascertaining an ever-more detailed geography of health and disease had clearly become a matter of state, pertinent to organizing the productive capability of the nation's population. But it also had other commercial and parochial uses, such as realizing the commercial potential of health 'resorts' and allowing insurance underwriters to formulate more accurate mortality tables. Furthermore, medical topography was a means for doctors to establish their professional reputations and bolster their standing in community medical hierarchies. Consider one representative example among a large corpus of highly local studies: Henry Tooley's *History of the Yellow Fever: As it Appeared in the City of Natchez, in the Months of August, September & October, 1823* (Tooley 1823). This description of the chief commercial town in Mississippi went through at least two editions, and at a time when the town contained no more than 3,000 residents (of which at least 312 died in the epidemic). Tooley prefaces his account of that devastating event with a detailed description of physical topography and town layout, then proceeds to plot the important spots of corporeal and moral decay. Although the dung and offal pit served as a 'hotbed of pestilence and death', equal if not more importance is given to disorderly taverns (the devil's churches), the theatre and circus (the devil's school houses), ballrooms and dance houses (the devil's banquet-houses), and dram-shops and porter-houses (the devil's hog-sites). Medical topography in this local mode spoke closely to the uses of community gossip and criticism. Yet Tooley also joined this rhetoric of moral condemnation with the specialist language of clinical symptoms, an account of fifteen dissections after death (the revelatory 'geography of the corpse') and a consideration of the specific location and uses of the temporary hospital in Natchez. As this example shows, the conventions of medical topography in practice worked across various scales and sites of public discourse as a means of constructing a useful image of place and health (explored in a number of essays in Dyck and Fletcher 2011).

It also reveals the still-active tradition of reading the medical environment to be part of the project of constructing political terrains and identities (Rupke 2000). Specific medical topographies informed new techniques and rationalities of rule dependent upon expanding geographic knowledge and relationships. Enlightenment-era thought aimed to see the healthy government of the city applied to the entire national territory. By extension, it also encouraged the 'worlding' of medical topography and emerged as a principal consideration of imperial administration. James Ranald Martin's influential treatise, *The Influence of Tropical Climates on European Constitutions*, explained that any general system of sanitary inquiry and improvement by the medical topographer must:

> . . . embrace information respecting the surface and elevation of the ground, the stratification and composition of the soil, the supply and quality of the water, the extent of marshes and wet ground, the progress of drainage; the nature and amount of the products of the land; the condition, increase or decrease, and prevalent diseases of the animals maintained thereon; together with periodical reports of the temperature, pressure, humidity, motion, and electricity of the atmosphere. Without a knowledge of these facts it is impossible to draw satisfactory conclusions with respect to the occurrence of epidemic diseases, and variations in the rate of mortality and reproduction.
> —Martin 1856: 102

The massive task of a detailed world atlas of health would be relational and comparative. As literary scholar Alan Bewell shows, Western medicine's representation of natural environments was put to use in modernity's radical collapsing of distances as well as in its careful articulation of differences (Bewell 1999). In one sense this proved completely instrumental, such as considering the specific regions that seemed to be inherently dangerous to European troops, administrators and settlers. Most of Africa, large parts of Asia and practically all of the West Indies were characterized as diseased environments possessing thick, sarcophagus-like air. This topography of natural fitness raised the prospect that such spaces might be 'improved' to an extent necessary to support the *life* of empire. Martin argued that making landscapes conducive to (European-style) agriculture would be conducive to (European) health. He observed that in India 'an atmosphere of death gathers over all the country':

> But what do not industry and perseverance accomplish? The marshes are drained; the rivers flow in their disencumbered channels; the axe and the fire clear away the forests; the earth furrowed by the plough is opened to the

rays of the sun, and the influence of the wind; the air, the soil, and the waters acquire by degrees a character of salubrity; and a vanquished nature yields its empire to man, who thus creates a country for himself . . . Agriculture must be much improved in Bengal before the European . . . can be said to have created a country for himself.

—Martin 1856: 21

Whereas unhealthy environments signify nature's empire over man, their transformation into healthy and productive places represented a turning of the table and the ability to 'create a country'. To be sure, plenty of persons had misgivings toward this sunny outlook, but detractors themselves participated in cementing a pervasive trope that mapped the world in such a way as to represent non-European environments as neglected and thus perilous to health. A successful colonial site would of necessity be in some way an *altered health landscape*. Mark Harrison traces how this colonial medicine came to be topographical medicine. Following upon more direct forms of territorial rule in the early nineteenth century, he writes, India and its environment became more alien and its climate more readily seen by British administrators as dangerously incompatible with a European presence (Harrison 1999). Medical opinion about 'climates and constitutions' thus played a key role in a process by which non-European spaces and peoples could be othered and pathologized – and increasingly figured as atavistic or even degenerate. While notions of environmental determinism were never absolute, these older ideas were taken up in the nineteenth century by a variety of theorists (such as colonial ethnographers) as a way to support new racial typologies, genealogies and hierarchies. So, for example, the belief that an environment moulded the characteristics of its people was central for writers such as Martin in upholding belief in the natural enervation and 'effeminacy' of tropical constitutions like Bengalis (Sinha 1995). To this was added what were believed to be new-found linkages between environment and heredity. To be sure, neither 'nature' nor 'nurture' were exclusively privileged in the rise of nineteenth-century racial thought (itself heavily shaped by early anthropology's preoccupation with spatial origins and physiological expressions). Rather, a blend of cultural and topographical typologies were interwoven with the new science of descent and destiny, as seen in the enthusiasm with which these ideas were adopted by medical proponents of slavery in the American South (Stowe 2004).

PLACING CHOLERA

Other concerns arose in regard to the geographic mobility of certain epidemic diseases. Particularly influential were the environmental imaginings of cholera, considered the 'shock disease' of the era. While its clinical symptoms were relatively new and dreadful to Europeans, the spatial itinerary of 'Asiatic cholera' proved equally startling and was ascribed tremendous importance. Indeed, there was an endless fascination with plotting, following and tracking its movement from its presumably ancient, natural 'seat' in the Ganges River delta to the civilized world (see Figure 1.1). Maps like this represent a deep appreciation of the global reach of sickness (a notion that was vaguely comprehended in earlier centuries' continental 'exchanges' of smallpox and syphilis). Many Western observers believed the primary lesson to be the worrisome linkages, routes and channels that had been forged to colonial environments, with the resulting impossibility of 'foreign diseases' staying in their natural places. Ultimately, this notion was capable of many different and competing meanings. For Irish poets John and Michael Banim, the advance of cholera in 1831 befitted the apocalyptic retribution due all oppressive empires:

> From my proper clime and subjects,
> In my hot and swarthy East,
> North and Westward I am coming
> For a conquest and a feast –
> And I come not until challenged,
> Through your chilly lands to roam! –
> As a bride ye march'd to woo me,
> And in triumph led me home!
>
> —Banim and Banim 1831: 3

A great number of medical writers indignantly insisted that cholera must be considered properly 'at home' in India, yet still capable of taking up temporary residence in the West. So said the author of *Cholera in its Home*, who explained that the disease always attached itself to particular places: riverbanks usually, especially those that were the most populous, crowded and filthy. He intended, not incidentally, to refute a wicked French notion that cholera was not naturally endemic to India but had been made so by British exploitation of the Indian people and their resulting moral and social 'dissolution' (Macpherson 1866).

That a disease could have an ancestral 'homeland' was at this time a conceit intrinsic to medical geography. It shaped theories about how a disease might visit (or 'invade') new lands and informed proposals for putting an end to these travels. As with the plague before it, cholera resulted in border quarantines and prompted states and empires to consider sundry rings of precautions that might delineate and demarcate the healthy inside from the unhealthy outside. Perhaps more so than other supposed 'imported' diseases of the age, cholera epitomized a natural violation of sovereign territory (as the Banim brothers ably commemorated). It also prompted new ways for Western publics to imagine their own medicalized homeland and the body of laws that might complement

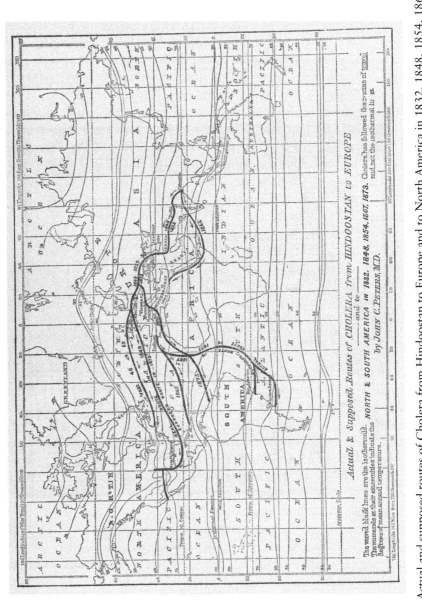

FIGURE 1.1: Actual and supposed routes of Cholera from Hindoostan to Europe and to North America in 1832, 1848, 1854, 1867 and 1873. John Peters, *A Treatise on Asiatic Cholera* (New York: W. Wood, 1885), btw. pp. 68 and 71. Wellcome Collection.

and protect the national bodily character. An 1832 broadside, *John Bull Catching the Cholera*, sketches a tale about the moral topography of Britain (see Figure 1.2). In the original print the turbaned cholera has menacingly blue skin and yellow eyes; he is only stopped by a rosy-cheeked John Bull commanding him by the neck and wielding a club labelled 'Heart of Oak'. Cholera has just

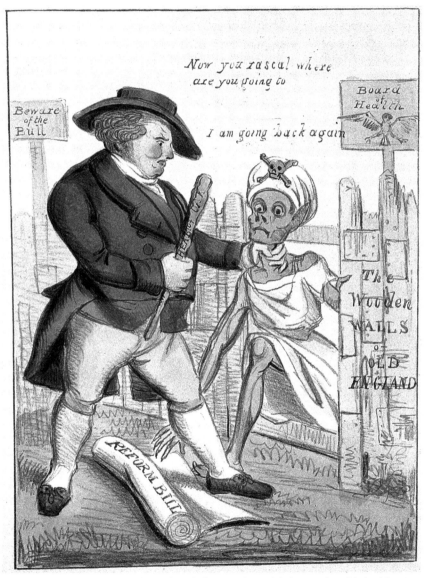

FIGURE 1.2: *John Bull Catching the Cholera*. Coloured lithograph published by O. Hodgson, London, *c.* 1832. Wellcome Collection.

slipped through 'The Wooden Walls of Old England' (a reference to the naval and commercial ships that long had shielded England from foreign threats but that also formed its link to the colonial world) and is reaching for a copy of the Great Reform Bill. The print seems to state that political stability and steadfastness of the people (symbolized in the figure of John Bull's stout 'constitution') was the true obstacle to cholera's entry. To 'catch' cholera at the border, as it were, is not to contract the disease, but rather to take it in hand and to restrict its spatial limits. Still, the broadside suggests some apprehensions about the ability to blockade the nation. It hints, for example, at an undercurrent of 'anti-contagionism' that had grown somewhat influential within anti-establishment medical thought and that Erwin Ackernecht classically argued was an expression of liberal mistrust of the system of ordinary quarantine (Ackernecht 1948). Cholera passed through England's 'Wooden Walls', after all. Whether or not believers in contagion, for a number of thinkers a key question was what sort of physical and moral environment diseases like cholera would find once they washed ashore – a throwback, to be sure, toward older ideas of 'epidemic constitution' and even more generally to medical topography's concern with the influence of atmospheres and predispositions upon 'prevailing diseases'.

Cholera contributed mightily to new postures of trepidation and fear toward urban environments already in the throes of radical change. Indeed, whereas in South Asia it was primarily a rural phenomenon, cholera in the West was seen mainly as a problem and an expression of cities. Historians Catherine Kudlick and Richard Evans provide classic accounts of how cholera gave rise to new strategies of meaning and cultural accommodation amongst the self-confident urban middle classes in Paris and Hamburg, respectively (Kudlick 1996; Evans 1987). These were in their own ways centres of liberal economic ascendency and emblems of the commercial and professional spatial hegemony rising in Western metropolises. Even though cholera's death toll was always lower than the commonplace fevers and dysenteries, it signified many of the broad bourgeois assumptions about the intrinsic unhealthiness of urban social environments. Above all, cholera was seen as an outgrowth of unnatural spatial compression. It called to mind an urban terrain too tightly crowded with the poor, with dilapidated housing and with an inexorable tide of human filth. These too were structured by increasingly stereotypical global juxtapositions of outcast and abject spaces (Marriott 2003). Cholera-afflicted spots seemed to share certain natural affinities with the backward East, and thus appeared like transplantations from far-off lands. Legends of the stifling alleyways of Jessore were linked with images of the 'Courts for King Cholera' to be found in the typical London slum (see Figure 1.3). John Leech's well-known and widely reproduced caricature gives these dirty poor people distinctively Irish physiognomies and thereby solidifies the association of dirty poor places with a

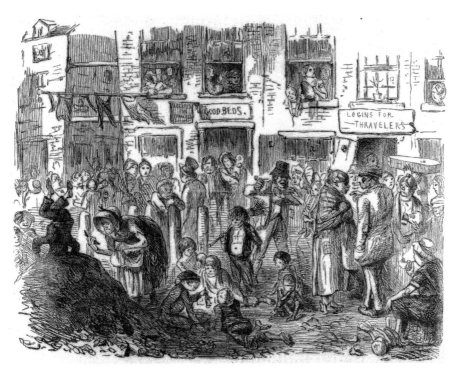

FIGURE 1.3: 'A Court for King Cholera', *Punch*, 25 September 1852, p. 139.
Wellcome Collection.

type of foreign contamination. And so while fear of cholera in the West was
always concerned with sites of entry, this fear itself came to be concentrated
upon the amassings and admixtures common to modern cities that held the
capacity to destabilize national and colonial boundaries. Indeed, for many
contemporaries, cholera legitimated and naturalized the overall context of
urban class conflict and blame – a well-established trope in British social history.
Stated a bit differently from the perspective of cultural history, cholera
functioned as a 'master referent for the condition of England debate [and] a
means of articulating concerns about the effect of the industrial revolution on
the English self' (O'Connor 2000: 28).

Similar statements could be made for other Western societies, which goes to
show how the most pressing questions of urban health served multiple,
interrelated layers of geographical meaning-making and accompanied the
spatial production of sanitary subjectivities. For instance, a growing number of
scholars have sought to feel out the emotional and sensory contours to this
cultural topography of urban modernity (Kenny 2014; Mack 2015). A classic
expression is Alain Corbin's *The Foul and the Fragrant*, which argues that it is

necessary to place smell historically and to trace the ways the olfactory register was both displaced and brought into play by bourgeois culture in the nineteenth century. As conventionally practised 'on the ground' and 'by the nose', medical topography's search for the spaces of disease necessarily involved a form of sensory assault and subjection – a fact that helps explain the urban middle class's heightened sensitivity to smellscapes as well as its steadily lowering threshold of tolerance for putrescent odours. Perceptibility of the environment was a key means for both demarking social status as well as publishing personal distinction (Corbin 1986; Drobnick 2006). So, for example, the denizens of King Cholera's court are morbidly 'at home' amongst their mounds of filth and not bothered at all by the obligatory stench – they are both disastrously subjected and perhaps also frighteningly immune to the effects of miasma. This seeming paradox comes up constantly in the 1842 *Report on the Sanitary Conditions of the Labouring Population of Great Britain* by Edwin Chadwick (he of 'all smell is disease' fame) and it hints at how the cultural construction of the olfactory environment was absolutely central to the spatial work of sanitary reform (Kiechle 2017; Reinarz 2014). Cholera was just one of many disease threats that, apart from encouraging the deodorization of cities, helped to circumscribe a 'civilizing process' whereby urban society invested and rewarded the possession of delicate and discriminating sensitivities. As two doctors investigating fever in London explained, 'Malaria being invisible and intangible, men in rude states of society are totally ignorant of its existence' (Arnott and Kay 1837–8: 68). This was the essential environmental backdrop for nineteenth-century osmology (a science and aesthetics of 'who smells'), itself necessary for George Orwell's mocking cliché that 'the lower classes smell' (Carlisle 2004; Orwell 1937/2001). Often enough it is this fascination with the symbolically low, rejected and peripheral that makes such objects culturally central to the bourgeois project of distinguishing itself (Stallybrass and White 1986). Such is the thrust of the multidisciplinary work, *Filth: Dirt, Disgust and Modern Life*, whose authors suggest that the construction of sanitary landscapes have been inseparably linked with the cultural production of repulsive landscapes (Cohen and Johnson 2004)

A notch below disgust, we can also think of the nineteenth-century city giving rise to medical discourses of sensory irritation and annoyance. Doubtlessly, the expanding variety and intensity of urban and industrial sounds created new environments of auditory disorientation, and at the same time they also fuelled a bourgeois culture of close listening and auditory regulation (Picker 2003). The shifting soundscapes of modern cities were in this way inseparable from the shifting importance of hearing and always involved efforts to redefine the proper location of *noise* – akin to filth, it is sound that is 'out of place' (Bailey 1996; Douglas 2002). Alain Corbin has famously traced the 'desacralization' of church bells in nineteenth-century France, a process during which their peals progressively lost the prophylactic ability to purify the air and to instil 'the peace of near, well-defined horizons' (Corbin 1998). It was a longer process than for stench, but by the end of the century *noise* was also substantially remedicalized – an accomplishment that went hand in hand with the commodification of silence and with attempts to rationalize the acoustic environment by creating fixed zones of auditory performance. Other historians suggest even more pointedly that we should be carefully attuned to the place of nineteenth-century medicine in the cultural production of quietude and its spatial meanings. The problem with noise gradually became a concern about mental stress and nervous diseases, which itself must be recognized as an outgrowth of changing ideas about modern urban life (Boutin 2015; Payer 2007; Thompson 2004; Bull and Black 2003).

Similar concerns framed the medicalization and spatialization of sight. While much of visual culture studies in the 1980s and 1990s initially focused specifically upon the representation and utilization of the body (propelled by Foucault's notion of the medical gaze; see Crary 1990 and Stafford 1991), historians have started to look more at the medical and cultural construction of nineteenth-century visual environments. Philosophical and aesthetic debates over modernity and its 'visual regimes' have tended to stress either the commercial practices of display and exhibition or the governmental geographies of inspection and surveillance. The technical and cultural history of lighting by Wolfgang Schivelbusch seemed so pioneering because it explored the productive interplay between spectacle and panopticism (Schivelbusch 1995). Meanwhile, Chris Otter's intriguing book on Victorian technologies of visuality seeks explicitly to challenge these categories. He is concerned with the messy process of organizing the visual environment, practically all of which compulsively intersected with concerns about public health and the limits of the body. The movement for smoke abatement and slaughterhouse reform, the provision of public lighting and road paving, the expansion of glass panelling – all are read by Otter as creating spaces for encouraging individual contemplation and self-judgement (Otter 2008). The medical privileging of sight therefore might also serve as a key political technology of nineteenth-century liberalism. In a very general way, then, the cultural study of the senses can usefully inform the ways that older concepts of environmental 'nuisance' came to be framed as medical matters. It also provides important opportunities for historians to examine the contingency and instability of sensory cultures, as well as how this structured the 'invention of pollution' in the nineteenth century (Thorsheim 2006; Taylor 2016).

Closely tied to tropes of urban disorder and crisis, cholera is especially connected (at least figuratively) with the nineteenth-century's major urban environmental reforms and sanitary infrastructure. Much of this was enacted juridically: laws that enabled local building codes, zoning ordinances, rules and procedures for removal of specific hazards, civil protections against the adulteration of foodstuffs, as well as the establishment of public health officials to oversee and inspect and manual workers to build and cleanse. 'Sanitationism' is perhaps best known for large projects of sanitary construction bringing about the material architectures of power. An important aim was to re-engineer city landscapes and thereby 'canalize' individual and social conduct in completely new ways. The result was fundamentally new (yet also problematic and contested) relationships between the city and its bodies, classes, populations and governances. This model was established by the comprehensive reconstruction of Paris's infrastructure initiated in the early 1850s under the Baron Georges Haussmann and his chief engineer Eugène Belgrand. *Haussmannization* put into practice the principles and objectives of circulation, both material and symbolic. These famously called for a convoluted sewer network and for the creation of wide, paved streets that would be more easily aerated and cleansed of filth (and, so it is said, of potential revolutionaries). These Parisian reforms, in part structured by the vision of a medicalized urban landscape, served to organize a new form of metropolitan experience, epitomized in the city's boulevard culture that merged flâneur aesthetics, commercial spectacles and bureaucratic scopic regimes (Harvey 2003; Reid 1991). In Britain the sanitary gospel resulted in a focus on slum clearance, an interest in water and baths provision and especially an instrumental enthusiasm for drains and sewers. Sanitary reform in London and elsewhere required the reconstruction and update of ancient systems of local governance, and thus in various ways Whitehall ran up against and had to accommodate the interests of urban elites. The *system* itself was one of negotiation and compromise, and shows the important connection between public health and the public sphere (each conceived, by the way, as spatial and environmental). A number of recent histories of health governance in Britain stress the extent to which sanitary authority was not imposed from outside and above but rather built up, assembled and self-limited from within an atmosphere of open debate and contestation (Newsom Kerr 2018; Crook 2016; Mooney 2015).

The emerging conception of the city environment suitably overlaid by toilets and underlain by sewers was one aimed at mediating the newly appreciated and subtly varied geography of health-endangering filth. One of Edwin Chadwick's informants mapped his district by the extent of privy accommodation and graded the latrines he encountered on a tour of a poor district thus: two were 'rather filthy', ten 'filthy', forty-five 'very filthy', seven 'exceedingly filthy', and twenty-six 'disgustingly filthy'. Chris Hamlin argues that this sensory environment led the British public (and many historians) 'by the nose' to the only conceivable answer: 'the small bore pipe sewer' (Hamlin 1998: 8, 11). Expressly medical responses initially played second fiddle to engineering solutions. It was, Hamlin contends, one of 'the greatest technical fixes in

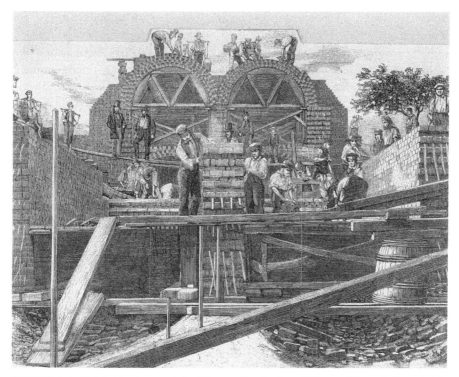

FIGURE 1.4: 'Main Drainage of the Metropolis. Sectional View of Tunnels from Wick Lane, Near Old Ford, Bow, Looking Westward', *Illustrated London News*, 27 August 1859. Wellcome Collection.

history' (15), which allowed policymakers to defer consideration of the social preconditions of epidemic events (such as wages, education, diet and so on). Poor people would continue to be essentially deprived and relatively hungry, but they could be less sick simply by breaking their physical connection to miasma. Although this focus on water and filth was believed to be ostensibly politically neutral, it nonetheless became an immensely significant technology of urban material culture. Systems of sewerage infrastructure were usually not aimed so much at completely redoing urban environments as much as adding a layer (or substrata) of access to 'the social' (Osborne 1996; Gilbert 2009). Or at least that was the idea in some of the most optimistic versions of sanitary systems. Infrastructural reform played out differently in many national and municipal contexts, but was everywhere a key part of the 'creative destruction' sweeping over nineteenth-century cities. Sewer construction could temporarily rent the urban fabric and expose to view the world beneath one's feet (see Figure 1.4). The scale of these public works dwarfed the human figure and human labour itself, and it effectively rendered the massive apparatus itself the operative agent of purification. Furthermore, and in actuality, there was constant struggle over the 'naturalness' of these sanitary systems. Literary scholar Michelle Allen traces some of the popular misgivings about a sprawling subterranean empire of filth. Instead of providing a neat image of containment, she writes, the sewer network was seen as '[drawing] together the individual and the mass, the poor and the rich, the diseased and the healthy' (Allen 2008: 43). Sanitary improvements were hailed as a piece with the monumentalization of imperial cities but just as often condemned for tearing down the eccentric old quarters of towns, disfiguring familiar environments and producing an urban landscape marked by a profound sense of disorientation and dislocation.

The reoccurrence of urban disease crises (as well as the steady toll of ill health perceived to be bundled in urban spaces) underscore the emergence of cities as terrains of problematic legibility. Indeed, it was the nineteenth-century city and its growing literate public that provided an ever-recomposing site of journalistic adventure and commentary. This at times vied with and at other times supported the perception of the city environment as a field for rational scrutiny and exact measurements. Indeed, although cholera and other epidemics were not directly associated with political revolutions, they undeniably triggered a wave of scientific and public investigations – and it was these observations that in turn sparked interventions (Hamlin 2009: 11; Evans 1988). One can clearly discern the rise of a new breed of urban explorers like Henry Mayhew, who insinuated that the 'localities of fever and disease' in London had become so well known that the metropolis could be 'mapped out pathologically, and divided into its morbid districts and deadly cantons'.

> We might lay our fingers on the Ordnance map, and say here is the typhoid parish, and there the ward of cholera; for as truly as the West-end rejoices in the title of Belgravia, might the southern shores of the Thames be christened Pestilentia. As season follows season, so does disease follow disease in the quarters that may be more literally than metaphorically styled the plague-spots of London.
>
> —Mayhew 1849

Mayhew's method, even though it conferred an air of objectivity around urban medical topography, nonetheless also relied upon startling narratives of his journeys into dark, dangerous, strange regions within London, penetrated with great difficulty and at high risk to himself. The sensationalism of filth rubbed off in some respects onto official investigations, which were sometimes anticipated as significant literary events. There was, for example, a palpable sense of eagerness about an imminent report by the City of London medical officer, in tabular form, on the results of a house-to-house inspection during the 1849 cholera outbreak. The London *Times* believed it 'likely to equal, in the fearful interest of its unvarnished disclosures, the vivid horrors of those fictitious chronicles, the *Mysteries of Paris* and the *Revelations of London*' (*Times*, 22 October 1849). The explosive growth of the amateur and official sanitary exposé as a genre bears many similarities with the mid-century emergence of detective fiction (having its own affinities with earlier forms of Gothic and serial crime literature).

By this time the urban environment had became something like an unruly text to be read, deciphered and recomposed in a coherent narrative – especially those 'plague-spots' that awaited illumination and articulation by heroic medical men. One example is Dr Hector Gavin's *Sanitary Rambles* through the London slum of Bethnal Green. To 'ramble' had been to undertake a pleasurable hike across country lanes and fields, akin to 'sauntering' without a definite goal; for Gavin and his contemporaries the urban terrain became knowable through the acts of walking, looking, discovering and reporting (Gavin 1848). Finding its limits, that form of narrative itself also involved a manoeuvre of containment: defining and marking out those dark, furtive, labyrinthine and exotic parts of modern cities that resisted intelligibility. This is the point that Susan Craddock makes about the official and amateur sanitary surveys of San Francisco's Chinatown from the 1860s onward. Kay Anderson in her analysis of Vancouver's Chinatown likewise argues that there was a propensity for nineteenth-century Western cities to create 'landscape types' for immigrants deemed too foreign to assimilate. Spaces of racial separation and distancing were discursively reproduced in texts that compulsively narrate an experience of difference, exoticness and pathologization. These were used to justify the near-place's continued neglect or even complete abolition. The genre is exemplified by Charles Warren Stoddard's 'A Bit of Old China', which takes the reader on a venture beyond and below the front streets of the 'coolie quarter' in San Francisco. He recounts being 'plunged' into a disorienting 'Mongolian' maze of catacombs and black holes:

> Between brick walls we thread our way, and begin descending into the abysmal darkness; the tapers, without which it were impossible to proceed with safety, burn feebly in the double night of the subterranean tenements. Most of the habitable quarters under the ground are like so many pigeon-houses indiscriminately heaped together. If there were only sunshine enough to drink up the slime that glosses every plank, and fresh air enough to sweeten the mildewed kennels, this highly eccentric style of architecture might charm for a time, by reason of its novelty; there is, moreover, a suspicion of the picturesque lurking about the place – but, heaven save us, how it smells!

Stoddard in his breathless adventure stumbles upon insensible opium smokers 'having the look of plague-stricken corpses', a small hospital 'smelling of punk and pestilence', and the city pest-house having a whole section set aside for Chinese lepers. 'China is not more Chinese than this section of our Christian city,' he wrote. Admitting that the journey produced more amazement than firm understanding, Stoddard deduces (in a significantly geographic manner) that 'it is but a step from Confucius to confusion' (Stoddard 1901/1912).

Indeed, the relentless confusion manufactured by the modern urban environment prompted many different medical projects of rationalization and various discursive strategies for producing clarity and legibility. Among the most important were efforts to map the city and its natural forces. Several literary critics have considered Victorian cartography's relationship to medical metaphors of circulation, to sanitary surveillance and to rational constructions of the social body (Nead 2005; Poovey 1995). Cholera was the disease that inaugurated some of the most important innovations in medical mapping. For many contemporaries, maps seemed to promise a health topography cleanly encoded by the cool, objective, surveilling eye of statistics and exact measurements. The powers of clinical observation, perfected on individual sick bodies, would be brought to bear upon afflicted cities and populations. The most persuasive maps, critical cartographers have argued, are those which deny the process of their own creation and which hold at arm's length the anecdotal and impressionistic mode of description that characterized the typical sanitary survey. A map's depiction of a space was supposedly more reliable than the narration of the same space – the map *is* the territory. Historians interested in the cultural context of scientific knowledge are quick to show that this vision of cartographic objectivity was actually highly contested; debates over the source of cholera for example were wrought with conflicts over the interpretation of map-images. To take the most famous example, John Snow's cartographic inscription of London cholera in 1854 often enough today serves as *the* exemplar of nineteenth century medical mapping, even though scholars in the field have shown the maps were something of an afterthought for Snow himself and achieved little at the time to advance his theory of waterborne cholera. The myth of John Snow is essentially the myth of his map (the 'ghost map', as it is hailed in a recent popular history; see Johnson 2007).

The overinflated importance given to Snow's map (not his epidemiology) can be chalked up to an air of objectivity that still accrues to statistics and to maps, and that arguably characterizes our own time even more strongly than the nineteenth-century. Today, as then, the focus on the reality of the thing represented has the effect of obscuring the modes and tactics of representing reality (a disconnect, by the way, that marks the essential difference between the methods and objectives of social history compared to those of the cultural history of medicine). As the literary scholar Pamela Gilbert deftly shows, Victorian medical mapmakers were always concerned with finding ways to successfully guide interpretation of their images and to gain respect for the

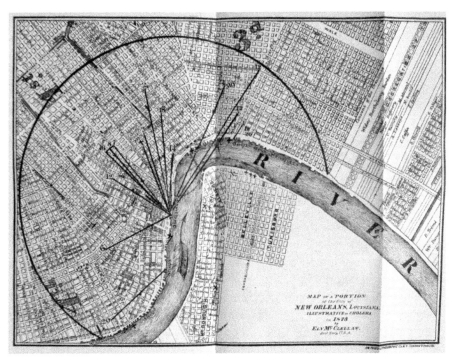

FIGURE 1.5: Map of a Portion of the City of New Orleans, Louisiana, Illustrative of Cholera in 1873 by Ely McClellan, Asst. Surg. U.S.A. John M. Wordworth, *The Cholera Epidemic of 1873 in the United States* (Washington: Government Printing Office, 1875), following p. 104. USA National Library of Medicine, Bethesda.

medical comprehension of urban environments (Gilbert 2004). An illustrative example is the study of the cholera epidemic of 1873 conducted for the US Surgeon General by Ely McClelland. His massive report featured a number of maps of affected cities along the Mississippi River and these were intended to refute the anti-contagionist doctrine of non-importation (see Figure 1.5). McClelland's map of New Orleans identified the residences of the first twenty persons to suffer from cholera and connected these with straight lines to their places of employment. Lines converged at a levee where steamships arriving from infected cities had docked. He also added a semi-circle to enclose the area of greatest prevalence (not coincidentally centred exactly around the levee), implying not a general diffusion of cholera but a circumscribed space of intensity that contained what McClelland had already argued were the primary means of transmission: the steamboat trade and traffic. The map proposes and inscribes a disease epicentre – an idea resisted by the city's own physicians, although they had been the ones to supply the data (Woodworth 1875; Koch 2005: 159–76). Quite unlike Snow, McClelland used cartography to make his argument about the movement of cholera being linked to the movement of people. His map takes a common visualization of the environment (an ordinary street map) and literally draws attention to certain instrumental spatial factors. The *evidence* that is produced is visual. The map itself in fact serves as an analytical space and is presented as a device for producing legibility, resolving doubt and rendering the disorderly life of the city calculable and probabilistic. It was often remarked that disease maps of this sort were more persuasive than several pages of explanatory text and narration, which underscores how cartography was rising to become a key representational tactic of modernity.

TUBERCULOSIS AND CURABLE GEOGRAPHIES

Whereas cholera was always linked in some way to medical geography within Western thought, tuberculosis is an example of a disease that gradually built a significant connection to the environment over the course of the nineteenth century. At the beginning of the period, few European doctors considered the possibility of consumption being communicable, an assumption that seemed to toughen by mid-century (in Italy, however, Fracastoro's concept of contagion continued to be followed). This, one of the most prevalent sources of mortality, was generally considered an inherited predisposition that could be activated by some 'intervening causes' such as damp indoor habitation and morbid mental state – 'sorrowful passions', Laënnec believed. As David Barnes shows, the epidemiological study of pulmonary tuberculosis arose alongside that of other diseases, but unlike with cholera this did not necessarily connect in any important way with theories of cause (Barnes 1995). French hygienists took the lead in recognizing that consumption could be mapped socially and geographically, which supported a notion of the unequal burdens of disease and the social determinants of health. Comparing the differential mortality in Parisian arrondissements, for example, Louis-René Villermé found the only significant variable to be wealth. The poor quite simply suffered more sickness and died earlier than the rich, and consumption was a key way this relationship was expressed. Although these insights informed debates about the 'social question' and promoted a statistical understanding of public health, they failed at the time to advance much of a corresponding medical programme for the prevention of tuberculosis.

Instead, shifting patterns of leisure and migration tended to intersect with new ideas about salutary climates and to engender the search for environmental treatments for consumption. An important piece of context was the reblossoming of European spa resorts after the Napoleonic Wars and the era's significantly changed distribution of wealth and power. For centuries spas had served primarily as sites for aristocratic sociability and the display of manners; they provided important scenes of classed and gendered self-fashioning rooted in medical and philosophical notions of therapeutic landscapes (Herbert 2009; Gesler 1998; Gesler 1992; Porter 1990). Similar thinking about the healing power of nature had also significantly shaped asylum design and hospital gardens (Moran et. al. 2011; Hickman 2013). Douglas Mackaman argues that, starting in the 1820s, spas helped the French bourgeoisie to create an acceptable and 'disciplined' practice of leisure on vacation. Key to this was the *medicalization* of spa treatment and the rage for a bracing, ascetic hydrotherapy regimen that architecturally and administratively exhibited virtues of privacy and respectability. With some variation, similar developments in health tourism were occurring across Europe, and these aided in constructing middle-class identity (Mackaman 1998; Anderson and Tabb 2002; Chambers 2002). This commodification of the spaces of treatment corresponds with the sentimentalization of consumption as a romantic ailment. The flushed, hectic expenditure of life force was now viewed as giving an air of languor that could be quite becoming. Consumption became a common index of the genteel and sensitive character, a trope for ephemeral genius and a sign of fashionable and refined sensibilities – at least for well-healed sufferers (Lawlor 2006). A romantic disease required suitably commensurate locations of retreat and treatment. At the turn of the century, Italy was the popular destination of wealthy English consumptives like John Keats. A treatise by James Clark, Keats's physician, recommended residence for some years in a mild climate as a means of alleviating symptoms but cautioned against expecting a cure (Clark 1829). This type of advice was integrated into older conventions of medical travel, yet also eventually made its way into rising enthusiasm for different sorts of therapeutic places.

Romantic faith in nature's healing powers tended to diminish the attraction of highly manicured spas and to elevate the importance of rustic, untrammelled lands. The new attitude toward a 'change of air and habits' is indicated by the naturally dramatic and lonely environments increasingly recommended: deserts and mountains. Starting in the 1850s, Hermann Brehmer advanced the somewhat heretical belief that consumption could be cured by proper diet, judicious exercise and above all plenty of fresh mountain air. In 1859, with the assistance of his friend, the explorer and geographer Alexander von Humbolt, he opened the first sanatorium for consumptives at Görbersdorf in Silesia (where his sister-in-law had already operated a successful hydropathic spa). Brehmer encouraged his patients to take their exercise in the form of uphill rambles. His faith in the healthful effects of crisp, high-altitude air never lacked in detractors, and in fact there were just enough emulators to start a small movement. A handful of spas catering specifically to consumptives opened in Davos, Switzerland, starting with the former mountain inn converted to this use by entrepreneur Willem Jan Holsboer and Dr Alexander Spengler in 1868 and operated on the medical principles set down by Brehmer. These *Kurhausen*

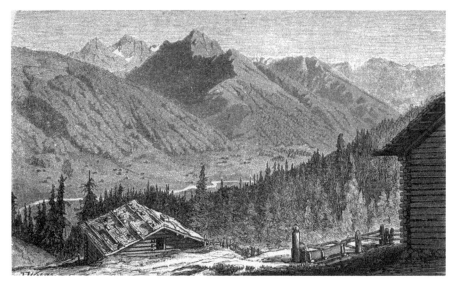

FIGURE 1.6: Rustic Cure-Site: The Schatzalp in 1878. Le Paysage de Davos: Station Climatérique pour Maladies de Poitrine, au point de vue spécial de la méthode thérapeutique suivie dans l'etablissement de cure. W. J. Holboer, *Guide Pour Medicins et Malades* (Zurich: Orell Füssli & Co., 1878), facing p. 34. From copy held in the Boston Medical Library in the Francis A. Countway Library of Medicine.

were surrounded by scenic-point trails and little mountainside outposts like the Schatzalp – 300 metres above Davos and at the time accessible only by foot (see Figure 1.6). The regimen was supposed to consist of patients engrossing themselves in the invigorating Alpine atmosphere, although it allegedly also took the form of lounging about the town's casinos, which must have been quite reminiscent of spa vacations.

The shifting medical geographies of consumption correspond to shifting destinations for treatment and to identities of sickness fashioned by these locations. The cultural meaning of tuberculosis was increasingly framed as a restless, searching subjectivity. Nowhere was this perhaps truer than in North America, where by the 1830s frontier settlement had coincided with a culture of *health seeking*. As described by Sheila Rothman, these sojourners were not looking momentarily to 'take a cure', but rather to fully take on a simpler, regenerative lifestyle. Westward expansion was partly fuelled by fantasies stoked in advice literature and popular anecdotes (bolstered first by trappers and pioneers, and later by city promoters and real estate adventurers) that the American Southwest and Pacific seaboard offered an Eden in comparison to the crowded cities and torpid plantation landscapes of the eastern states. One magnificent tale of the healthful environment involved a 250 year-old man who had to return east to die; alas, when his corpse was returned to California for burial, it leapt up again with the vitality and beauty of youth (Rothman 1994: 134)! Slightly less incredible stories (sometimes told in all earnestness) no doubt impelled some health-seekers, and they are in some way indicative of the general professional attitude toward the dry and mountainous frontier environment. In 1915 some four-fifths of the members of the Colorado Medical Society reported that they had come west for their own health (Rothman 1994: 132). Medical topography was the prevailing frame of reference for American physicians' professional writing in the first half of the century; this clearly retained its appeal and came to shape the gendered and patriotic stakes of health-seeking. A cult of wilderness-shaped manly virility reached its apogee in figures like Teddy Roosevelt, who provided a moral legend about camping, hunting and roughing one's way to health. The type of image he emulated and cultivated was popular enough to eventually fuel a backlash of sorts. The fear of being awash in consumptives led to attempts to limit the migration of 'lungers' to places like Los Angeles at the end of the century (Abel 2007; Ott 1996).

That is because the connection of tuberculosis with the environment was again being geographically transformed by treatment practices and new understandings of etiology. In America, this had started with the transcontinental railroad and the growth of towns marketed as meccas for consumptives. Medically-prescribed locations for consumption were becoming significantly less rustic and self-sufficient, significantly more systematic and institutional. Reflecting what has been called the *incorporation* of American society and culture (Trachtenberg 1982), medical thought shifted toward upholding the necessity of careful observation and physician-administered treatment regimens. These developments changed the spatial and cultural meaning of sickness; they converted consumptives from independent *health-seekers* into *guided passengers* and *submissive lodgers*. At the same time, climate in and of itself, though still important, was receding as a primary element of treatment – a reconfiguration of the place of the environment undoubtedly also linked to Robert Koch's discovery of the tubercle bacillus in 1882. The emerging bacteriology of tuberculosis seemed to signal an end to the romantic conception of consumption. It pushed most sanatoriums to conform to the more enclosed and controlled hospital architecture reminiscent of laboratories. Understanding tuberculosis as an effect of a pathogen also shifted the spatial rationale of the sanatorium in some degree toward isolating infected sick persons from vulnerable, germ-free people. It is in this context that Flurin Condrau writes of the 'interdependence of medical institutions and the production of stigma' towards tuberculosis (Condrau 2010: 85). Alison Bashford notices how a 'culture of confinement' had always more or less been a part of the sanatorium, but this was increasingly accentuated in specifically medicalized ways – even while the experience continued to be more like a health retreat for the rich and more a hospital for the masses (Bashford 2003: 133).

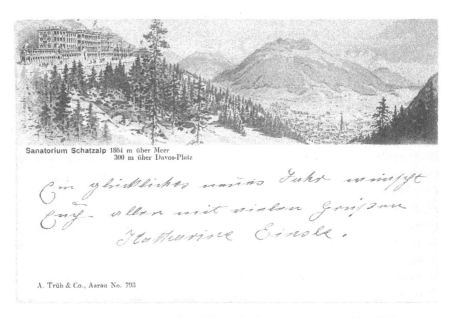

Sanatorium Schatzalp 1864 m über Meer
300 m über Davos-Platz

A. Trüb & Co., Aarau No. 793

FIGURE 1.7: Institutional Cure-Site: Schatztalp Sanatorium, opened in 1900.
Postcard in author's (MNK) possession.

In this light, the cultural history of tuberculosis is a relatively clear example
of the interlap of modern spaces and modern identities. As the geography of
tuberculosis shifted once again, so did its mode of therapy – from plucky
restlessness to sedentary 'rest cure'. At the turn of the century the mantra was
'open-air' treatment: a form of accessing the healing effects of the 'outside'
from nominally 'inside' places such as verandas and balconies. The central
questions of this treatment were more architectural than topographical – a
matter of what benefits can accrue from the built environment rather than from
the natural environment. The sanatorium of the turn of the century was a
machine for extracting what was needed from the normal climate (light and
air), maximizing its effects and training bodies to comport themselves in a more
healthy manner. This shifting spatiality of cure was demonstrated at Davos,
which had become a sanatorium town dominated by large institutions. Holsboer,
who had for decades been charmed by the rugged and remote Schatzalp,
constructed a large new institution there and connected it to the town by high-
grade funicular railcars (see Figure 1.7). Patients were no longer encouraged to
hike the hills on their own, but they were allowed walks in the woods if
prescribed by the physician. The Schatzalp Sanatorium is the only sanatorium
mentioned by its real name in Thomas Mann's *The Magic Mountain* (1924),
and is indicative of the modernist sensibility incubating within turn-of-the-
century sanatoria. Architectural historian Beatriz Colomina argues that 'the

architecture of the early twentieth century cannot be understood outside of tuberculosis' (Colomina 2007: 156). Design historian Margaret Campbell contends that the social functionalism and open-structure hygiene of these sanatoriums directly shaped early twentieth-century modernism (Campbell 2005). A curious artefact is the upholstery-eschewing *chaise longue* – the 'cure chair' also known as the 'Davos Couch' – which epitomizes how the consumptive body was to be moulded into new postures of aseptic consciousness and relaxful self-inspection (Campbell 1999). This was one way that, as Graham Mooney shows, the distinctive technology of the sanatorium could be resited and rescaled for the home environment in the form of commercial products and medical appurtenances for maintaining good health (Mooney 2013). As these examples suggest, tuberculosis had over the course of the century gained a completely new geography of meaning and reference.

MALARIA AND TROPICAL MEDICINE

The rising spatial modernity of tuberculosis in the nineteenth century may be placed in contrast to the geographical anti-modernity that malaria acquired over the same period. By the time the consumptive had comfortably settled into a chaise longue for civilized rest, the malaria victim was in essence viewed by Western medicine as a negative symbol of cultural and racial laggardness. As was well known, *ague* or marsh fever (as it was called then) had been endemic in parts of England and France up until the eighteenth century, when the maximization of agriculture caused large expanses of low countries to be more effectively drained and cultivated. The ebbing of malarial fevers was noticed at the time and served to confirm the ancient fear of marshlands and their attendant miasmas. In American medical writings of the early 1800s, malaria constituted a group of 'chill-fevers' or 'remittent fevers' accompanying the early stages of settlement in the western interior – places like Missouri and Illinois, whose debilitative environments were memorably depicted by writers such as Mark Twain and Charles Dickens. Malarial disease seemed to affect freshly penetrated and still-marshy frontier regions, not the established towns and cities that according to lore more typically suffered yellow fever (Humphries 2001: 30–6). The cultural connotations of malaria therefore came to be geographically imagined as places in a rude or primitive state of development. New arrivals to that environment were in for a period of 'seasoning'. Importantly, it was *malaria* (from the Italian, *mal-aria*, or bad air arising from decaying animal or vegetable matter) that was the *cause* of these fevers, not a synonym for them. Only later in the century did the term for malaria's origin become the name of a disease itself.

The idea is expressed in Antoine-Auguste-Ernest Hébert's painting, *La mal'aria*, which received extraordinary acclaim at the Paris Salon of 1850 (see

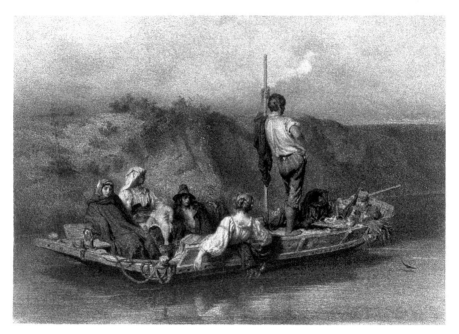

FIGURE 1.8: Antoine-August-Ernest Hébert, *La mal'aria*, 1850. Lithograph.
Wellcome Collection.

Figure 1.8). Set in the Pontine Marshes south-east of Rome, it depicts the sickly
atmosphere that for centuries had ravaged and practically depopulated the
region (interpreted in Victorian Britain and elsewhere as a poor reflection upon
backward-looking Catholicism). We find a group of classically picturesque but
disturbingly languid persons in a shallow punt. The Italianate peasantry was a
very popular iconographic genre that refracted the essential elements of upper-
class portraiture. Here, though, the passengers possess an eerie *excess* of repose.
What they lack is any clear aim and purpose, as though they are destined to
remain in that boat forever. A latter-day ship of fools, the party provides an
object lesson comparable to the one previously told about madness. Hébert's
painting, however, is less about the people than their environment. The title is
a reference to the dreamy, hazy, lethargic landscape – a marsh lacking all virtues
of depth and profundity claimed by the ocean, a blurred terrain-aquatic
completely unlike the relatively sharp margin of the seashore. This sense of
indistinctness is compounded by an overall atmosphere of low-lying stagnancy
and apathetic motionlessness. For the bourgeois and elite art world, as well also
for medical and social thought, malaria was read almost exclusively as a sort of
moral terrain lending to sickness. The French novelist Edmond About teasingly
chided Hébert for cultivating disease as others cultivate health: *La mal'aria*

gave the viewer an unwholesome flush to contemplate and represented a style not safe to carry to excess. If he had one of Hébert's pictures in his room, About famously remarked, he could not help but look at it frequently and catch fever. Like the medical topography of colonial spaces and colonized people, this was a land that had been disastrously neglected and imperfectly utilized. Hébert's peasants are not sick with malaria as we would say today; rather they are afflicted by a malarial environment. And so these are not just places on the front edge of development; they are also places left behind by modernity, which could be read as either picturesque or primitive, but not both.

This freshly imagined geography of malaria contributed many layers of meaning to the global capabilities of environmental mobility and management touted by empire – a relationship that was powerfully expressed by shifting quinine networks in the nineteenth century. Long before the identification of malaria plasmodium, this extract from the cinchona tree had been recognized as a treatment for fever-induced shivering. Cinchona bark was native to the hilly upland Andean forests of western South America and had been taken up by apothecaries in Rome as early as 1631. Quinine, the active component, was first extracted and isolated from cinchona in 1820 – an achievement that raised the stakes around obtaining greater yield of the alkaloid and improving techniques of cinchona cultivation. Criticisms arose about the harvesting methods allowed under the Peruvian government, but these controversies mainly stemmed from the newfound strategic importance of this natural resource. Several Western nations sponsored missions (some more covert than others) to buck the Peruvian monopoly and smuggle not cinchona bark but rather its plants and seeds out of the country. One was an 1859 British expedition having the aim of starting plantations in South Asia. Cinchona was first cultivated near British hill stations in southern India and later alongside tea plantations in Ceylon. These operations were profitable until undercut by competition from Dutch cinchona plantations in Java (Veale 2010).

Much has been said of quinine as a 'tool of empire' in a straightforward practical sense. It helped preserve the health of troops and colonizers and made the western African environment in particular seem not quite the 'white man's grave'. Many others have noticed quinine's place in the commodity culture of empire and in colonial health rituals – that is, taking it in wine or gin prophylactically. Rather less attention has been paid to quinine as a device of colonial environmental discourse. In this sense, we may say that the history of cinchona plantations, and quinine itself, exemplify practices of imperial *transplantation*. It was a relationship casually represented in an 1862 print depicting the ceremonial planting of the first cinchona tree in the summer-capital region of British India (see Figure 1.9). The ground has been prepared with plots and perfect rows – an industrious gridding of the colonial landscape to support colonialism there and elsewhere. There is one remaining strip of yet

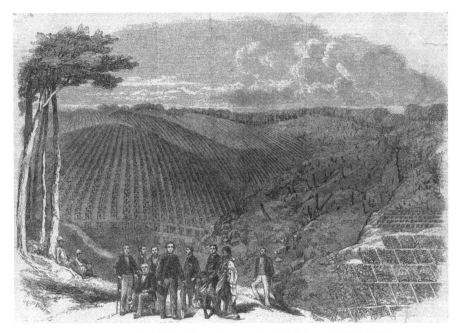

FIGURE 1.9: 'Peruvian Bark Tree Plantations in the Neilgherry Hills, India', *Illustrated London News*, 6 December 1862, p. 592. Wellcome Collection.

uncleared and disorganized stumps as well as a smattering of native lookers-on, including ones with machete and axe. Meanwhile the Governor of Madras, Sir William Denison, holds a shovel. He directs the cultivation of a natural cure for a disease arising from untamed nature. Mobilizing the broader aims of medical topography, the image suggests some of the ways that the civilizing mission was imagined as an environmental project. It instantiates how the comprehension of climate and natural habitats both grew out of and supported the command of those terrains. Furthermore, it supposes something about the perceived strategic interchangeability of climate regions. The British imagined the Neilgherry Hills to be reminiscent of Alpine resorts, as did the French of their hill-stations in Indochina (Jennings 2011). In both cases these were the colonial and environmental antitheses of Pontine marshes and torrid zones.

Without a doubt, relocating cinchona production away from South America was a means of shoring up spaces of medical vulnerability and securing the health of Europeans. But this was in the context of eliciting and organizing environmental knowledge – a context that becomes better appreciated by recent cultural histories of the connections between medicine and botany on the one hand and mercantile and commercial empires on the other. An incisive example is Londa Shiebinger's work on the legacy of 'colonial bioprospecting' undertaken by European naturalists and explorers in the eighteenth-century

Caribbean. Botanical classification constituted a form of 'linguistic imperialism', she argues, and the organization of male-dominated medicine constrained what could be asked and said about women's health and methods to control fertility (Shiebinger 2004). With cinchona we find a nineteenth-century convergence of medical topography and botanical conceptions of a suitable climate – a convergence that itself helped construct entirely new geographical technologies of rule. Quinine became an imagined and useful (and usefully imagined) product of the imperial environment. It involved the transplantation of a profitable plant, but unlike other cash crops cinchona was freighted under the medicinal symbol of empire-building.

So, malaria was a disorder of the environment before it was a disease of the body. Nonetheless, it was these environmental imaginings and discourses that shaped how bodies were utilized in relation to imperial projects and raced in furtherance of their designs. As Megan Vaughan has argued regarding Africa more generally, 'the power of colonial medicine lay not so much in its direct effects on the bodies of its subjects . . . but in its ability to provide "naturalized" and "pathologized" accounts of those subjects' (Vaughan 1991: 25). This notion is echoed in David Arnold's work on colonial India, which traces the role of epidemic disease in constructing political narratives of subjection and hierarchicalization (Arnold 1993). To be sure, nineteenth-century colonial medicine offered a number of different and competing responses to problems like malaria. Moreover, the specific problem of malaria only gradually became seen *primarily* as an imperial concern. And yet this itself reveals much about how empire was reimagined as an environmental struggle against ill health, corporeal decay and even degeneration. As Arnold observes, Britain had essentially given up on substantial white settlement in India by the 1870s, and this change resulted partly from medical justifications being added to and informing the accumulating difficulties of direct rule. While the specific effect of malaria on empire-building is still debated, there should be little doubt that it eventually came to occupy the centre-ground of how that project was culturally framed for Westerners. The medical construction of malaria is a crucial part of how entire sections of the earth and their inhabitants were judged to be naturally peripheral and primordial. Indeed, malaria was *made exotic* and the archetypal malarial landscape was thus prepared as an imperial project.

It is in this way that Nancy Leys Stepan writes about the naturalization of 'the tropics' – an imagined and constructed place, she argues, as much as a physical location. Western medicine played a crucial role in manufacturing the tropical environment as a cultural trope. Stepan focuses on nineteenth-century Brazil and the pictorial and narrative conventions used by explorers and scientists to construct a powerful impression of the tropical setting as an abundantly perilous health environment. Given the imperial context, the accumulation of knowledge had the effect of making such places less a geographical type and more a geographical novelty (Stepan 2001). The trope of the tropics, founded so closely on contradictory myths of health and disease, aligned closely with myths about empire and Western masculinity as well as myths about the hallmark abnormalities of colonized peoples. In other words, medicine was called upon both to naturalize certain environments and to pathologize their 'natural' inhabitants. 'Tropical disease' and 'tropical medicine' were both a creation of this fascination with fantastic environments. They each worked to signify the temporal backwardness of places and the backwardness of people stuck in a wayward historical era, people who lose history and are thus excluded from the events of modernity. Colonized peoples were mired in space and therefore mired in an earlier time. Their heightened placedness and timelessness had to be set against the essential placelessness and highly specific forward temporal position of colonial knowledge. This task was aided by links forged between conventions of the older medical geography and tenets of the newer physical anthropology – links that contributed to and were perhaps essential for 'dying race theory'. Ultimately, most iterations of the imperial mission intended to render the environment of little importance while also at the same time seeking to take advantage of those people who could not similarly transcend their natural environment. And so questions of *place* continued to be central to colonial medicine in ways no longer very important to medicine practised in the West. One could argue that medical topography as an identifiable discipline was reduced by the end of the century to almost nothing more than 'tropical medicine', which itself started to refer less to the tropics per se and more to all those diseases properly located outside the temperate climates native to Western man. It was finally possible for malaria to be substantially made into a tropical disease. In the end, the cultural construction of the tropics – alongside and in hand with the scientific construction of tropical medicine – raises the question of whether the medical management of empire was ever separable from the medical construction of race.

While there has been a good deal of critical attention given to the tropics as a key category of Western imagination (as well as some interest in the arctic as a site of exploration and cultural assembly), less consideration has been paid to the concurrent medical construction of the temperate environment as an effect of the West's newly-forged relations to the colonial sphere. This is notable and surprising, given the influence of the 'new imperial history' and that school's contention that empire organized projects of self-exploration and shaped formations of domestic, normal, fit and familiar space. Some of these insights have been brought to bear in the seminal work of Warwick Anderson, who seeks to show that Western medicine's interaction with exotic climates and locales was central to the intellectual and popular construction of whiteness. His earlier groundbreaking work on the sanitary governance of the US-administered Philippines focuses on how tropical medicine gained for itself a vast medical laboratory in which to elucidate the connection between hygiene and race and to modernize the colony by means of pacifying, purifying and civilizing what was considered a contaminated environment (collected in Anderson 2006). In *The Cultivation of Whiteness*, Anderson brings a close reading to nineteenth-century discourse of medical geography and traces the ways it was employed toward the goal of securing a white nation in late nineteenth- and early twentieth-century Australia (Anderson 2002). Fears of white degeneration in the antipodean environment, which settlers found imminently weird and exhausting, intersected and deeply inflected how germ theories of disease were incorporated into medical theory and practice. These themes are echoed by Alison Bashford, who argues that Australian public health was completely infused by a preoccupation with whiteness, with fitness and with the creation of spaces for the protection of both (Bashford 2004). Anderson, however, further asks how the new disciplines of bacteriology and parasitology – so crucial to the formation of tropical medicine – reshaped the geographical understandings of disease. Anderson suggests that the rise of laboratory knowledge invariably shifted the meanings of environmental knowledge; there was not so much a decline of geographical perspectives on disease and colonization, but definitely a repurposing of them. For example, tropical medicine's valorization of the pathogen placed assumptions about pathological environments in a new light and led many to come around to an idea of the white man's basic suitability to the tropics.

The mercuriality of this notion of environmental adaptability points to tropical medicine's connection with eugenic thought and underlines how it contributed to broader scientific narratives of racial origins and destinies. These narratives were in reality constantly being adjusted to new geographical problems and political circumstances – and to new etiologies. As Arnold's writing about India shows, Ronald Ross's identification of the malaria parasite and mosquito-transmission at the end of the century displaced earlier vague beliefs about malarial climates. Malaria truly became a bodily disease instead of an environmental quality, but this too was used to supplement and support already prevalent interlinkages of diseased environments and racial stagnation. Ross and others concluded that a previously vigorous 'Aryan' civilization had become moribund by its centuries-long contact with malaria and that this in itself possessed great lessons for India's new rulers (Arnold 1999). The immediate significance for Ross was the need for specific spatial and environmental strategies, such as racial segregation of residences. As Alexandra Minna Stern argues, these sorts of actions must also be traced to beliefs that arose about racial immunity to diseases such as malaria, sleeping sickness and syphilis. She shows that, specifically regarding yellow fever, American public health officials attempted to leverage these conceits regarding variable susceptibility into a tool for the medical management of Cuba and the Panama Canal Zone (Stern 2006). Few historians indeed have committed the mistake of thinking that the discovery of microscopic pathogens erased the significance of the environment, but perhaps we would be better served by even more closely considering the ways that environmental discourse continued to feature at the end of the century as a key signifier for the new scientific culture of germs. It has already started to yield important insights upon the medical construction of place and race.

It seems appropriate to conclude this chapter by suggesting that it is in this way that a critical cultural history of the environment is an area ripe for further research in the medical making of the age of empire. The era brought about a fundamental reimagining of the 'natural' environments of health and disease. It was undoubtedly a time in which ideas about healthfulness and diseasedness underwent tremendous geographical shifts, both locally and globally. The care and maintenance of the body was resited by medical discourse and re-placed into newly significant physical and cultural topographies. It is not controversial at all nowadays to suggest that the natural environment has historically shaped the cultural environment, and vice versa. Probably this was never in question. But it seems to still be a different order of criticism to say that the natural environment *produced* the cultural environment, and vice versa. We need more serious consideration of the *place* of medicine in that process of cultural production.

CHAPTER TWO

Food

VANESSA HEGGIE

Western medicine made its break with humoral theories definite in the nineteenth century, but at least one of the non-naturals – food – remained a core element of healing practices and disease theories. From 1800 to 1920, food and eating were rewritten into new theories of biomedicine, while at the same time maintaining strong socio-cultural meanings, leading to complex identities for individual foodstuffs, specific eating habits and even practices of preparation and storage. Building on older, empirically-focused studies of what, when and how much people ate (Burnett 1966), social and cultural historians interested in the interactions between nineteenth-century science and food practices take one of two paths: first is a concentration on the intersection of public health – another nineteenth-century preoccupation – and the analysis of foods, as demonstrated by the pure food movements and by campaigns and scandals about the adulteration of foodstuffs. Laboratories for the analysis of foods (including, sometimes, drinks and drugs), some state-sponsored, others the function of private or philanthropic interests, were established across Europe and to a lesser extent in North America in the nineteenth century (Hardy 1999; Oddy 2007; Scholliers 2007; Heirholzer 2007; Stanzaiani 2007; Horrocks 1994). At the same time, legislation about pure foods, adulteration, fraud and public health was passed, again much earlier in Europe than in North America where strong pro-trade and pro-commerce interests delayed federal intervention until the early twentieth century (Guillem-Llobat 2014). Notably, European historical accounts emphasize the positive public health aspects of this work, while American historians are more sceptical, seeing the hand of monopoly-seeking big business and elite professional interests at play in legislation that restricted commercial freedoms (Goodwin 1999).

Secondly, historians have noted that foodstuffs were part of the so-called 'laboratory revolution' in medicine in the nineteenth century (Cunningham and Williams 1992). While more recent works have begun to re-emphasize the role of field and clinical sciences, it is clear that Western scientific practice was industrialized, professionalized and constructed as an object of both social and political value through the nineteenth century (Heggie 2016). Practices of standardization, mass production and the creation of expert knowledge followed through into many areas of everyday life, including diet (Dierig 2003). Foodstuffs were analysed as part of a drive to discover the basic elements of nutrition, and from that to better understand the human machine: what were its essential needs, its minimum inputs and maximum outputs? These were questions that were particularly explored in military and penal contexts (Milles 1995; Treitel 2007). This push was partly a consequence of the changing research-scape in medicine, but, as with the drive to analyse quality, it was also a response to the extraordinary socio-cultural changes of industrialization. An urbanized, high-density population had fewer opportunities to grow and make its own food and was likely to be more distanced, literally as well as figuratively, from food producers. Long trains of food supply from rural areas and from overseas into the cities led to multiple opportunities for corruption and contamination. Even if apparently pure food could be brought into the city, the conditions of slaughter, process and packing often left much to be desired; the homes of consumers in the new cities frequently lacked the space or sanitation to keep food safely once it had been bought (Horowitz, Pilcher and Watts 2004). This distance between manufacturer and consumer led to an increased reliance on 'middle-men' – in this case shopkeepers and retailers – and of course the 'guarantee' of branded products (more on this below); a process of creating a consumer society that was certainly not new in the nineteenth century, but was accelerating (Trentman 2004). Layered over these problems were European and colonial conflicts and of course a civil war in North America, which disrupted supply and led to control policies such as the Corn Laws and other forms of economic manipulation. As theories of political economy and statistical analysis became more influential, the facts and figures of food mattered more and more: whether at the macro scale – how much bread did the country need? – or at the micro – how much nitrogenous food ought we to allow per prisoner or workhouse inmate (Carpenter 2006)?

To these two traditional approaches – the histories of food analysis for adulteration and for efficiency – we can add a third, which is histories that attempt to establish the impact of changing food practices on the lived experience of people in the nineteenth century. Consisting of analyses of recommended diets, comparisons of imports and exports, and calculations of mortality and morbidity, these histories also form part of the ongoing debate that was sparked by Thomas McKeown's work on the relative role of personal wealth and public intervention on the health of Victorians and has subsequently evolved into a broader discussion of the modern rise of population (Harris 2004; Oddy 1983). Likewise there have been significant attempts to answer the question 'Were hunger strikers really hungry?' (Williams 1976) through empirically focused studies of food and diet (Oddy 1983; Fogel 2004). More cultural approaches exist: for example, James Vernon's (2007) history of hunger as a concept, which looks to the successful ending of hunger as a routine – possibly essential – feature of human experience in Western Europe and North America, and its subsequent reinvention as a moral failing (of individual or government) and as a mechanism for exerting political pressure. Vernon's work has received some criticism for apparently ignoring the work of empirical historians (Oddy 2008) and emphasizing hunger as something that is culturally constructed, rather than being 'solely the consequence of the objectively measurable lack of food' (Scholliers 2012: 1937). This approach certainly has its problematic features: for example, for Vernon it is twentieth-century science, particularly the discovery of vitamins, that splits hunger into two forms – *mal-* and *under*nutrition, where the latter indicates a simple lack of quantity, while the former is a more complex problem of variety and quality. Vernon claims this distinction occurs only after 1920, outside the remit of this volume, but it is apparent from other research that the mal-/undernutrition distinction occurs much earlier: it is clearly present in the *Report of the Interdepartmental Committee on Physical Deterioration* in 1904 (Heggie 2008), and traces of it can be found even in very early nineteenth-century work into, for example, the proportions of protein needed to keep prisoners fit while working the treadmill (Chapman 1967). Clearly a combination of traditional, social, economic and cultural approaches provide a better overview of complex issues such as hunger, taste and nutrition in the nineteenth century.

Mal-/undernutrition is also a mechanism for allocating the blame or responsibility for poor diets, and it is in this division that the gender tensions of changing food practices become apparent. Food occupies a liminal space between the public and private spheres, and as a substance is frequently the responsibility – from purchase to preparation – of the female members of a household. What was the point of enacting restrictive legislation or raising worker's wages, when this could be undermined by ignorant housewives choosing, storing and preparing food inadequately? Here too the anxieties about female emancipation, through work and education, are absolutely clear, as sanitary societies, heath visitors and later compulsory domestic education sought to remedy the apparently negative effects on food skills caused by female employment.

The 'rise of the laboratory' in food history also masks a slippery relationship between the socio-cultural and biomedical identities of foods, and indeed the positive or negative contribution of the laboratory to food itself, as site of purity assurance and of adulteration (Ferrières 2006). While 'purity' (and possibly 'authenticity') remained a generally positive food attribute, it was not consistently associated with other binaries, particularly natural/man-made or natural/ chemical. At times the man-made, the chemical, the rational was the marker of purity and safety; at others, and particularly towards the end of the century in the work of food reform organizations, the man-made and chemical stood for the artificial and adulterated, and it was the 'natural' and 'simple' that construed food purity (similarly, provenance as a marker shifted in meaning across the century, so that at some periods the 'Frenchness' of a wine was a sign of quality, while at others it was a foreign substance to be actively avoided in favour of home-grown alternatives). Those who thought, wrote and campaigned about food in the nineteenth century were acutely aware that food had multiple identities, and that no scientific investigation or health reform would succeed if it took cognisance of just one of these: at a pragmatic level, reformers repeatedly pointed out that domestic education had to be tailored to the realities of working-class lives, and incorporate only the utensils, storage and cooking techniques available in 'poor cottages'. Likewise, the most rational, thoroughly studied and carefully designed prison dietary would still result in underfed, malnourished prisoners if it was not made digestible and attractive. For example, despite the exhortations by reformers about the economic and nutritional benefits available to those willing to eat horsemeat, the hippophagy movement remained a failure in the UK – while becoming an extraordinary success across the Channel (Otter 2011). Although this discrepancy has some of its explanation in economic and local political differences, the fact that the French ate horses and the British did not knowingly became a self-fulfilling cultural conceit.

Clearly a marker for gender and class identities, food has been widely studied as an aspect of regional identities, which could be supranational, racial or extremely localized. By the nineteenth century, food cultures had been deeply impacted by the expansion of European empires, and most of Western Europe was saturated in a globalized food culture, with 'local' foodways unimaginable without tea, coffee, sugar, spices, tomatoes, opium, and so on. Rather than being a century of new food encounters, what is perhaps more characteristic of the nineteenth century is that it is a time of new food transport and processing. Although this may seem a less exciting historical strand, the ability to ship vast quantities of meat from one hemisphere to another meant that Argentinian or Australian food policies could effectively break a food strike by miner's wives or lead to the production of one of the most famous medical foods (and also, incidentally, the first food to sponsor an Olympic event: Oxo). Canning, freezing, drying and condensing food also provided new ways to provision armies and exploratory teams; although doctors still recommended shifts in diets for those travelling from temperate to tropical regions – after all, the act of 'seasoning' could mean acclimatizing to a new environment as well flavouring or maturing a foodstuff – guides such as Galton's *The Art of Travel* included tips on making a passable cup of tea in remote locations (including how to drink it 'Paraguay style' with a reed straight out of the kettle if there was no teapot available) (Galton 1855: 53).

This chapter will highlight some of these global threads, track the slippage between man-made and 'natural' purity and add a socio-cultural angle to the existing meta-narratives about food quality and quantity in the nineteenth century. Although this story will range over dozens of foodstuffs, multiple foodways and through many countries, one food ties all these themes together, and that is milk. Much historians' ink has already been spilled on this subject, but this chapter will go beyond the usual discussions of adulteration and urbanization, because milk is a deeply symbolic foodstuff: it represents the demographic disruption of industrialization and urbanization; it is a rhetorically domestic substance, associated with family and home, and therefore highlights the tensions between public science and private lives; it is, extraordinarily, a foodstuff made by human animals, and its feminine identity acts as a way to understand the gendered practices of food science and medical reform.

FOOD ESSENCES: CONCENTRATION, RATIONALIZATION

Food was always a part of the urge to create the reductive, analytical understandings of the human machine that proliferated in the nineteenth century, from Liebig's analytical chemistry through to (Wilbur) Atwater's comprehensive analytical tables of food around 1900. This story of nineteenth-century experimental physiology and metabolic study is well explored elsewhere (Heggie 2016) and can be briefly summarized: a research trend that prioritized calculation, the discovery of basic or atomic particles, and mathematically-expressed natural laws, focused attention on the 'parts' of food, of finding and applying fundamental physical laws of motion and energy to the human machine. Socio-politically, these themes resonated strongly with industrializing countries, where the metaphors of human workers as machines and steam engines promised efficient management and improved productivity – the growth potential essential for capitalist societies, literally reading food as fuel for the human machine (Milles 1995; Wise and Smith 1990; Rabinbach 1992). At the same time, at least in Europe, the social uncertainties caused by conflict, by the revolutions of 1848 and by similar demands for enfranchisement and social reform in the 1830s and 1840s elsewhere meant that governments were also pushed to look to reform of their institutions for war and welfare. 'Scientific' and 'rational' dietaries were presented as fair and humane, whether for a conscripted soldier, an asylum inmate or a citizen in a workhouse.

This is not to say that consensus was reached on the minimum needs or most efficient feeding of the human body. The invention of the food calorie at around mid-century provided a standardized quantification of the inputs and outputs of the human (mostly adult male) body (the identity of the 'true' inventor of the calorie is heavily disputed: Hargrove 2006). But humans proved to be extremely variable in their metabolism and energetic activity, and the technologies of measurement remained experimental through the nineteenth century. Furthermore, although some agreement could be reached on the need to match gross input to gross output, a more detailed *ideal* diet remained a point of dispute: in particular the relative roles and importance of even the basic food groups – proteins, fats and carbohydrates – was not established until well into the twentieth century. For Western Europeans and North Americans, protein – at least in the form of meat – was strongly associated in popular consciousness with masculinity and strength (Carpenter 1994; Spiering 2006). While this could include a negative association with, say, violence, intemperance or particular diseases such as gout, it meant that when Liebig asserted in the 1830s and 1840s that protein ('nitrogenous matter') was the source of motive energy for the human body, his scientific conclusions squared perfectly with socio-cultural assumptions. Although evidence that carbohydrates and fats were more important to the energy requirements of the body than proteins built systematically through the nineteenth century (Fick and Wislicenus 1866), a prejudice towards protein – specifically animal protein – remained difficult to counter. In part this was due to the relative expense of meat; even with rising standards of living, meat, particularly cuts of red meat, was often a drain on middling and working-class incomes. Food for the poor, in state welfare institutions or philanthropic spaces such as soup kitchens, was frequently characterized by a low proportion of animal protein; in the UK, early school meals tended towards the vegetarian – not only because of their sponsorship by food reform societies, but also because bread and coffee, or bread and pea soup, turned out to be the most economical way to put calories into children on a massive scale.

In this context it is not surprising that concentrated meat tonics could become a popular and pervasive home treatment for sickness and fatigue. Combining the promise of efficient, industrial, scientific rationality and the popular association of meat with strength, meat tonics were a modern answer to an old prejudice. One of the first, and certainly the longest-lived, was that developed by Justus von Liebig. Liebig's Extract of Meat – later to become the contemporary brand Oxo – was the reason a meat processing plant was built in Fray Bentos in 1863, as the site in Uruguay was able to supply meat and labour cheap enough to turn a significant profit. Somewhat ironically, Liebig's extract contained relatively little protein, and after several challenges its marketing was shifted consciously from an efficient provider of *nutrition* to an efficient provider of *flavour*, and its consumer refigured as the busy housewife, rather than the sick nurse – mirroring a move from medicine to food seen in the marketing of other products, like drinking chocolate and other liquid tonics. Such medico-foods often went through a phase of claiming, if not strictly *curative* properties, then that they were specially (often 'scientifically') prepared for easy assimilation and digestion, or, they were extremely nutrition dense and therefore *efficient* forms of nutrition; examples would be Plasmon and Protene, both products made from dairy protein (dried casein from milk), which were marketed for invalids, but also for travel and exploration (Guly 2013; Steinitz 2017). And, of course, alcohol maintained a similarly ambiguous position as stimulant, tonic and poison into the early decades of the twentieth century.

So initially Liebig's extract of meat was explicitly a medical product: beef tea made to his recipe, published in 1847, was added to the Bavarian and German Pharmacopeia, and by the early 1850s British doctors were urging for *extractum carnis* to be added to the London Pharmacopeia to allow British pharmacists to manufacture a product used to treat everything from fatigue to tuberculosis and typhus (Finlay 1992). Liebig's beef tea was made by 'soaking lean raw meat for several hours in cold water, adding salt and [hydrochloric] acid, and straining', and as such could be made in small batches by doctors and apothecaries, but was not efficient enough a process initially to turn a commercial success, not least due to the expense of beef in much of Europe – made worse in the UK by an outbreak of cattle plague in 1865. The southern hemisphere therefore offered a ray of hope: Australian and South American beef herds were by mid-century touted as sources of cheap meat for the working poor in industrializing Europe. Liebig partnered with George Giebert, a German railway engineer working in Brazil, who bought the land in Fray Bentos and with Liebig exported the industrial machinery needed to reduce hundreds of thousands of Brazilian cattle into a thick brown paste for shipping to Europe.

Liebig's Extract is a master class in the selling of drugs and foods; building on a trade card and advertising tradition that had proved successful in the eighteenth century, for patent medicines and 'irregular' doctors as well as other commercial products (Barker 1989; Porter 1989), the company used highly coloured and narrowly focused advertising to promote meat extract as flexible, desirable, respectable (Finlay 1995). Liebig's name and reputation stood for the scientific validity and rationality of the meat extract, his signature on labels often acting as a guarantee of purity and authenticity in an uncertain marketplace (Finlay 1992; Bickham 2008). The company produced cookbooks and collectible advertising cards, and solicited hard for testimonials (which is why Florence Nightingale was sent samples – Finlay 1995: 59). The success of these manoeuvres is evident as the brand flourished despite the fact that medical support for the specific curative claims about Liebig's extract waned almost as soon as it hit the commercial market beyond Germany (Finlay 1995: 60). Even when it no longer claimed to cure disease, Liebig's Extract still benefited from the popular belief that meat was strength. The company diversified, into tinned meat under the Fray Bentos brand (1873) and further into an explicitly domestic cookery context as a cheaper meat extract was produced and sold (from 1899) under the brand name Oxo. (Oxo was effectively the first commercial sponsor of the Olympic marathon, providing runners in London with free Oxo – hot and cold – suggesting it still valued the connection between strength, sport and meat.) Liebig's Extract of Meat Company turned to medicine again in the early twentieth century – slightly outside the remit of this volume – producing an extract, Organoid, from 1924, latching on to a contemporary trend for hormonal medicine (Krementsov 2008) (see Figure 2.1).

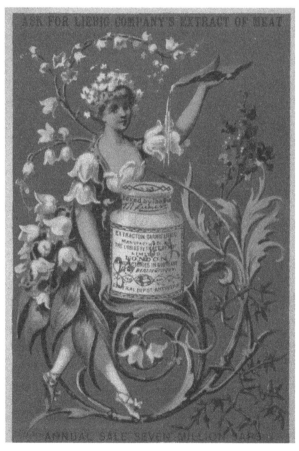

FIGURE 2.1: Advert for Liebig's Extract of Meat, *c.* 1890. The 'purity' and 'authenticity' of the extract was 'certified' by Liebig's signature across the jar's label. The British Library.

There is no doubt that the sophisticated marketing techniques, particularly the visual advertising, used by the Liebig business empire helped its products, especially the extract of meat, successfully transition from medicine to cooking ingredient. But it also benefited from a specific set of food cultures and social apprehensions: on the one hand the many values associated with animal flesh – a food that shifted from a luxury to an expected necessity, or at least a marker of the wealth of a civilization (did its poor eat meat?) over the nineteenth century. This was bolstered by the veneer of a scientific justification for the prejudice towards meat flesh: the ongoing association of animal protein with vigour and exertion (and masculinity) persists through to the twenty-first century, even while Liebig's assertion that protein was essential to provide motive power did not survive as a theory beyond the nineteenth (Carpenter 1994; Heggie 2016). Building on eighteenth-century understandings of stimulating and non-stimulating diets, systems using a bewildering range of terminology (low/high diets, non/phlogistic diets, etc.) fundamentally assumed that animal products and proteins were invigorating and exciting, and suitable only for certain patients (Worth Estes 1996). Therefore a second intertwining of lay and scientific thought that was also key to the success of meat extracts was the notion of tonics, essences and efficiency. 'Tonics' in a variety of forms have long been part of healing practices, and they remain remarkably persistent; one adaptation of Liebig's extract was Wincarnis, a tonic alcoholic drink invented in Norwich in 1881, which was eventually exported to the Caribbean and South East Asia. The brand survives in these areas into the twenty-first century with the same name, a contraction of wine and the Latin term *carnis*, although the tonic no longer contains meat extract.

Despite the long-standing and resilient cultural appeal of tonics, in the context of the nineteenth century the inventors of scientific pharma-foods looked to new theories in physics and chemistry to bolster their reputations. Whether it was cells, atoms, economic laws or the 'essence' of foodstuffs, the scientific project to reduce and simplify the natural world, to break it down and reorder it into efficiency, had clear rhetorical appeal to societies expanding due to industrialization, mechanization and rapid transport. Essences promised efficiency – providing the quintessence of a substance without all the unnecessary fat, offering the stereotyped time-poor housewife a quicker way of creating healthy, tasty meals: all in all a very modern promise. It was not just the reduction to an essence that appealed, but also the idea of concentration – of getting more for less (less cost, less space, less effort), as in the much repeated claim that 34lb of meat was condensed into 1lb of extract. Just as, a century later, TV dinners and other 'convenience' foods would be sold as modern and time efficient, so tinned, processed, dried and particularly *condensed* food was sold as a marker of food civilization in the mid-nineteenth century. (For other markers of civilization and particularly gentility in foodways, at least in the

Western anglophone world, see Young 2003.) While in the case of Liebig's extract its (supposed) origin in the laboratory of a famous scientist, and in the global networks of food that sent protein from the southern to the northern hemisphere, was celebrated, other foodstuffs had their origins effaced in order to recreate them as modern.

One such reinvented food turned up in the lists of substances analysed by the Analytical Sanitary Commissions organized in the UK by the *Lancet*. One of the earliest indications of the nineteenth-century's burgeoning obsession with food adulteration, the *Lancet*'s project was founded in 1851 by radical, campaigning editor Dr Thomas Wakley to investigate the purity of common household foods in order to reveal the extent of adulteration and put pressure on the government for intervention and reform (Smith 2001). As we might expect, the Commission studied coffee (its most tested substance), bread and tea, but its analysis of tinned foods was dominated by a less well-known commodity: pemmican (Smith 2001: 175). Pemmican is a food designed for efficiency, usually prepared with beef, but, unlike Oxo, does not originate from a laboratory: instead this combination of dried (often powdered or ground) meat and fat was used as a travel food by several First Nations peoples in North America. It was rapidly assimilated into the diet of European settlers and colonialists, and by the early nineteenth century, the Hudson's Bay Company and its larger rival the North West Company were using between 70 and 80 tonnes of pemmican every year to fuel their canoeists, trappers and hunters (and these figures would more than double by the end of the century – Ray 1984: 271).

Pemmican was imported into Europe as a military food, and this is the context in which it was analysed by the *Lancet*. Victorian naval recipes included added sugar and dried fruit, and in some countries it was known by Europeanized names, often variants on 'meat biscuit'. Various entrepreneurs tried to reinvent and profit from pemmican-like substances, so, for example, a commercialized 'meat biscuit' was developed in the 1840s by an American inventor – Gail Borden – who cited Liebig's theories about food to reinforce his claims about the nutritional benefits of a dried meat product that could be turned into soup. Based on dried bread and meat rather than fat and meat, it would, he said, preserve the health of seamen (not least by preventing scurvy), prove a flexible foodstuff for convalescent homes and hospitals, and also be 'convenient' for families (Borden 1850). The US Army did not adopt this home-grown efficient food (Borden turned instead to another efficiency project – condensed milk), but European armies, and particularly the British Royal Navy, used pemmican variants in their rations throughout the century. This was part of an ongoing attempt to use theories from physiology and nutrition to create efficient, and physically robust, military forces.

By the early twentieth century, pemmican was more of an 'emergency' food than a standard ration – often appearing in the packs of explorers. Despite

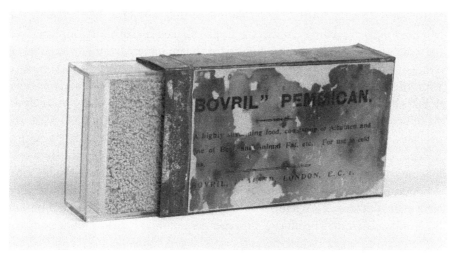

FIGURE 2.2: Pemmican packet. An opened packet of Bovril brand pemmican; the paper label claims it as a very 'nourishing' food. Dundee Heritage Trust (Photo Collection Item).

being part of encounters with the wild, pemmican was thoroughly Westernized and domesticated. Throughout the nineteenth century it was reinvented as a rational, scientific foodstuff, analysed in laboratories and repeatedly adjusted, tweaked and reworked by inventors and scientists; by the end of the century it was also a commercial product, neatly wrapped and portioned and marked clearly with the domestic brand names such as the UK's Bovril or (for the fancier canned version) Danish 'JD Beauvais' pemmican with dried fruit' (see Figure 2.2).

The branding, the canning, the chemical analysis, all seem to have entirely stripped away the indigenous origins of pemmican, leaving only a rational Western food that provided meat (and therefore health) to men – an essence of nineteenth-century food science. Throughout the nineteenth century, colonial and imperial medicine also worked to figure the meat-heavy diet of Western Europe as intrinsically superior to consumption patterns found in other nations. The relative worth of all kinds of basic foodstuffs, such as potatoes, bread, manioc and rice, was debated and settled into a hierarchy that started with the foods of Europeans and worked 'down' to those of the indigenous and the colonized (with internal gradations, for example prioritizing 'British' bread over inferior 'Irish' potatoes).

Condensing meat achieved a lot of cultural work: satisfying Eurocentric food preferences while emphasizing scientific civilization, rational masculinity and industrial efficiency. It was also a highly gendered food and it had a direct feminized corollary: milk. Perhaps even more than was the case for meat, urbanization and industrialization disrupted milk supplies, both human and animal; longer travelling distances and middle men meant more opportunities for cow's milk to become adulterated or contaminated; and in parallel as women increasingly worked outside the home, human milk was substituted with animal milk, pablum and pobs, stupefying tonics, and, of course, *condensed* milk. Milk and meat were indivisible parts of the same story of analysis, synthesis, economic disruption and cultural norms: Liebig developed what was probably the first commercial baby formula product in the late 1860s, and Borden, one of the first (would-be) commercializers of pemmican, shifted to making condensed milk when the US military proved disinterested in his meat products (Mepham 1993). The domestic sphere remained a problem for food reformers, doctors and scientists to solve: however pure, efficient and perfect the food was that they produced, however certain their figures about calories or carbohydrates, ensuring the nation was well fed fundamentally required the cooperation of women.

PUBLIC HEALTH IN PRIVATE KITCHENS

Across the Western world, and indeed in many other cultures besides, the procurement and preparation of food is a female task. There are some institutional exceptions – religious brotherhoods perhaps being the obvious one, along with the armed forces, who often contributed ex-staff to medical and welfare institutions such as prisons, workhouses and hospitals. But even in all-male institutions women were frequently involved in food preparation and cleaning even if they took no other part in the life of the institution and did not run the kitchen (Hawkins and Tanner 2016). By and large, then, most men were fed by women – by wives, daughters, mothers, landladies, canteen workers. In wealthier households this activity may have been carried out by servants rather than family members, but even here the success (and economy) of a cook still reflected on the feminine achievements of the lady of the house, a hierarchical model of class and gender also explicitly replicated in hospitals through ladies' committees, matrons and nursing personnel (Davidoff 1974). Just as they had advised on regimen in the humoral era, so doctors in the nineteenth century thought they needed to influence the purchase, storage and preparation of daily meals to ensure the health of a population, and that this had to be done through women.

One method of getting public science into private rooms was to use women themselves as go-betweens. By the middle of the nineteenth century, initiatives to send out women as 'sanitary missionaries' into the homes of the poor were already underway in the first industrial cities, in London, Liverpool and Manchester (Heggie 2011a). Although these were not food-focused specifically, providing advice on the rational purchase, sanitary storage and healthy preparation of food was part of a remit of 'evangelizing' a sanitarian vision of clean living in the slums. These organizations were female-led, and often female-funded, usually organized by local 'ladies' who may have visited the poor themselves, but frequently found that a trained 'respectable' working-class intermediary got better traction amongst the tenements than the erstwhile 'lady bountiful' (Howse 2006). Men were present, however, as experts – often providing biomedical training (including in food science) to the home visitors, or writing and advising on informational leaflets to be handed out in lieu of personal instruction. The shape of female visiting societies obviously varied across nations according to local contexts, as well as the pace of industrial and urban change; but even where food and feeding were at best only a marginal concern, such as in the attempts at 'racial uplift' by African-American female philanthropists at the end of the nineteenth century, women remained a way to bridge the domestic and the public; to ensure that individual households participated in progress at the same pace as whole societies (Perkins 1983).

Throughout the nineteenth century, and into the twentieth, concerns about domestic food preparation and about women's participation in food commerce acted as ciphers for concerns about women's role in the public sphere. While doctors and reformers cited poverty and ignorance as the reason for unhealthy food choices, at the same time it seemed clear that women's absence from the home while at work or at school posed a threat to the health of a domestic economy. Women's employment remained an intractable problem (and more on this below), but the introduction of compulsory (state) education offered an opportunity as well as a threat – if girls were not being adequately trained in domestic tasks by their mothers (and were being kept out of the home by schooling), domestic education might provide a way to create a new generation of rational, scientifically-literate, competent home cooks (Lieffers 2012). And, it was often hoped, they might even be able to transfer these skills to an older generation who had not had the benefit of a compulsory education.

Specific systems of domestic education obviously varied, although most Western nations sought to ensure that girl children were taught domestic skills as part of compulsory education, while also supporting welfare and philanthropic interventions to provide these skills outside of formal schooling. In England a specific grant (initially 4 shillings per pupil aged over twelve taking at least forty hours of cookery lessons) was made available from 1883 onwards to support the teaching of cookery in schools, and by 1911 there were grants available for 'combined domestic subjects' and 'housewifery' (Bourke 1994: 183) (the 4 shilling grant was introduced into the Education Code for 1882; Sillitoe 1933: 35). While it is the case that economy, nutrition and the health of the nation were used to varying extents as the justification for such schemes, food was also a useful 'way in' to the domestic lives of citizens. Domestic education celebrated

– possibly co-created – an idealized middle-class form of femininity, and in some cases it is clear that domestic education for the working classes was hoped to provide a solution to the 'servant problem' of the middle classes, rather than improving the meals of the poor. In addition, the demand for 'trained' teachers of domestic education, and for 'experts' who could write not just recipe books but guides to hygiene, home decoration and domestic economy, provided a useful career option to middle-class women (Leavitt 2002: esp. chapters 1 and 2; Heggie 2011b).

Philanthropic and campaign groups, including national organizations like the British Association for the Advancement of Science and professional organizations such as the Association of Teachers of Domestic Science, campaigned for reforms to school-based domestic education; at the same time, early feminist campaigners pushed back against a segregated and gendered education system (Manthorpe 1986). In Manchester, the first industrial city in the UK, the only female member of the Manchester School Board was Miss Lydia Ernestine Becker, who fought hard from the 1870s against 'intellectual segregation', worrying that the demands of domestic education crowded other subjects – notably the sciences – out of girls' curricula (Parker 2001). Domestic education was a double-edged sword; it could lead to the segregation of women in formal education, but campaigners like Becker also attempted to use it as a 'Trojan horse', putting science education at the heart of a feminized curriculum by concentrating on exactly the reductive, analytical, chemical and physiological work that so characterized the intersection of food and science in the nineteenth century.

The amount of domestic education available in schools, as well as the level of scientific content included in cookery and nutrition lessons, reflected local socio-cultural expectations of class and gender; likewise it varied due to expense – cookery, as a practical science, required some investment in specialized teaching spaces and equipment. Consequently school domestic education often occurred against a backdrop of, or in conjunction with, philanthropic activities. To continue with the example of Manchester, while the two local school boards (Salford and Manchester) struggled with funding and argued over the detailed curriculum content for their domestic education schemes, the city also had no fewer than three charitable organizations dedicated to teaching the art of cookery. In 1876 a school of cookery was founded in connection with the YMCA, and for a few years offered fee-charging cookery lessons; in 1880 a School of Domestic Economy was founded, initially as a franchise of the better established Edinburgh School of Cookery, and this offered fee-charging cookery classes and teacher training that was supposed to subsidize free or low-cost cookery lessons for the poor; finally the 'Domestic Institute' based in the Jewish and Irish slum area of Cheetham Hill offered education, charity and social space for the poor (Heggie 2011b).

Almost all of these interventions – and those like them elsewhere – were dually justified on health and welfare grounds: to provide women and girls with the skills necessary to produce *economical* as well as nutritional meals for men and children. But, as one might expect with a complex socio-cultural object such as food, a series of conflicting aims and expectations shaped food and cookery education. One, mentioned above, was the level of scientific content taught to girls; as nutritional science and metabolic studies became a well established part of contemporary physiology, cookery education was a space where tensions between women's idealized traditional roles as homemakers and their increasing participation in formal education and paid employment could be played out. That women needed scientific education in order to feed their families could be used as leverage for better technical and scientific education for women; conversely, it could result in women only being taught a circumscribed and applied science curriculum, whose content was dictated by the expectations of household management and motherhood. Turning domestic skills into something that needed to be formally taught by experts, rather than learnt at home from family, also created new jobs for women, now able to take diplomas in cookery education. Class-based tensions manifested in criticisms of the content of domestic education courses. These were criticized for being unrealistic, using equipment and ingredients that were not available in the average working-class or slum home – which was particularly significant as the 'professionalization' of the housewife and introduction of expert texts, mentioned above, meant there had been an increase in the use of gadgets and equipment in middle-class and/or urban households which were not matched with the extremely basic stove-and-pot or open-fire-and-cauldron kitchens of the poor household. This disconnect between nutritional ideal and lived reality was therefore partly due to the gentrification of cookery teaching, but sometimes because some cookery education was also intended to provide servants for the middle classes, and their modern kitchens, not nurturing mothers for the poor.

Domestic education, whether based in formal (state) education or via (semi-) philanthropic interventions was also part of a wider economy of food culture and health practices. In schools, cookery lessons for older girls could be used to provide school meals for younger pupils, free or for a small fee that then subsidized the cookery lessons. Lessons might be provided as part of a broader network of educational activities, taking place across working men's institutions, YMCA branches, temperance coffee shops, cooperative and union associations and other socio-cultural spaces. Often, advice on food – its selection and preparation – was part of a broader scheme to educate citizens in 'health' in general, with nutrition and cookery taught alongside first aid and domestic and personal hygiene (Heggie 2011b). Advice on food and feeding could therefore enter a home through many passageways: from children who attended a lecture in order to get their free school meal of pea soup and bread; from talks given to mothers at local mother and baby groups; from health visitors; from male family members who had attended a working men's evening lecture or union educational meeting. (This pattern occurred in other countries too: Apple 1995.) This is, of course, in addition to the nutritionally focused advertising and branding material already in the pantry on tubs of Liebig's extract, and similar products, or contained in books of household hints and tips. Much of this information came freighted with moral and social values: *The Frugal Housewife* (1829) is usually credited with being the first American work of domestic expertise, and the subsequent boom in this literature across the Western world in the nineteenth century carried with it a varying and culturally-specific baggage of economy, efficiency, good taste, exclusiveness, artistry and so on – health was another moral value amongst many (Hollows 2008).

PURE AND AUTHENTIC

The web of food cultures that included school meals, soup kitchens, food reform organizations and laboratory-based physiologists configured food as both the essence of health (when selected in a modern, scientific, economical way) and as the source of sickness, contagion and misery. Some foodstuffs dramatically occupied both categories, and for Western medicine it is probably milk that most obviously exemplifies this, from 'breast is best' to 'white poison'. Milk's domestic, feminized identity no doubt added to its cultural power, alongside the fact that it is, uniquely, a product of the human animal. So while food reformers and nutritional scientists engaged with school meals for younger children, domestic education, lectures on nutrition and cookery instruction for older children and adults, they also targeted new mothers and infants.

It is the French doctor, Pierre Budin, who is usually credited with founding the first milk clinic/depot in 1892; by asking women who gave birth at the Charité hospital to attend an outpatient's clinic he was able to institute a regime of education and health propaganda, as well as weighing and measuring the babies (Dwork 1987). Breastfeeding was firmly encouraged, but where it was not sufficient, sterilized undiluted cows' milk was offered. Two years later (and independently of the Parisian developments) Leon Dufour opened a *goutte de lait* in Fécamp (Normandy) offering much the same mix of education, instruction and surveillance. By the turn of the twentieth century there were around two dozen *consultations de nourrissons/goutte de lait* in Paris alone (Dwork 1987). Milk depots and related institutions are excellent ways to make international comparisons between food and health culture; while extremely successful in France, *gouttes de lait* were tried in England (the first in St Helens in 1899) but never achieved the same results or popularity. This was in part due to attitudes to welfare; for example, the English institutions tended to charge a flat – and relatively high – fee, while Budin's institutions used a sliding scale of contributions. It was also a reflection of differing infant feeding cultures; Budin and Dufour's schemes were part of a long-running socio-medical campaign against wet-nursing, once the prerogative of the social elite, but becoming an option increasingly chosen by struggling working women in industrializing French cities in a way that was not prevalent among the British poor (Paul 2011: Chap. 5).

Systems for analysing the success of infant foods also varied heavily according to national cultures of health-care provision: Lawrence Weaver (2010) highlights three such systems: the 'gravimetric', 'caloric' and 'volumetric'. So, as we have seen above, in France studies of feeding and survival were based out of the maternity clinics of hospitals for the poor, and so systems of success measurement remained simple – weighing, construction of growth charts, a practice spearheaded by Budin and Gaston Variot. In contrast, German systems of infant feeding analysis grew out of specialist clinics in hospitals with strong university links, so that researchers favoured the 'modern', high-tech methods pioneered by Liebig – the calorimeter and related technologies. Meanwhile, in the USA it was private physicians with strong maternal and paediatric practices that began to publish on ideal diets and growth rates, representing food in a 'pharmaceutical approach' that focused on milk formulas (Weaver 2010: 322).

Cultures of childcare and infant feeding helped to shape the medical interventions around milk – both human and animal. Although, generally speaking, Western medicine largely favoured breastfeeding over most of the alternatives, this still varied by specific circumstance; where breast milk was scanty, supplements were recommended, and advice about the right time to wean or add other foods was inconsistent. The debates about what was right – medically and culturally – for the baby and infant were inevitably coloured by asymmetrical comparisons. 'Scientific' preparations, whether that was chemically analysed formula or condensed milk (spiked, if necessary, with Liebig's beef concentrate) may have led to babies that gained weight more quickly than those fed on breast milk alone – but again, as campaigners themselves pointed out, if *mothers* were underfed, were in employment out of the home and unable to regularly feed, or were alcoholics, the success of artificial foods was more about the poverty of the individual breast than its inadequacy as a food in general. Likewise, although it was known that cows' milk differed in nutrients from breast milk (leading to attempts to 'humanize' it) (Mepham 1993), it was nonetheless a crucial basic foodstuff for infants and young children. But were the dangers from milk inherent to the nutritional quality of cows' milk, or to the risks of infectious and contagious diseases it contained, or to contamination during transport into the swelling cities, or to domestic sluttery on the part of mothers who used filthy, unsterilized rubber teats on bottles?

The complexities of milk have proved a rich ground for historians: it neatly brings together the key health and social concerns of the nineteenth century – urbanization, changes in gender roles, capitalism, state (non-)intervention, the increasingly political role of laboratory science, the intractable connection between medicine and welfare, the social challenges of capitalist economies, the drive for efficiency (Valenze 2011). Some of the standardization and analysis of milk can be rewritten as a masculinization of this problematic, fluid foodstuff; not only were most of the roles involved – farmer, milk entrepreneur, analyst, doctor, veterinarian – male-dominated, but as Block has shown for Progressive-era urban America, even the imagery around milk could be designed to disguise the 'female' origin of the food. Making something 'scientific' often meant making it 'rational', and by implication *male* (Block 2005).

Unsurprisingly, then, blame for poor food was consistently placed on women. It is in the debates over milk, and more broadly the feeding of infants and young children, that we find the clear distinction between *mal*nutrition and *under*nutrition. An infant, weaned early onto scrapings from its parents' plates was not being *under*fed in terms of strict calories, or simple want of money: it was being given a badly chosen, unbalanced and inappropriate diet. Philanthropists, reformers, politicians and doctors around 1900 were very clear that the drive for education was about preventing this sort of hunger. While school meals, soup kitchens and state-funded analysts could feed the genuinely desperate, provide outlets for the meals cooked by girls in school and ensure the safety of products on the shelves, time and again the problem recentred on the housewife, her choice of food, her ability to balance a budget, and her cooking skills; failure in these areas was due, at best, to ignorance and at worst to laziness (Heggie 2011b).

At the absolute core of this problem was female employment. Although working women themselves emphasized the importance of the additional income they brought into the home in terms of the total domestic economy, for those outside the working class (and for some within it, notably in the trade unions), women's labour could only occur at the expense of domesticity: the consequence was that children went unfed to school, babies were left at nurseries, and men came home from work to find nothing on the table. In a familiar refrain, reformers also worried that a higher family income merely meant spending on 'convenience' foods – tinned meats, over-stimulating relishes, and fried fish from the local chip shop (Davin 1996).

Imbricated into these economic anxieties are concerns about the 'natural roles' of men and women in newly-reorganized societies. Amongst the desire to be modern, scientific and efficient was also a thread of arguments that turned to the natural as justification for social reform and economic change; increasingly couched in biomedical and evolutionary terms, the structures of society – whether the presence of poverty, gendered divisions of labour, or racist and imperial conceptions of superior and inferior peoples – were both scientifically rational and dictated by the 'natural' laws uncovered by scientists. This potential tension – the natural and artificial, the pure and the constructed – is clearly present in food cultures and anxieties and has been part of food history in particular since Mary Douglas's (1966) seminal work on dirt and taboo. Away from food's role in health and disease, modern food fashion, as Ken Albala (2014) has shown, revolves around two positions, one combining artifice and expense, the other authenticity and simplicity. Likewise the healthiness of food (or otherwise) was usually linked to its purity, but whether that purity was a 'natural' product or one created only through man-made interventions shifted through the nineteenth century (Waddington 2003).

Concerns over food adulteration illustrate this change. As we have seen above, the earliest interventions – such as the *Lancet*'s study of coffee, milk, tea and pemmican – figured adulteration as a form of deliberate deception: the substitution of cheaper and possibly dangerous substances to bulk out products. Liebig's signature on a label was there to guarantee its *purity* not in a strict chemical sense but rather as a mark of *authenticity* – this was *truthfully* Liebig's beef tonic, and contained what Liebig's beef tonic claimed to contain. While scientific processes could create these pure foods – as we have seen above, often through concentration or the creation of 'essences' – they could also act as threats to authenticity, as producers used 'artificial' means to bleach, flavour and enhance their products. At the extreme, food producers found ways to chemically mimic natural process, leading to some rather philosophically challenging debates about what authentic food could be; a classic example from the mid-nineteenth century would be the new deacidification technique invented by Ludwig Gall. Gall's intervention could make cheap wine taste like more expensive wine, infuriating producers whose cachet and profits depended on their expensive terroir, which as well as being a marker of provenance, also created 'naturally' deacidified wine. Gall's process baffled analysts, who were unable to distinguish between the 'natural' and the 'artificial' process in the final product (Goldberg 2011).

Chemical intervention therefore retained a dual position as protector of, and threat to, food – and, by implication, health. But as the nineteenth century progressed, food reformers began to worry about other contaminants, and increasingly these were *natural* products that posed a risk to human health: germs. As miasmatic theories of contagion gave way to germ theories, 'impure' food could now mean food containing a disease-causing payload, rather than one admixed with water or charcoal, or bleached. In these situations it was only (bio)chemical analysis, or microscopical and microbial inspection, that could determine if a food was pure and healthy or diseased and dangerous. Likewise, being 'natural' was no longer a marker for being 'pure' or 'healthy' – milk here being the key example, rendered safe by scientific examination and chemical treatment, from pasteurization to condensation.

There were those who continued to assert the superiority of the 'natural' for promoting bodily (and social) health. While artificial intervention was necessary to purify milk, water and other nutritional substances, it was still possible to argue that the corruption present in these 'natural' substances was itself a consequence of modernity, more specifically of the 'unnatural' way human beings had ordered their society. This is clearly visible in the discussions about milk, outlined above – what made milk toxic was, perhaps, poor farming practices, bulk production, long-distance transportation, artificial feeding systems, crowded urban living and, most importantly, modern women's apparent failure to 'naturally' breastfeed their infants. Or, to take another example, there was the problem of arsenic: although not strictly a foodstuff, arsenic was a widely used medical preparation, found in tonics and face creams alike; by the early nineteenth century it had become a lucrative industrial product, used to create brilliant dyes. While sometimes a straightforward contaminant – as a white powder, arsenic was easy to confuse with flour and other ingredients – it was also a deliberate addition to brightly coloured foods, in particular to sweets and cakes. Multiple cases of fatal poisoning, often from coated sweets or from highly coloured confectionary used to decorate grand feasts (e.g. green marzipan candlesticks), occurred across Europe and the USA in the middle third of the nineteenth century, as this 'Sugared Death' killed children in particular (Vernon 2007; Whorton 2011: Chap. 6). While there was some resistance to the idea that this 'natural' medicinal substance could be so toxic, the controversies about it played into familiar dichotomies: after all, it was chemical analysis that protected the public and it was often foreign (in London, Jewish) retailers at fault, or later decadent wealthy urbanites paying the price for their fashionable wallpaper and bright ballgowns. Even as the toxicity of the substance was gradually accepted, it could still be used to tell moral stories about consumption – or rather, non-consumption. In 1900 there was a sudden outbreak of neuritis, thought to be the result of overindulgence in alcohol, in Manchester and the neighbouring city of Salford (Copping 2003: Chap. 1). Eventually the disease was traced to a batch of arsenically contaminated sugar used in brewing. As the *Jewish Chronicle* proudly noted

> [T]here have been at least 20,000 cases of poisoning, in not a single one of these instances was the victim a Jew, the Jewish population numbering 25,000 souls having apparently entirely escaped the calamity. Explanation of this remarkable phenomenon is probably to be found in the proverbial sobriety of the Jew.
>
> —Anon. 1901

Purity was therefore not just a chemical characteristic of food, but also a moral human virtue, and the two senses of the word are almost inextricable when we look at the cultural role of food in health and medicine in the long nineteenth century.

MODERNITY AND MODERATION: GLOBAL FOOD CULTURE

Nineteenth-century food reform societies have proven a popular topic for historians (see above); meanwhile the literature on the role of taboo in food cultures is vast, and yet the two have not significantly intersected. This is despite the fact that the major cultural responses in the West to changing ideas of biology, medicine, health, society and consumption appear to be in the form of rejection – and specifically of rejection of the very foods included in histories because of their strong socio-cultural significance: meat, milk, beer and bread. Purity, moral and bodily (and often both at once), is a central justification for the vegetarian and temperance movements, and is littered throughout the propaganda of virtually all the food reform societies that rose and fell in urbanized, industrialized societies between 1800 and 1920.

While these movements aimed for purity, their embrace of 'natural' ways of living did not extend to a robust rejection of the chemical analysis and nutritional science that this chapter has shown was a key feature of food history in the nineteenth century. Allison's bread, Graham's crackers and Kellogg's cornflakes all relied on (semi)-industrial processing and all turned to analytical chemists to quantify their fibre, calorie and mineral content, as they would later do for vitamins. Many food reform movements also relied heavily on biomedical claims – for example the Uric Acid diet, popularized by London-based hospital consultant Alexander Haig, who argued that excess uric acid in the bloodstream caused a host of diseases and a restriction diet could be used to restore health (Barnett 1995: 164–5). Uric-acid forming purines are present in a large number of foods, and while Haig initially, in the 1880s, recommended a general reduction, by the early twentieth century he was pushing for complete dietary purity, and abstention from 'All meat, meat extracts, gravies, fish, fowl and the yolk of egg. All the pulses . . . Mushrooms, asparagus, pistachio and cashew nuts. Oatmeal, entire wheat meal and brown bread, containing any husk. Tea, Coffee, cocoa and chocolate' (Haig and Haig 1913: 2).

This is not to say that all these diets and eating practices were unproblematically accepted – there was of course much debate over the merits and demerits of the systems. Some seemed based on solid theories, but resulted in impractical living in the 'real world', such as Horace Fletcher's Chew-chew scheme, which instructed participants to chew their food until it was completely liquefied, possibly hundreds of times (Barnett 1997). Even more controversial was the brief popularity of the 'no breakfast diet' in the US and UK. Aside from the lack of metabolic evidence for the healthiness of the diet, commentators pointed out that plenty of people already went without breakfast –albeit from necessity not desire – and that this did not seem to provide them with any particular health advantages. That there might be a *moral* advantage to routine deprivation, however, was less controversial. Vernon (2007) has suggested that as Western society became less accustomed to periodic famine, hunger was itself reframed both as a political failing and as an aesthetic moral choice. His examples are most obviously hunger strikers, whose self-deprivation is a representation of an individual famine designed to draw attention to a political or social wrong, but similar processes of control through denial can be seen in other, often marginalized, groups in the long nineteenth century.

The self-deprivation of the vegetarian and temperance food reform groups, and perhaps less dramatically in all rhetorics of moderation in relation to consumption, are expressions of the importance of *control*. It is a truism in contemporary psychology that food is a locus of struggle for control, but for consumers in the nineteenth century it was often also a moral virtue in its own right, frequently displayed in contrast to the gluttony – for food, novelty and stimulation – of a new modern era; as such, it is intimately associated with fears of decay and degeneration. The physiologists who meticulously measured human intake and excretion to calculate the biochemical and energetic properties of food were fascinated by the side-show performances of nineteenth-century 'Hunger Artists' (Nieto-Galan 2015). Usually men, these were performers who claimed to survive long periods of fasting; not always total deprivation, but sometimes surviving on their own patent tonics (available to purchase, of course), or more eclectic sustenance, including their own urine (Atwater and Langworthy 1897: 92). Reaching a peak of popularity at the end of the nineteenth century, this form of deliberate bodily control, clearly gendered male, seems quite different to responses to the 'Fasting women' of the early part of the century, whose ability to survive without food, and importantly to go hungry *without suffering*, was far more often part of a religious and miraculous articulation of denial and purity (Gooldin 2003).

That the refusal of food was interpreted and represented so differently for men and women is a difficult inheritance for historians of conditions such as anorexia; it is deeply problematic to retrospectively diagnose a disease that is so intrinsically cultural and gendered. That said, given the valorization of the mother and wife who 'went without' to feed husband and children, and the relative lack of autonomy nineteenth-century women experienced, it is easy to see how food control could become a crucial part of female identity and self-expression. Women's responsibility for the choice, purchase and preparation of food may have been a burden when they were being critiqued for making unhealthy or uneconomic choices, but it was sometimes possible for women to use it as a form of socio-political activity. It could, of course, be a deeply personal political decision, as evidenced by stories of female slaves resisting pressure to eat well and reproduce liberally (Berti 2016). It could also be a community activity: when the rising price of meat began to cause problems for poor households in the mining communities of Durham and Northumberland in the 1870s, local newspapers blamed women for poor choices and bad cooking. But the women responded with action: they organized, set an acceptable price, boycotted butchers and vendors who tried to charge higher rates, and punished – with violence on occasion – 'blacklegs' who continued to buy at higher prices (Mood 2009).

We can read the meat boycott as a (rare) expression of female political power, and of the relationship between the politics of the family and of the trade unions; but for this chapter it is also a dramatic demonstration of the globalization of food. The meat boycott was essentially broken by the work of the Australian Meat Agency, who heavily promoted cheap, imported tinned meat, which proved an acceptable alternative to expensive fresh meat for the boycotters – helped no doubt by the attendance of the mayors of both Newcastle and Gateshead and 'a number of the most prominent ladies connected with the food agitation' who were all invited to a banquet in Gateshead funded by the Australian Meat Agency (Mood 2009: 421). Canning, refrigeration and the creation of shelf-stable meat extracts all encouraged meat importation – changing not only the economic and food landscape, but actively interacting with ideas of health and the production of 'medical' foods such as Liebig's extract and the many imitations that followed.

International trade, in people and ideas as well as objects, had an influence on many areas of the interaction between food, health and medicine. Pemmican may not have had as dramatic a transformative effect on food culture as the transportation of pasta, potatoes or tomatoes, nor was it as socio-economically consequential as the international trade in spices or sugar, but it is indicative of the ways food changed with travel. Chemical analysis and commercial branding allowed a food created from centuries of expertise of wild travel in North America to be refigured as a food of empire, a military staple, a health food, a tonic for invalids. Other foods underwent similar transformations: when, at the very end of the nineteenth century, the American chemist Atwater (1844–1907) published his extraordinarily comprehensive literature review of all the works he could find relating to metabolism, the foodstuffs considered were not confined to traditional European fare (Atwater and Langworthy 1897). Although milk, meat, bread and beer dominate, there are also studies of soy, rice and tofu. This is in part due to the 'educational exchange' between Japanese and German researchers in the 1870s and 1880s under the Meiji regime's attempts at modernization, which resulted in an interest in Japanese diets (and some Japanese researchers) in the German nutritional and physiological laboratories. Atwater also emphasized that crucial work was being done in

Russia – well away from the traditional centres of physiological and biochemical laboratory expertise in Western Europe.

Like pemmican, soy became inscribed into Western health practices, nutritional science and food culture through a process of analysis and effective 'rebranding' as 'scientific' and 'rational' – the markers of 'modernity' repeatedly found at the intersection of medical and food practices in the early twentieth century, at the end of the period considered in this volume (Teuteberg 2007). For example, it was used in the twentieth-century reform of the German sausage. As early as the 1870s, Europe and American commentators in the scientific and popular press could refer to German soldiers as 'scientific' partly due to their biomedically efficient rations, whose key feature was the Erbswurst, or pea sausage (not that this necessarily persuaded British consumers to buy them: Waddington 2012). Very similar in concept to pemmican, as it happens, these sausages constituted mostly of animal fat, bulked with pea flour, and were usually sliced up and used to make hot soups (Anon. 1877). In an unexpected encounter between science, culture and food, a major innovation involved the use of gelatine and bichromate of potash to make casings when animal organs were in short supply, a technology borrowed directly from the fashionable new art of photography. Faced with a more dramatic shortage of all kinds of meat during the First World War, the mayor of Cologne, Konrad Adenauer, developed a sausage-making process that replaced the pea flour with soy flour – a deliberate attempt to get people to eat more vegetable protein by 'disguising' it as meat (Anon. n.d.).

There is, however, a much darker side to the story of German wartime sausage-innovation. While Adenauer promoted his (rational, scientific, healthy) soy sausages, the national approach to food shortages was dramatic: *Schweinmord*, the slaughter of around 9 million pigs in the spring of 1915. The justification for this – from the official report of the 'Eltzbacher Commission' (named after Paul Eltzbacher, law professor and chair) – was the work of physiologist and metabolic researcher Nathan Zuntz. Zuntz had been measuring his bodyweight since 1888 as part of a lifelong metabolic experiment, and noticed he rapidly lost weight as wartime food restrictions came in (Gunga 2008: 84). He recommended the slaughter of pigs in order to free up grain and potatoes, arguing that it was more *efficient* in terms of hunger and calories for people to eat vegetable food themselves rather than to 'convert' it by passage through livestock. The slaughter did not resolve Germany's hunger crisis, and consequently later anti-Semitic commentators pointed to Zuntz's ethnicity as evidence that the entire enterprise was a Jewish plot to destroy German agriculture and the German economy.

The strong connections between ethnicity and food culture meant that nutritional science could not escape the effects of evolutionary ways of thinking, of racial science and even eugenics. Assumptions that the middle and upper classes 'needed' refined foods while the labouring poor could make 'rougher' food suffice, or that particular races and ethnicities (black slaves, the Irish, Jewish immigrants) could survive on fewer calories, less digestible and more adulterated foods, were often supported (and rarely challenged) by scientific investigation. Indeed, the Liebig-ian prioritization of animal protein as a source of vitality was used as evidence that the proportion of a population that regularly ate animal flesh was effectively a marker of civilization (Neill 2009). Yet there were circumstances, which we briefly encountered above, in which the meat-centric diet of Western Europeans was constituted as medically inappropriate – that is, when they travelled.

Just as food circulated the globe, so the nineteenth century saw a huge increase in Western European people travelling worldwide. Whether engaging in colonial appropriation, economic exploitation or missionary work, white Europeans found themselves in increasing numbers in Indo-China, Africa and around the Pacific rim. Historians of acclimatization have demonstrated a distinctive shift in ideas of human acclimatization through the long nineteenth century, from a confidence in the adaptability of the white body, to a fear that prolonged inhabitation of the tropics led to (racial) degeneration or death (Anderson 1996a; Anderson 1996b; Osborne 2014; Livinstone 1999; Harrison 1996). With the invention of tropical medicine at the end of the nineteenth century, many pathologies of white travellers were reinvented as forms of infectious disease, but this did not preclude the idea that changes in diet might also prevent the deterioration of health overseas. In particular, and with remarkable consistency through the nineteenth century, travellers to the tropics were advised to take up a reduced-meat diet – that is, to follow the 'non-stimulating' diets sometimes recommended to invalids, hospital inmates and so on. (See the specific appeal to Liebig's theories about the role of animal protein in stimulating the body by Dutch colonials in the East Indies: Pols 2012: 132–3.) Almost regardless of the medical theories of diet current at any time, red meat has been strongly associated with colder, temperate climates, while vegetarian diets, especially those veering towards vegan, involving pulses and legumes as key protein sources, have been regarded as the 'natural' food of the tropics. Likewise, alcohol remained a food for North and Western European climates, leading to disease, laziness and degeneration when consumed in the heat of the equatorial regions.

Post-Darwinian theories of human evolution caused climate and constitution to blur: a non-temperate environment led almost inevitably to 'less civilized' cultures, to a 'less industrious' population than the temperate zones of Europe and North America, and the common diets of these zones were part of this inadequacy. While there were situations in which it was appropriate to copy local diets (or other behaviours), such food cultures – including vegetarianism – remained controversial and non-ideal in the temperate regions. Although colonial countries often developed a taste for the food cultures of the nations they occupied, most notably Victorian Britain's embrace of curry, these were usually redefined and redesigned for European palates, and clearly figured as exceptional, not routine, eating (and not always appropriate for the sick or weak body). Meanwhile many guidebooks and handbooks offered colonials advice on trying to prepare 'home comforts' while overseas, perhaps most emphatically in the case of the French, for whom an elite food culture was a crucial aspect of national identity, and one that had to be maintained in internationally visible sites, even if that resulted in unlikely dishes such as boiled hippopotamus' feet with a traditional French sauce (Neill 2009: 15). As mentioned above, pursuing his early career as an African explorer, eugenicist Francis Galton's *Hints to Travellers* contains many pages of 'shifts and contrivances' for making good tea in non-European conditions. Such advice often emphasized hygiene; the creation of tropical medicine as a specialism at the end of the century re-emphasized the tropics as sites of particular danger with regard to contagion, but likewise, public health reforms in European countries meant that the potentially contaminated water and food of 'foreign' countries were increasingly emphasized in *contrast* to the safe, hygienic conditions of food and water, milk and meat 'at home'.

The advice 'not to drink the water' is an indicator of a binary in consumption: us/them, civilized/barbaric, safe/risky, healthy/unhealthy. Modernity and urban 'civilization' did not always mean healthier food – as this chapter has shown they could also be associated with decadence, degeneration, adulteration and 'unnatural' foods. But by the early decades of the twentieth century there was a new confidence, certainly within Western medicine, that the fundamental principles of 'scientific nutrition' were understood, and that through social and political reform the cultures of eating amongst a population could be shifted into healthier (and more economically beneficial) consumption patterns. Diets could be clean, modern and rational; but, of course, that required people to be clean, modern and rational too, a demand that perhaps proved unrealistic through the century that followed.

CHAPTER THREE

Disease[1]

BERTRAND TAITHE

Any cultural history of disease after 1800 has to begin with the visit to the hospital wards. Hospitals more than any other structures were designed to contain, classify, understand and display diseases. In 1800 most remained the object of containment rather than effective treatment yet the visit to the hospital served a range of cultural purposes. One of Napoleon's early propaganda paintings by Antoine-Jean Gros of 1804 thus represented the future emperor visiting his soldiers sick with the plague of Jaffa in 1799. The general was portrayed reaching out and touching their buboes in a gesture reminiscent of the royal touch which was meant to cure scrofula in an earlier period (Grigsby 1995: 1–46; Outram 1988).[2] The painting conveyed the French leader's personal courage and Christ-like thaumaturgic powers (see Figure 3.1). The truth had been rather different and Napoleon had not performed any miraculous healing touch, yet it mattered that a ruler should be represented confidently facing a deadly disease (Kelly 2010).

Around the same period, Michel Foucault argued in a key text of 1963, hospitals and wards were reorganized according to disease classifications (nosology). In Paris, hospital specialization enabled the concentration of cases which early medical specialization required. Overcrowded wards offered to the medical gaze of trainee doctors the full 'natural history' of illnesses, from early symptoms to their final manifestations (Foucault 1963). According to Foucault, these teaching hospitals represented an opportunity for a radical 'epistemological break' in medical ways of knowing. On the one hand, it enabled new systems of knowledge to appear (epistemic systems) and, on the other, it allowed new forms of authoritarian and dehumanizing treatment of patients. Medical knowledge in hospitals and medical structures congealed

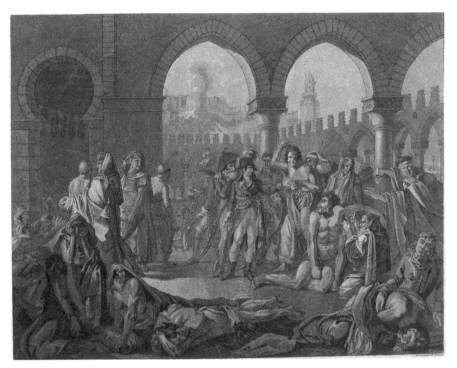

FIGURE 3.1: *Napoleon Bonaparte Visiting the Plague-Stricken in Jaffa*. Aquatint by G. A. Lehmann after Baron Gros. Wellcome Library.

around diseases, Foucault argued. These developments encouraged specialization and a Copernican break with a more discursive approach to the body (Jones and Porter 2002). A generation later, according to the philosopher Georges Canguilhem, the work of Claude Bernard and experimental work on animals enabled medical specialists to test to destruction individual organs – distancing physiology further from patients. Experiments on animals enabled the scientist to push the boundaries of what could be seen in a disease. Through experiments and induced ailments, a scientist could reproduce in a laboratory how a disease might begin and end, how organs and life itself could extend the boundaries of what could be normal in response to disease (Coleman and Holmes 1988). Claude Bernard's argument that medicine was no longer a bedside science, but one which was situated in laboratories and based on observations and experimentations – thereby isolating diseases from patients – inflamed the imagination of a range of artists. In literature the naturalists who followed Émile Zola's injunction conceived the novel as a form of laboratory suited to the observation of hereditary and social diseases (Bernard 1865; Zola 1880).

If at first enunciation, disease might seem an obvious cultural category – the absence of disease defining health[3] – it proved difficult to narrow down and define in reality. The attempts at definitions published in 1900 in the *British Medical Journal* by Sydney Wilson Macilwaine were somewhat circular even though they claimed to represent a major advance on previous approaches: 'the sum total of the pathological consequences resulting in a patient from the interference with his [sic] physiological state from a disease cause' (Macilwaine 1900: 1703–4). The author then proceeds to list intrinsic (for instance, wear and tear or insanity), external (microbes) and indeterminate causes (as yet not understood) which might indeed interfere – only to leave open the idea that a disease was what made you unwell (exhibiting pathological symptoms). Many dysfunctions could coexist in one person and indeed be an expression of a perverted physical vitality. As early as 1800, Bichat had argued that organs were defined by their instability (Canghilhem Xavier 1965: 156; Pickstone 1981, 1999). Cancers grow and thrive (Hayle Walshe 1846), and illnesses were now understood to be produced by the body against itself as well as in response to external threats.[4] Building on natural science systems of classification, medical observers refined their approach to the symptoms and nature of ailments, and their classification of diseases branched out and grew dramatically in the nineteenth century. First concentrating on organs, then tissues and so on, they observed chronic ailments created by lifestyle or work (diabetes, heart diseases, lung diseases), epidemic and pandemic diseases which shook the world (cholera in 1830–2, 1850 and 1866;[5] influenza in 1918), shameful ailments like syphilis or other sexually transmitted diseases, intractable mass killers like tuberculosis (Bryder 1988) or 'hidden' diseases like cancer (Pinel 1992; Moscucci 2005).

Each of these ailments has a cultural history of its own (Le Goff and Sournia 1985; Rousseau, Gill and Haycock 2003), and much of the scholarship has indeed been devoted to the contested definitions and various treatments and representations of one or another ailment. Diseases have a history even in the way they were defined or named by scientists. Medical practitioners invariably described diseases through literature reviews of previous clinical observations and sought to make sense of them in historical terms. In the footsteps of medical practitioners themselves, often reliant on their stories, professional historians have often claimed particular primacy or cultural significance for their pet disease. Some have claimed that syphilis haunted fears of racial decline (Parascandola: 2008), that cholera echoed revolutions (Kudlick 1996: 176–211), that tropical diseases and their treatment conditioned the growth of empire (Curtin 1998; Anderson 1996: 94–118; Curtin 1961, and 1990: 63–88), or that the madness of a king cast new lights on nineteenth-century notions of the self (Scull 2005; Micale and Porter 1995). Many of these claims are indeed grounded, and diseases have been a prime cultural anchor point for the history of medicine and medicalised history more broadly.

To engage with different cultural meanings of diseases in the long nineteenth century, this chapter seeks to propose that diseases can indeed be considered in relation to cultural understanding of the self, of the social and the global, and that this shift reflected growing alienation, distance and loss of control over the cultural meanings of disease (Joyce 1994). Cultural in this sense retains a profound political significance, albeit one in which debates often remain embedded in narrative forms which are not openly about political choices (Chartier 1988). The chapter will thus engage with diseases through patient-centred narratives, illness as metaphors (to borrow from Susan Sontag's famous formulation of 1978) for the woes of society and understanding of biothreats in the era of nineteenth-century imperial globalization. It will end with the concept of diseases of civilization – in the literal eugenic sense arising from new ways of writing global history and engaging with the growing scale of disease-related concerns. It follows that a wide range of chronological frameworks might apply. From a purely medical science perspective, one can follow the shift from clinical- to laboratory-based medical work on diseases (which is of course incomplete and supplementary; laboratories grew alongside clinical practices, and clinics themselves increasingly adopted technological modes of gazing at and into the body, such as x-rays or new laboratory tests such as the much lionized Wassermann test for syphilis) (Lawrence 1985). From the professional point of view, one witnessed the increased professionalization of medical sciences which grew from humble apprenticeships and competing medical schools into elitist pursuits (Weisz 2003; Bynum 1994). Across the West and even in colonial empires, the nineteenth century is an era during when medical doctors managed to isolate and marginalize less university qualified competitors, in which nurses became essential actors in the struggle against orderlies or nuns, in which dentists and pharmacists graduated from the commercial sphere into a scientific establishment (McClelland 2002; Lewenson and Herrmann 2007). Each profession created cultural institutions, academies and societies patrolling the borders of their professional territory (see also Michael Brown's chapter in this same volume; Weisz 1995).

Each country has its own trajectory, but international emulation played a crucial part in shaping this evolution (Léonard 1978). From the patients' perspective, of course, the growth of hospital medicine and complex treatments increasingly undermined whatever control and understanding the sick might have had over their own ailments. Finally, diseases played a key role in public discourses on government, the rule of law, democracy and the redistribution of resources within societies and across empires (Wilson 2004). One could add a chronology of the growth of mass media, with newspapers becoming ubiquitous from the 1840s, film from the 1900s, and radio towards the end of our period

(Lupton 2012). Within this realm of cultural production, novels became a dominant form of storytelling in the first half of the nineteenth century, and many authors focused their plots on the threat or course of diseases (tuberculosis being a clear favourite), matching or mapped on characterization (Barnes 1995). Periodization is therefore context related and dependent on specific bearings one might chart a path with.

These layers of complexity notwithstanding, this chapter will argue that the shift from the self to the social and to the global can be mapped out on most of these spheres of cultural production. Though it would be foolish to divide the period into three equal phases of forty years, there are some valid arguments to suggest that each period represented an acute moment of expression and fresh articulation of these concerns for self, society and global perspectives on diseases. Finally, building on the work of Foucault, Sontag and social historians of medicine, diseases exist as manifest symptoms, visible and experienced by people, as risks expressed by groups anticipating ill-health (sometimes experienced as a risk worth taking or an unpredictable danger) and as metaphors, ways of representing through disease cultural, social and political change.

DISEASES AND THE SELF

Being ill was a quotidian preoccupation of nineteenth-century humans. Diaries attest to the frequency of attacks, bouts, weaknesses, fevers or recurrent ailments while seldom mentioning health, as if the absence of ill health alone could define pleasurable life. Diarists such as the British political economist Harriet Martineau or the French novelist Alphonse Daudet could chart the progress of their diseases (probably cancer and syphilis respectively) and the nature of the treatments and cures they had to endure. They also concerned themselves with the manner in which disease changed them as persons (Daudet 2003). They chronicled how their interaction with their loved ones could be altered by their unceasing pain, by their demands on their time and attention, not to mention the costly drain a chronic ailment presented to a family unit. Martineau teased out how fraught relationships became when disease became the object around which everything revolved:

> Going back to the days when I, myself, was the sympathiser, I remember how strong is the temptation to imagine, and to assure the sick one, that his pain will not last; that the time will come when he will be well again; that he is already better; or, if it be impossible to say that, that he will get used to his affliction, and find it more endurable. How was it that I did not see that such offers of consolation must be purely irritating to one who was not feeling better, nor believing that he should ever be better, nor in a state to be cheered by any speculation as to whether his pain would, or would not become more

endurable with time! Exactly in proportion to the zeal with which such considerations were pressed, must have been the sufferer's clearness of perception of the disguised selfishness which dictated the topics and the words. I was (as I half suspected at the time, from my sense of restraint and uneasiness) trying to console myself, and not my friend; indulging my own cowardice, my own shrinking from a painful truth, at the expense of the feelings of the sufferer for whom my heart was aching.

—Martineau 1845: 27

The consoler anticipating disease projected her fears on the sufferer. Words not only failed but shielded the spectator from the inevitability of future pain. While disease could not be avoided if one lived long, one could attempt to deny its hold on others. Culturally, diseases could be framed as an absence or a silence, as Charles Rosenberg pointed out (Rosenberg, Golden and Peitzman 1992; Aronowitz 2008: 1–9). There was little heroics in a slow and painful illness. The sordid nature of a body drenched in sweat or releasing excrements and other fluids[6] challenged romantic notions of the self (Porter 1997).

In the face of disease, self-pity and awareness could be expressed equally clearly and clinically. Daudet could thus suddenly embrace the rapid onset of his tertiary syphilis (or *tabes dorsalis* according to the latest nineteenth-century French classification) (Nitrini 2000: 605–6; McIntosh et al. 1913: 1–30; Waugh 1974): 'In my cubicle, in the shower baths, in front of the mirror: what emaciation! I have suddenly turned into a funny little old man. I have vaulted from forty-five to sixty-five. Twenty years I haven't experienced' (Daudet 2003: 3.) Disease became 'I' in Daudet's case and rhythmed his remaining years with a bewildering range of symptoms until his death at the age of fifty-seven.

Of course, such diaries tended to have survived most when they were the product of significantly wealthy individuals equipped with the leisure and desire to bear witness to the manifold effects of diseases, yet literary expressions of disease seem to have had a cross-class currency. Thus a few of the working-class diaries collected in Britain by Burnett, Vincent and Mayall also show similar concerns (1984). The harrowing autobiography of a Glasgow working-class woman, Elizabeth Storie, poisoned as a child in 1823 by the experimental mercury treatment prescribed by her physician Robert Falconer, testified to her anger at the dramatic alteration to her physique (her jaws fused by mercury) or inability to speak (but not to litigate) (Storie 1859; Boos 2013: 251–69). Her life, as she narrated it, consisted of a series of frustrating legal claims and lawsuits, rejection from her Kirk and community, defrauding by lawyers and medical obfuscation in acknowledging gross negligence. This legal case echoes the earlier case of *Priestly vs Fowler*. Her disease was intrinsically medical (an iatrogenic disease caused by medical interference). In her case, the intervention was, she argued, a callous act of experimental malpractice which various operations on her jaws could never correct.[7] Notwithstanding the stigma attached to many ailments, the voices of sufferers often denoted struggles and resistance.

Historians of the self have tended to take a rather positive position on these writings; some like Miriam Bailin arguing that the sick room represented a strategy of control for women in particular – a space within which being ill could become a technology of the self (Bailin 2007). Florence Nightingale herself did indeed retire to the sick room while embodying reforming in nursing. For an intellectual like Nightingale, the sick room could be used as 'a room of one's own'[8] from which the invalid could issue sharp commentary on the world around them (Nightingale 1990). The diseased self could thus acquire a centrality of a sort in the domestic arrangement through the identification of a sick room in a home. The sick room was a privilege which quarantine policies could enshrine and recognize. Bye-laws on the notification of highly contagious diseases in the late nineteenth century would, for instance, acknowledge the middle class's ability to look after its own in private sick rooms – away from the unwashed crowds of the fever hospitals (Mooney 1999: 238–67). Testimonials from working-class men witness – either in the clinical cases doctors published of their lives prior to their internment in hospital structures or in diaries – how radically diseases could affect their circumstances as income earner, their families and indeed their masculinity (Bederman 2008). The historiography of masculinity has often concentrated on the healthy and sporting body produced in schools and middle-class education. By contrast, the diseased male body appears in the historiography as impaired and de-masculinized (Forth 2008).

Diseases of the mind among the poor and the rich similarly had very different trajectories. Since the pioneering work of anti-asylum inspired historians, a multitude of more detailed studies such as the work of Robert Ellis have shown how mental illness among the poor could lead to a range of social agents taking over responsibility for the survival of the sick patient, shifting them from poorhouse to asylum to home according to resource transfer logics which could remain totally unreadable to the patients (Ellis 2006). The 'humane' treatment of the mad, focusing on controlling their mind rather than restraining their bodies, was indeed a nineteenth-century development but it was not rolled out universally or evenly outside Europe.

The diseased were not simply engaging with health care structures, domestic or institutional, they were consuming goods, techniques and drugs developed for them and sold according to evolving cultural norms by a growing industry focused on diseases (Marcellus 2008). As Graham Mooney has shown in relation to the material culture that grew around tuberculosis, this consumer culture responded to convergent attempts to control the domestic world of the patients while patients sought to regain some control over their disease (Mooney 2013). The development of the pharmaceutical industry as a business based on other sciences like chemistry or biology and engaging through experimental medicine in what has become known as translational medicine (from the laboratory to the bedside) began in earnest in the long nineteenth century. It assumed and conditioned a range of cultural shifts in the patients themselves. While patients had long been self-prescribing and keen purchasers of well-advertised patent medicines (arguably the back bone of the advertising market in Europe and the USA in the nineteenth century) (Jackson 1983: 1–38), drugs with genuinely active ingredients required posology, control and self-control. The growth of the pharmaceutical industry in the nineteenth century relied on a chain of production and delivery which included the patients themselves.

Patients had to engage with their treatments – change their diets, posture, physical and bodily regimen, monitor their excretions, fluid intake, sleep patterns or desires. Medical regimens from dieting, to rubbing ointments, to taking an expensive water cure could shape the day or planning of the year (Gilman 2008). A veritable cacophony of claims to authority presented alternative paths to health – making being diseased a particularly testing customer position. Historians of medicine have been keen to challenge simplistic professionalization narratives in order to extol the virtues or variegated nature of the medical marketplace. Patients had choice according to their education, wealth, social connections and networks. Some could engage with the new sciences which flooded the marketplace. The sick could turn to techniques originating from afar, such as acupuncture, which reached the West in earnest in the nineteenth century (White and Ernst 2004; Bivins 2000), sciences that made a more holistic sense of their self such as phrenology (Cooter 1984), or even the contrarian logic of watered down treatments of infinitesimal dosage like homeopathy (Warner 1998: 5–29; Baschin 2016).

Truth be told, the struggle for market-shares in the long nineteenth century had primarily been studied by historians concerned with debates about professionalization or medical power. Patients faced with diversity and costs, medical fees and charitable provisions had to navigate the extent to which they could afford their autonomy. As accurate medical diagnosis greatly predated effective medical treatments, facing disease was primarily to seek a counsel of despair and face dilemma. Medical culture proved difficult to decipher and engage with. Gustave Flaubert lampooned naive, self-taught medical amateurs in his novels and in particular in his masterly lampooning of petit bourgeois stupidity in *Bouvard et Pécuchet* (Flaubert 1881: 247–53; Sugaya 2010). In this satirical romp, the heroes' alternate treatments on themselves and others, jumping from one false remedy to another, leave behind a trail of bewildered patients and doctors. Flaubert equally lampooned the naive and the positivists whose trust in science betrayed cultural ineptitude and narrow-mindedness.

In the face of incurable diseases, what made one experimentalist a pioneer and another a dangerous quack was often the result of how well integrated the practitioner was in the networks of science and influence. An experimentalist such as the Parisian self-experimentalist Auzias Turenne, who attempted to treat syphilis through a multitude of injections and reinjections of pus (an experiment he conducted on many patients as well as himself), could claim that his method, 'a saturation' of the body with a poison, offered good results (Taithe 1999: 34; Dracobly 2003). That the disease itself, syphilis, was then discovered to have active phases separated sometimes by many years of inactivity undoubtedly lent his experiment some credibility. Patients could indeed walk symptom free for a long while. In fact, diseases were seldom observed free of treatment to the point that one had limited knowledge of what syphilis was or could do until the Tuskegee 'bad blood' experiment after the Second World War (Jones 1993). Treatments with mercury, and later arsenic based Salvarsan and Neo-Salvarsan, would produce such side effects that it became impossible to determine which made the patient most unwell (Brandt 1987).

Other diseases lent themselves to radical changes of climate and lifestyle – creating veritable communities of sufferers assembled in sanatoria. Pulmonary tuberculosis made the fortune of seaside resorts like Berk sur Mer, mountain refuges, rivieras in the south of France, Italy, North Africa and Egypt, where patients sought drier and warmer air as their lungs or bones struggled to cope (Woloshyn 2013: 74–93).[9] Thomas Mann's *Magic Mountain*, begun in 1912, provides an iconic portrayal of the communities of sufferers created by tuberculosis in luxury resorts (in this case the sanatorium of Davos).[10] Health tourists were thus often pioneers in a burgeoning international leisure industry and involved in the origins of sunbathing for instance. Their needs shaped and favoured the development of resorts which included casinos, promenades, gardens, cultural and social life conditioned by their seasonal presence (Gordon 2012). Water cures in Budapest, Bath, Baden Baden, colonial spas or Vichy, addressed digestive complaints, gout or skin disorders of various kind while hotels and resorts offered entertainment and fine dining (Jennings 2006). If pure air could not be sold to those who could not afford a lifestyle change, however temporary, waters and mud could be bottled and purchased and became prime commodities at the margins between medicine and luxury goods by the end of the nineteenth century (Hamlin 1990: 16–46).

Ultimately, disease always triumphed – short of an accidental death. Historians of death and mourning, such as Julie-Marie Strange and others (Strange 2005; Laderman 2003) have pointed out the depth of this fatalism and the cultural significance given to death and the 'good' death. The sick room could easily convert into the waking room – much to the chagrin of medical experts who sought to isolate and remove contaminated matter from the social environment.

DISEASES AND THE SOCIAL

The work of Michel Foucault has played a very significant role in shaping the social and cultural historiography of the nineteenth century. Most of his work began with the observation of social responses to diseases: a classificatory gaze in his work on systems of thoughts, a coercive approach to the deviant or sickly in his work on prisons or sexuality. *Discipline and Punish* (1975), which arguably most influenced the historiography until the rediscovery of his work on governmentality (Foucault 2012; Foucault 1991; Rose 1999), began with a discussion of torture and rehabilitation. In his view, practices to force the body into a shape or a disciplined posture or to inculcate moral norms through physical regimens echoed a new attitude to power – one in which the body became the centre of attention of government and modes of government. In that perspective, diseases acquired particular significance as the evidence of bad government or bad behaviour, poor policing (in his broader understanding of the term) and failing governmentality. Historians of governmentality then explored further this conceptual framework to expose the governmental logic in every aspect of public health policy (Crook 2007; Crook and Esbester 2016).

Foucault's argument echoed the pioneering work of Susan Sontag. His concepts revisited Marxist approaches to social reform and gave a range of deeper and sometimes sinister meanings to the deployment of the public health enterprise throughout the nineteenth century. Public health experts concerned themselves with groups rather than individuals – they enquired and portrayed the spread of diseases across society, rural and urban, the range of infectious and epidemic ailments afflicting developing societies (Hardy 1993; Aisenberg 1999; La Berge and Fowler 2002). As the introduction of this book points out, from the 1820s onwards, epidemiologists and public health statisticians converted what had been primarily a personal experience of ill health into a pattern of ill health – determined by factors such as housing, water supplies, wind and bad air (miasma), and later on, germs and contaminating agents which dominated the second half of the nineteenth century (Worboys 2000; on the agency of germs, see Latour 1988). The ambitions of statisticians were hubristic. Nothing would escape their observation: food consumption and its impact on localized diseases such as the deficiency induced ailments, for instance the disease caused by an over-reliance on maize in northern Italy (pellagra) (Mariani-Costantiniand 2007: 163–71), lack of fresh fruits at sea (scurvy) or salt in the Alps, as Jonathan Reinarz points out in the introduction (Droin 2005: 307–24).

Some diseases were redefined as evidence of cultural backwardness, such as Alpine cretinism, while others were evidence of modernity. Among the latter, 'railway spine' or fashionable ailments like kleptomania emerged in direct response to new ways of living and consuming (Harrington 2003; O'Brien 1983). Overcrowding and industrial slums were represented as breeding grounds for disease and as evidence of the need for systemic reform – primarily through changes of circumstances and the provision of clean water, food and air; but also through matching reformed behaviour through the inculcation of discipline, hygienic attitudes, washing, compartmentalized spaces for bodily functions and physical distance between the sexes. Alain Corbin showed how the stench of the urban environment came to signify profound obstacles to progress (Corbin 1986). This rhetoric of a diseased social body could take many forms and have many objects, from the health of the elderly to the feeding of infants, but it implied – rhetorically if not in action – authoritarian interventions and coercion. The paradox of this moralizing disciplinarian perspective on disease (which began by reproving prostitution and alcohol, but also later smoking, fatty food, inactivity, masturbation and a wide range of widely indulged pastimes) was that it took place in an era of increased democratization.

Politically most European or American societies paid at least lip service to male representation and suffrage from the 1840s onwards, with some societies introducing female suffrage towards the end of the century. Mutual societies and trade unions blossomed across urban societies, to the point of becoming emblematic of the health of civic life. Many social organizations and charities were concerned with diseases, their prevention and their cure. Visitors and new social sciences, from the mid-century onwards, shaped a perception of the healthy body as Mary Poovey argued (Poovey 1995). Slum narratives of depravity and squalor became a genre in itself and all emphasized the abnormal, the deficient and the diseased as Seth Koven showed (Koven 2006).

The paradox of such fervent denunciation was of course that the range of solutions always paled in comparison with the brutality of the diagnostic. The diseased social body was intractable. There were a few mythologized interventions, such as Snow's removal of the handle of a contaminated water pump, but few quick fixes could be applied when it came to cultural approaches to the body and health. When solutions existed, for instance the preventative vaccination against smallpox – one of very few genuine protective measures available in the early nineteenth-century medical arsenal – they faced bewildering resistance. This resistance is echoed today in the violent attacks against vaccinators attempting to eradicate polio in Africa and Parkistan. As Nadia Durbach has shown, resistance to vaccination reflected profound anxieties about power relations over the body and a widespread desire to remain in control. Anti-vaccinators connected their resistance to a hegemonic medical discourse and the struggle against slavery for instance (Durbach 2004: 83). Much of these anxieties were absolutely rational and reflected genuine and well-grounded fears that, as governmentality theorists would argue, public health was about the protection of society rather than individual welfare. Other regulatory attempts at managing the spread of diseases were nakedly exposing forms of systemic violence. The regulation of prostitution enshrined, often at a municipal level, gender and class inequality in the name of the control of illnesses.[11] In countries where the debate was most vociferous, opponents of medically sanctioned policing or the broader notion of medical police denounced how one disease or another could become the cover for exploitation and authoritarianism.

The deployment of diseases to justify policies of social and cultural segregation was often most stark in social contexts lacking strong organized opposition. The colonial context in this respect proved a particularly obvious field of experimentation, as Warwick Anderson clearly demonstrated in relation to US experiments in the Philippines (Anderson 2006). The empire could become a space in which the regulation of 'contagious diseases' (read STD) could be fostered even though similar legislation had been abolished in the metropole of the British Empire (Levine 2003). Following from the pioneering work of Frantz Fanon (1952), who noted how colonial psychiatry enshrined racial difference through a multitude of segregated diagnostics (Keller 2008; Keller 2001), historians of empire have, fifty years hence, engaged in a thorough deconstruction of medical practices in the imperial domain. Medical research and Pasteur institutes could promote aggressive campaigns against all forms of diseases and challenge the local cultures which had tolerated them (Laberge 1987: 274; Vaughan 1991; Arnold 1993; Petitjean, Jami and Moulin 1992).

While much of the colonial world remained under some form of militarized control (directly through occupying armies or through authoritarian forms of indirect rule), public health policies could be applied authoritatively rather than through convoluted political negotiations. Health policies could affect the design of colonial cities, keeping bad air and natives away from the white settlers, shaping unequal health provisions and segregating colonial subjects from their masters in the name of health (Deacon 1996). High mortality rates among the colonists justified these policies, which played a significant role in shaping racialized medical discourses. It was a paradox that the conquerors should prove so inept at staying alive in new climates (Arnold 1996; Anderson 1997; Crozier 2007; Curtin 1989). The climates themselves were blamed for the toll they extracted from colonial staff. Debilitating and morbid, they were deleterious to the European frame and revealed an unsuspected weakness in their constitution. Some empires resolved the issue by allowing or even encouraging the development of racial cross-breeding – along the lines advocated by the French governor of Senegal Louis Faidherbe in the 1850s (H. Jones 2005: 27–48) – but most of the colonial regimes which advocated a 'modern' approach to their empire ended up segregating intensely and policing the racial divide with great energy (Acevedo-Garcia 2000; Njoh 2008).[12]

The development of racial ideology was not only an export commodity. It had applied domestically to class and as Louis Chevalier showed for France, or as many others have shown in relation to migrant groups in Europe and

America, the newcomers or the less settled became closely associated with
diseases and racial specific traits favouring the spread of diseases (Chevalier
1958). The Irish in the Anglo-American world, the Poles in Germany and, as a
rule, any poor and culturally ill-integrated group became the bearers of diseases,
social as well as moral ailments (Maglen 2005: 80–99). As Nyan Shah shows in
relation to Chinatowns in San Francisco, diseases were essential ingredients in
the negative portrayal of new immigrant groups (Shah 2001). Of course, all
discourses and cultural representations based on diseases and bio-risk were
contestable and contested. Throughout the nineteenth century, a wide range of
campaigns and lobbies attempted to demonstrate the logical errors at the heart
of any swift generalization. Interestingly, many of these campaigns took an
international form in the second half of the nineteenth century. This evolution
reflected the fact that major public health debates on a variety of issues from
alcohol to sexually transmitted diseases were now the object of international
exchanges of information and practices (Sakula 1982: 183–90; Packard and
Brown 1997: 181–94; Harrison 2006: 197).

DISEASES AND THE GLOBAL

The dissemination of information on diseases and their risks took several forms.
Towards the end of our period, from the 1880s until 1920, actuaries and
insurance providers were keenest in the pursuit of data that would enable them
to establish with a degree of certainty the exposure of their funds and those of
mutual societies. Any financial institution claiming to offer some financial
protection to the sick and disabled had to understand in great detail the nature
of the risk (the odds of granting cover) and exposure (the likely duration of the
financial loss) they might entail. Diseases became economic agents in their own
right and actuaries had to understand them on a rather different basis than
statisticians of the earlier period. While individuals had increasingly insured
themselves against inevitable expenditure (funeral insurance), they had also
increasingly bought into health insurance which might cover some of the costs
of more expensive treatments or disability. From the 1870s onwards, states had
themselves invested in safety nets of variable elasticity and robustness to provide
for paupers in the first instance and more universal coverage by the 1920s.
Many of these initiatives were provided in a context of international exchanges
and networking. While historians have paid most attention to the scientific
networks themselves – focusing typically on the transmission of ideas and the
dissemination of practices – they have paid less attention to the financial
technologies which underwrote medical provisions. The international gathering
that took place in San Francisco in 1914, 'a city built on insurance' following
its destruction by earthquake and fire in 1906, attempted to pool a wide range
of help societies, rescuers and epidemiologists – all people whose work would

feed a world of insurance solidarity grounded in the knowledge of diseases.[13] Mass organizations devoted to first aid and health prevention, as well as wartime relief, could develop their mandate in relation to civil and industrial accidents and define them afresh as global humanitarian concerns.[14] Building on fifty years of social redefining of diseases as 'social diseases', humanitarian actors such as the Saint John Ambulance or the Red Cross movement could embrace 'social prevention' (prévoyance sociale) as a humanitarian pursuit and join in global gatherings mixing policymakers, insurance brokers and health providers.

The internationalization of these networks of insurance provision and response to a variety of risk (among which diseases were not necessarily the dominant ones) built on a century of globalization in which epidemics and pandemics had played a considerable part. Even arch imperialists understood that global reach entailed a global understanding of disease that challenged stable categories of foreign (tropical) and domestic concerns. Colonial empires had built a system of exchange which traded goods, people and diseases. Some diseases proved more apt at crossing cultural and geographical divides and were the object of surveillance and fears, as shown by Alan Kraut (1995). Diseases became emblematic of the fears of miscegenation – contamination became a way for racists to highlight the dangers presented by different groups to their own community. Yet, contrary to widespread fears, northern ailments travelled more readily than southern ones which could not thrive in the wrong climate. Traditional methods to fend off new arrivals like quarantine were ill suited to a trading culture reliant on speedier travel. William Coleman showed well how the sudden but short-lived incursion of yellow fever in the north gave rise to contrasting methods of containment in France and Wales (Coleman 1987). Others, on the contrary, benefited greatly from the new exchange networks empires and trade routes created. The great pandemic of cholera, a water borne disease, thus logically followed the water routes across Europe all the way from India via Russia between 1829 and 1837. As Evans and Rosenberg note, the reporting of the disease's journey built up an expectation of its ineluctable march which no quarantine proved able to block (Evans 1988; Rosenberg 1966). The international reporting of the progress of new diseases or the recurrence of ancient nightmares such as the plague (unseen in Western Europe since 1720, but chronic in the French colonial empire or in the Middle East) occupied some important cultural space – it was a regular feature in the press and in travel narratives. The global recurrence of the disease in 1850 and 1866 only added to its status. If the first response to the epidemic in the 1830s had included a day of public atonement in the United Kingdom, the correlation between the disease and water made it an indicator of the quality of infrastructure and of the need for public health reforms (Hamlin 1998).

The great pandemics of the nineteenth century were thus spectacles in their own right – and cholera in particular had considerable echoes in a wide range of cultural media. It gave some phrases to various languages – in French a 'peur bleue' refers directly to the blueish tinge of cyanosis at the last stage of cholera, while choleric referred to the excess of bile associated with the disease. Debates on free trade and quarantines agitated commercial and medical circles throughout the period. To understand diseases as the inevitable corollary of free trade was to recognize a fact and to balance the benefits brought about by the international trade in commodities, including foodstuffs, with the dangers epidemics might represent.

If major colonial powers rejected any prolonged quarantine, they nevertheless imposed controls and restrictions on their imperial subjects' travels. In particular, the great Hajj and pilgrimages in general presented acute risks of mingling diseases from the entire world in one site and all became the object of strict epidemiological observation and control (Harrison 1992; Low 2008: 269–90). Though empires were built around notions of circulation and exchanges – at least within them – imperial powers feared the horizontal flows which might spread ailments and ideas around the world. Tropical diseases became an object of investment and enquiry, with Pasteurian medicine taking a keen interest in the various cycles at the heart of malaria – by then a declining disease in Europe – and new diseases such as sleeping sickness, which the colonial powers encountered in West and Central Africa. The former was identified and some of its ecology became more clearly associated with the mosquito as the vector and stagnant waters as the breeding ground for the parasite. Sleeping sickness was also clearly associated with a parasite which thrived on animals and humans living near waterways (Lyons 2002). If Europeans were unequal in addressing the personal risks presented by malaria, they all tended to engage with major developments of the spaces in which they worked and lived. For sleeping sickness, the matter was more complex, and as the historiography has shown, its prevention and treatment were contrary to development and irrigation policies promoted by colonial authorities (Osborn 2004).

Diseases of development could thus have complex relationships also found in Western work culture. One cannot overestimate the beneficial impact of modernity on health. Industrial processes worldwide revealed 'new' 'industrial' diseases which from 'phossy jaw' for matchmakers working with phosphorous material (Harrison 1995) to the miner's silicosis were recognizable conditions provoked by working conditions. Some of these diseases were gendered like 'phossy jaw', which affected women workers, while others were deemed necessary attributes of dangerous trades as pointed out by Peter Bartrip and Sandra Burman (Bartrip and Burman 1983). As 'soldiers of industry', workers faced dangers like soldiers in war and with the same fatalism. Workers' diseases affected the artisan hatter using mercury in their effort to shape beaver fur into hats or anyone using heavy metal based paint in the workplace (Hamilton 1908: 655–8). As the US statistician Frederick Hoffman pointed out in 1909:

The common-law doctrine of the complete assumption of industrial risk by the workmen employed in more or less dangerous trades, excepting gross negligence on the part of the employer, is no longer tenable, and gradually a policy of labor protection is being perfected, which, in addition to a more or less clearly defined employers' liability, includes community responsibility for the social consequences of industrial accidents and industrial diseases.

—Hoffman 1909: 567

Hoffman then proceeded to describing the range of diseases affecting a variety of trades and the statistical proportion of death by consumption among workers in particularly dusty trades like weaving (50%) or instrument making (56%) (Hoffman 1909: 573). Such rates of disease in the productive force of the nation represented, according to Hobson, one of the major liberal economists of the era, an unsustainable drain on national resources and made no economic sense. Within the era of international trade and exchanges, diseases represented a significant financial and social liability not only for the employers – increasingly at risk of prosecution for negligence – but for the nation at large. Hoffman, like many of his contemporaries, argued that preventable diseases would ultimately greatly diminish: 'a considerable proportion consists of diseases and deaths which, in their nature, are more or less preventable. In fact, it is not going too far to say that the causes responsible for industrial diseases are much more subject to control and gradual elimination than the causes and conditions responsible for industrial accident' (Hoffman 1909: 573). A culture of risk-taking was, he argued, about to be transformed.

Workers themselves were aware of the significant risk of disease they faced in their chosen trade, but the terms of that choice were often restricted to the point of not being a choice at all. When various mines directly recruited their workers from the schools of mining communities, they offered terms in which lung diseases and death by suffocation did not feature heavily. Though most of the young men recruited would have encountered someone barely able to breathe as a result of silicosis, they were not in a position to reject offers of employment. Mining was not merely a high-risk form of employment; it was a holistic cultural environment from which it was difficult to escape. Key analysts of industrial diseases followed the path of Florence Nightingale when they analysed exposure to preventable illnesses as negligence. Like Nightingale, they challenged assumptions that some losses were 'natural' and could not be alleviated through better care or preventative measures.

Cultural intolerance to risk was broader and also targeted products of mass consumption such as alcohol and tobacco. Though an element of choice was undoubtedly the focal point of various temperance campaigns, often under religious leadership, much of the argument was that the industrial circumstances of the modern world shaped consuming patterns and the ineluctable diseases that ensued. Alcoholism (coined as dipsomania in 1819 and alcoholism in 1849; Holt 2006; Sournia 1990) became a disease of civilization itself – which, combined with other acquired hereditary traits, could threaten the fabric of society (Müller-Wille and Hans-JörgRheinberger 2012).

The historiography of eugenics has long focused on the development of theories of heredity and on the relationship between theories of evolution inspired by Lamarck and Darwin and new concerns for racial purity (Adams 1990). The Eugenic Society created in the UK by Charles Darwin's cousin Francis Galton may have been at best a small focus group of highly privileged individuals, but it nevertheless articulated common concerns arising from an increasingly globalized competitive environment. The idea of race related directly to prevalent diseases across society. With the rise of new humanitarian organizations such as the Red Cross, tuberculosis became naturally a concern of humanitarians in peacetime. They could project onto the disease the same rhetoric of mobilization that they would later employ in wartime. The American Red Cross thus resourced in 1908 the 'struggle against tuberculosis' through thirty-two sanatoria – ten in the state of New York alone. This global effort against what the Red Cross called a 'social disease' was matched by the Swedish Red Cross in 1881, Hungary (1895), Germany (1896), Belgium (1908), Greece (1909), Spain (1912), Japan (1914) and Romania (1919). A matching effort was devoted to a communication campaign aimed at prevention. In Austria, the Red Cross could project the same rhetoric against alcoholism and anaemia in 1897, while the Italians identified malaria as a key 'humanitarian' target from 1899.[15] Other diseases such as smallpox, typhoid and diphtheria were the object of shorter-term campaigns as and when epidemics occurred (1879, 1883, 1884, 1896 for diphtheria in Russia for instance; for typhoid, 1881 in France, 1889 and 1896 in Denmark, 1903 in Spain and 1908 in Uruguay).[16]

The notions of diseases of civilization was not one that affected only the working class: ideas of degeneracy could be deployed at both ends of the social spectrum. Literary scholars have thus echoed the fin de siècle spirit which found its best embodiment in the ambiguous writings of Joris-Karl Huysmans. Huysmans' work *Against Nature* (*à rebours*) belongs to a category of literature that pushed the boundaries of acceptable representation. Within the text, Huysmans placed considerable emphasis on the role of disease – in particular syphilis (Szreter 2014) – imprinting itself on civilization in a hallucinatory pattern of decline and corruption. The disease acquired agency:

'All is syphilis,' thought Des Esseintes, his eye riveted upon the horrible streaked stainings of the Caladium plants caressed by a ray of light. And he beheld a sudden vision of humanity consumed through the centuries by the virus of this disease. Since the world's beginnings, every single creature had, from sire to son, transmitted the imperishable heritage, the eternal malady which has ravaged man's ancestors and whose effects are visible even in the bones of old fossils that have been exhumed. The disease had swept on through the centuries gaining momentum. It even raged today, concealed in obscure sufferings, dissimulated under symptoms of headaches and bronchitis, hysterics and gout. It crept to the surface from time to time, preferably attacking the ill-nourished and the poverty stricken, spotting faces with gold pieces, ironically decorating the faces of poor wretches, stamping the mark of money on their skins to aggravate their unhappiness.

—Huysmans: 1884, Ch 8

Huysmans echoed contemporary metaphors that diseases might possess a kind of destructive willpower and grow throughout civilization. Wider cultural concerns with the decline and fall of empires were largely a product of a tradition of historical writing on a grand scale. From Henry Thomas Buckle's study of civilization in England in 1857 to major comparative history projects, such as Arthur de Gobineau's racial theory (Boissel 1993), intellectuals chartered the course of cultures and that of the diseases which brought about their downfall (Crook, Gill and Taithe 2011). In this politico-historical register, ideas themselves could feature as diseases of civilization. Collective psychology developed in the late nineteenth century by Gustave LeBon and echoed later in Freud's psychoanalysis medicalized some of the political concepts which had been applied to describe revolutionary fervour (Freud 1921). For instance, the revolutionary spirit of the Commune of Paris in 1871 was regularly assigned to a form of obsidional fever ensuing from the harsh conditions of the siege during the Franco-Prussian War (du Camp 1878–80; Legrand du Saule 1896; Lidsky 1982). Metaphorical uses of disease in political discourse entailed swift and simplistic answers such as quarantine or radical treatment. The mass murder of communards was thus a 'purge', while racists and anti-Semites from 1900 onwards used disease metaphors to invoke radical action. The cultural meanings of diseases had developed a life of their own and they fuelled discrimination and removal of minorities from public life.[17] By the early twentieth century, global order diseases of the modern environment, decline of the race and even the spread of germs of revolutions could all become pandemic and apocalyptic.

CONCLUSION

By the outbreak of the First World War, discourses making heavy stock of disease metaphors evoked the regenerative and purgative potential of violence in class or national war, but the cultural hopes raised by such a purge were dashed in the bloodletting. In the post-war order, international approaches to diseases appeared to triumph. Debates at the League of Nations, international and national mobilization and humanitarian work included wars on diseases and the restraints on actual war, compensating pacifism in the political sphere with militancy in the struggle against diseases. Diseases no longer belonged to the individual sufferers and their carer-takers, they were the object of national and international initiatives. The aftermath of the war itself revealed large-scale suffering in Eastern and Central Europe, the Middle East and Russia. The end of the war had been combined with the largest influenza epidemic recorded in history in 1918 (Johnson and Mueller 2002; Phillips 2014), an epidemic that still haunts public health discourses today – each flu episode raising the prospect of a return of the virus which allegedly killed as many people as the war had done. Arguably the recent response to COVID-19 in the West has paid too much attention to this ill-fitting historical precedent (Javelle and Raoult 2020). Yet in contrast to the visit of Napoleon to his sick soldiers, diseases in 1918 no longer called for *mise en scène* for propagandistic purposes. There are no widely circulated images of Douglas Haig or Philippe Pétain visiting the influenza wards, and no paintings of the politicians of 1918 touching those sufferers adorn the Louvre today.[18] By 1920, there was no longer much cultural and political stock to be made from an individual facing modern plagues in person (Honigsbaum 2016).

NOTES

1. This article was written during a residence in 2017 at the Fondation Brocher, Geneva, which must be thanked for the ideal working conditions it offers.
2. http://www.louvre.fr/oeuvre-notices/bonaparte-visitant-les-pestiferes-de-jaffa-le-11-mars-1799.
3. This is of course a very contested definition of health, challenged from 1948 by the World Health Organization and revised in more positive terms by WHO in its Ottawa charter of 1986 (Huber, van Vliet, Giezenberg et al. 2016).
4. See for instance the debates on eczema which was defined by the absence of obvious causes (Freeman 1900: 398–401). Freeman, a skin specialist from the Reading dispensary, tended towards an unknown external cause rather than accept that the body might generate the disease spontaneously in certain circumstances.
5. Cholera recurred throughout our period in more regional outbreaks, for instance in 1881 in southern France; in 1883 in Egypt, Greece and Russia; in 1884–5 in France and Spain; in 1892 in Hungary in 1894 in Russia; in 1896 in Austria; in 1910 in Austria, Spain, Italy and Russia; in 1911 in the USA and Lybia in 1913 in Romania; and in 1918 in the USA and Palestine. This list is not exhaustive and reflects internationally significant responses. Archives du Comité International de la Croix Rouge (henceforth CICR), A, CR 103-1, *L'oeuvre de la croix rouge en temps de paix* ; Delaporte 1986.
6. Excrements also served as metaphors for social diseases. See Corbin 1986: 209–19.
7. The classic denunciation of medical diseases was produced by Ivan Illich, under the title 'Medical Nemesis', in 1974.
8. Virginia Woolf's *A Room of One's Own*, published in 1929, built on this tradition of literary uses of domestic surroundings.

9. As Woloshyn argues, sunbathing goes further back than the historiography had previously suggested.

10. Thomas Mann, *The Magic Mountain* (*Des Zoberberg*) was written between 1912 and 1924. Its impact has been reflected in the history of medicine ever since (Bryder 1988).

11. There is a prolific historiography on this topic, though it is clear that in France for instance the policy was first and foremost intended to contain prostitutes to an invisible margin of society and only later became primarily about health; in Britain it emerged as part of a health agenda (Walkowitz 1980; McHugh 1980; Mort 1987; Smith 2006: 197–215). For pioneering work on continental regulation, see Corbin 1996.

12. Njoh contrasts French (social) and British (medical) segregation policies to conclude on their hygienic convergence over time (588–9).

13. CICR, A, A, AF/24, 6 *Exposition de San Francisco*

14. CICR, A, CR 103-1, *L'œuvre de la Croix Rouge en temps de paix, prévoyance sociale.*

15. CICR, A, CR 103-1, *L'œuvre de la croix rouge en temps de paix.*

16. CICR, A, CR 103-1, *L'œuvre de la croix rouge en temps de paix, épidémies.*

17. See, for instance, the attributions of some ailments to specific groups as explored by Shelley Z. Reuter 2006.

18. Arguably one has to wait for princess Diana visiting AIDS patients to see a revival of the royal touch and its iconic power. Gill Valentine and Ruth Butler 1999.

CHAPTER FOUR

Animals

ABIGAIL WOODS

As illustrated in a sister volume to this work, *The Cultural History of Animals in the Age of Empire* (Kete 2007), the period 1800–1920 saw animals transformed physically, conceptually and in their lived relations with humans. In 1800, they were understood through the prism of natural theology as part of a nature perfectly designed and sanctioned by God, in which humans held an exalted place. Subsequently, evolutionary ideas devised most famously but not exclusively by Charles Darwin changed understandings of the kind and degree of difference between human and non-human animals, and attributed them to natural forces (Ritvo 1995; Farber 2000). Concurrently, the bodies of domesticated animals were reshaped by the rise of pedigree breeding as a fashionable pursuit (Ritvo 1987; Derry 2015), and their lives and health altered by changing husbandry practices (Beinart 2007; Woods 2016). Hunting animals became a popular recreation, particularly in the colonies where hunted populations were shrinking noticeably by 1900 (MacKenzie 1988). In the West, pet keeping expanded, and the predominantly rural societies in which humans had lived in close proximity with nature became more urbanized. City populations of horses and livestock first expanded to keep pace with inhabitants' demands for food and transport, and then declined, as horses were displaced by the internal combustion engine and livestock removed by environmental health campaigns (Atkins 2012). Zoological gardens were founded as symbols of imperial conquest and sites of scientific enquiry, public education and entertainment (Rothfels 2002; Baratay and Hardouin-Fugier 2002). They were supplied by an expanding body of collectors who scoured the colonies for animals that they sold also as dead specimens to private collectors and the growing number of natural history museums (Murray 2007). Most notably in

Britain, this period also witnessed the rise of humanitarian concern for animals that produced the first laws to prevent animal cruelty (Harrison 1973).

Meanwhile, as documented in this book, medicine underwent its own transformations. In 1800, it constituted a broad epistemological domain, incorporating a range of enlightened activities pursued also by polite society, such as botany, mathematics, philosophy, agriculture, natural history, farriery and comparative anatomy. Subsequently, it became a more specialized, bounded, vocational profession, with its own educational pathways, institutions and collective orientation (Brown 2011). Veterinary medicine and biology peeled off from human medicine and developed their own, not entirely distinct identities and trajectories (Pauly 1984: 369–97; Nyhart 2009; Woods 2017a). The boundaries between qualified and unqualified, orthodox and unorthodox healers hardened. Surgery elevated its status from that of manual craft. The development of 'hospital' medicine, 'laboratory' medicine and public health introduced new medical ideas, practices, cultures and careers, while imperial conquest provided new opportunities for medical research, practice and government service (Bynum 1994; Risse 1999; Crowther and Dupree 2007).

As a consequence of these shifts, the relationships between animals and medicine also changed (Kirk and Worboys 2011; Woods 2017b, 2017c). Existing literature suggests that during the age of empire they developed in three distinctive ways, as illustrated in Figures 4.1, 4.2 and 4.3. Figure 4.1 shows men standing helplessly on the South African veldt in 1890, surrounded by the bloated carcasses of cows killed by the highly fatal, contagious cattle plague or rinderpest. It represents 'veterinary medicine', or the *medicine of animals*. Historians portray this as an activity conducted by vets and lay animal healers who aimed to advance animal health as an end in itself. Cattle plague

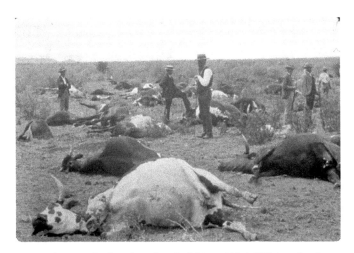

FIGURE 4.1: Rinderpest Outbreak in South Africa, 1896. Wikimedia Commons.

was a key stimulus and shaping force. Its devastating effects in eighteenth-century Western Europe influenced the creation and evolution of the first veterinary schools in Lyons, Alfort (Paris), Vienna, Dresden, Hanover, and London (Wilkinson 1992). Facilitated by colonial conquest, the liberalization of trade and the development of railways and steamships, cattle plague returned to Western Europe in the 1860s then swept through South Asia. Entering Ethiopia in 1888, it spread to southern Africa, causing transport and livestock economies to collapse, and depriving indigenous peoples of fuel, fertilizer, food, clothing, draft power and currency. National and colonial governments responded by attempting to control this and subsequently other major contagious animal diseases. Their interventions elevated veterinarians by awarding them roles as advisors and executors of policy, and establishing laboratories for their research (Woods 2016).

Figure 4.2 is an 1832 painting of a writhing dog, straining helplessly at the ropes that bind it to a table while a group of unconcerned men witness its vivisection. It represents animal experimentation, an activity which many historians regard as synonymous with the history of *animals in medicine*. Although animal experiments had a long history, they were performed more frequently as

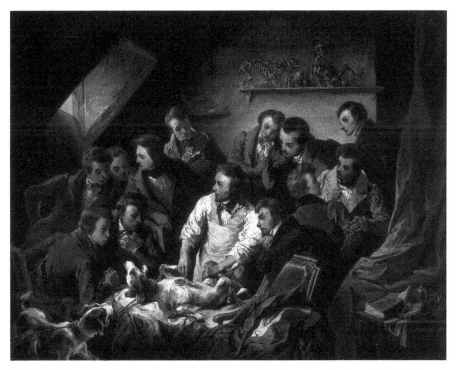

FIGURE 4.2: *A Physiological Demonstration with Vivisection of a Dog*, 1832. Oil Painting by Emile-Edouard Mouchy. Wellcome Collection.b

the nineteenth century progressed, with medical scientists in Germany and France leading the way. Dogs, monkeys and rodents were particularly common subjects. Operating as proxies or models for the human body, they contributed to the development of experimental physiology – which aimed to work out bodily functions – and bacteriology, which sought to identify the microbial causes of disease and develop protective vaccines and sera. Their use was associated with the wider adoption of experimentation as a dominant 'way of knowing' in science and medicine, and was pursued within universities and dedicated medical research institutions which were invested with national pride. Usually justified in terms of the human health benefits that would follow, animal experiments provoked considerable controversy, particularly in Britain where concerns about the motives of experimenters and the cruelty inflicted resulted in the regulation of experiments under the 1876 Cruelty to Animals Act (French 1975; Rupke 1990; Bynum 1990; Guerrini 2003; Franco 2013; Pickstone 2000).

Figure 4.3 depicts Louis Pasteur vaccinating a sheep donated by local farmers in the small French village of Pouilly-le-Fort in 1881. It represents the coming together of *animals in medicine* and the *medicine of animals* in the investigation and management of diseases that transmitted across the species divide. Pasteur was conducting a public trial of his new anthrax vaccine, which he had developed in response to the discovery that the diseases known in humans as 'malignant pustule' (a skin disease) and 'Woolsorters disease' (a frequently fatal respiratory condition of wool workers) had the same bacterial cause as anthrax, which led to sudden death in livestock. Commercialized and sold around the globe, the vaccine proved extremely effective in protecting cattle and sheep from infection, so preventing disease spread to humans (Latour 1988; Cassier 2005; Jones 2010). Anthrax was just one of several diseases (now known as zoonoses) that were identified in the late nineteenth century as transmissible between animals and humans (Woods 2016). Typically explored within histories of public health, their incidence was increasing owing to expansions in the livestock trade, meat and milk consumption, horse transport and pet-keeping. Vaccines offered one solution, which Pasteur applied also to rabies. Others included state-led sanitary controls over meat and milk, and the diagnostic testing of animals followed by the slaughter or quarantine of those infected. The development and application of these controls involved vets, public health doctors and medical scientists like Pasteur. At intervals, controversies broke out between them over the nature of disease, responses to it, priority for scientific discoveries, and the respective jurisdictions of medical and veterinary experts (Waddington 2003; Jones 2003; Lee 2008; Mitsuda 2017; Haalboom 2017).

While these three types of relationship between animals and medicine certainly existed historically, their elevation and representation in existing literature is not a straightforward reflection of the past, but it is mediated by historians' priorities and perspectives, which have skewed understandings of

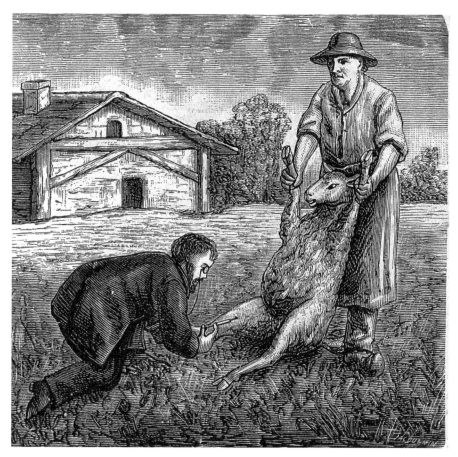

FIGURE 4.3: Pasteur Inoculating a Sheep against Anthrax, 1883. Wellcome Collection.

the subject in important but largely unrecognized ways. Existing narratives focus particularly on developments in Western Europe during the last third of the nineteenth century. These have attracted scholarly attention on account of their perceived significance for the development of modern medicine, or their status as precedents to present-day concerns surrounding animal experimentation and the global resurgence of animal plagues and zoonotic diseases. The relationships between animals and medicine in other parts of the globe and during the earlier age of empire are relatively neglected, as are knowledge-practices that were important at the time but have no obvious present-day equivalent.

A second problem with existing narratives is their tripartite framing of the subject, which follows an outdated disciplinary tradition in which 'it is automatically assumed that a "historian of medicine" is a person who works on the history of *human medicine*' (Porter 1993: 19). This approach positions animals as relevant to medical history only because of their impacts upon human health. Animals whose health was perceived as a problem in its own right are typically located within the parallel field of veterinary history, and those suffering from zoonotic diseases at the intersection of these domains. Implicit in this compartmentalization is a mapping of the professions: *animals in medicine* were the concern of doctors; the *medicine of animals* fell to veterinarians, while zoonoses constituted a site of inter-professional collaboration and conflict. However, analysis of original historical source materials shows that while such distinctions may have applied in certain times and places, in others they did not. Historians' adherence to them has therefore resulted in a somewhat ahistorical and anthropocentric perspective on the evolving relationships between animals and medicine.

In tackling these methodological weaknesses, the remainder of this chapter presents fresh insights into what constituted 'animal medicine' in the age of empire. Departing from the standard historical practice of taking pre-defined medical problems, people or institutions as the starting point of enquiry, it turns instead to the animal subjects of medicine. Historians of animals have pointed out that, as non-verbal creatures, animals leave no texts. Nevertheless, it is possible to access embodied traces of their past lives (Benson 2011). These exist in the verbal descriptions and engravings of animals that feature in medical textbooks and journals, in statistical accounts of their diseases contained within institutional and government records, and in the material specimens of their bodies that were preserved and displayed within medical museums. Exploring the nature of these embodied traces and the circumstances of their creation provides a new perspective on the places, purposes, subjects and investigators of animal medicine. Departing quite substantially from the story outlined above, it reveals the richly zoological nature of human medicine, its interpenetration with veterinary medicine and the importance of non-experimental modes of medical enquiry into animals (Woods et al. 2017).

Owing to the novelty of this approach and the variable extent to which animal traces were created and preserved, it is currently not possible to offer a broad international account of this 'animal medicine'. Although this chapter extends the chronological frame back to the early age of empire, its findings relate particularly to Britain, the subject of the author's own research. Developments in other countries are touched upon, but merit more dedicated attention from future scholars. It begins by describing the interlinked histories of human and veterinary medicine, locating them within a wider tradition of medical enquiry into animal bodies and diseases. It identifies key sites – including the veterinary schools – in which doctors pursued these enquiries. The second section explores the ideas and practices of this 'animal medicine' and the language used to describe it. It reveals the importance of observing animals in life, dissecting them after death, and reasoning by analogy. The final section draws on these insights to reveal how, in encouraging doctors to think about and investigate disease as a cross-species phenomenon, this long-standing zoological tradition shaped late nineteenth-century experimental medicine, public health and veterinary–medical relationships (an observation made in passing but unfortunately not developed by two seminal articles on the history of human/animal health: Bynum 1990; Hardy 2003).

THE PLACE AND PERSONNEL OF 'ANIMAL MEDICINE'

Animals as medical subjects long predated the age of empire. However, they became increasingly important from the later eighteenth century, and especially to surgeons, who viewed the investigation of animal bodies and diseases as a means of elevating their personal and professional status. In Britain, a number of these men worked to refashion farriery from an empirical practice into a polite, gentlemanly art, and to found schools and infirmaries for the purpose. Many others engaged with animals via natural history, which was a popular gentlemanly pursuit, took up comparative anatomy, which was a cutting edge mode of enquiry, and continued the long-standing tradition of experimenting upon animals. Inspired by physiocratic ideas in France and gentlemanly agricultural improvement in Britain, they also turned their attention to cattle plague and other animal diseases. On account of these interests, certain medical men came to play important roles as founders, teachers and pupils in the early veterinary schools, which were established across Western Europe in the late eighteenth century. Historians have tended to interpret their participation as a necessary, but temporary, step along the road to an independent veterinary profession that would deliver much-needed improvements in animal health (Wilkinson 1992; Hannaway 1994; Hubscher 1999; Mitsuda 2017). However, recent research shows that the individuals concerned did not set out to create a new veterinary profession, but rather to promote and develop their existing interests in studying animal bodies and advancing animal health (MacKay 2009; Woods 2017a).

In France, the Alfort veterinary school was reshaped in the late eighteenth century as a site for research and education in a unified vision of human/animal medicine advanced by physician and professor of comparative anatomy, Vic D'Azyr, who led investigations into cattle plague on behalf of a French government commission (Hannaway 1977). Subsequently, Alfort became an important site for the development of early experimental physiology, not least because of its plentiful horse bodies. Francois Magendie carried out experiments there in the 1820s (Elliot 1990: 50–4). In Britain, medical men were well represented amongst the governors and vice-presidents of the London Veterinary College (LVC, est. 1791). For nearly forty years the school was directed by a surgeon, Edward Coleman, who was appointed on the strength of his comparative anatomical and experimental research on animals. Students attended medical lectures and read medical literature, and exams were conducted by a 'medical experimental committee' populated wholly by doctors. Surgeons and apothecaries were well represented among the early pupils (Woods 2017a).

The authority that medicine wielded over early veterinary medicine in Britain was acknowledged by influential veterinary commentator, Delebere Blaine. He described the latter as 'a branch that has sprung from, and must grow with medicine as its parent stock', in which historical advances had been achieved 'usually by the exertions of some enlightened physician or surgeon' (Blaine 1802: xii, viii). He recommended surgeons to attend the LVC because they had already 'travelled three fourths of the road towards making a good veterinarian' (Blaine: 107–11). His contemporary, the vet and surgeon, William Percivall, acknowledged that 'so much analogy is there throughout between the structure and economy of the horse and those of the human subject' that 'the theory of medicine in the human subject is the theory of medicine in the brute; it is the application of that theory – the practice alone that is different . . . the laws of the animal economy are the same in all' (Percivall 1823: xiii–xiv).

This notion of the unity of medicine began to break down in Britain during the 1820s and 1830s, as vets who had qualified from the London school and earned their living in veterinary practice began to group together and follow the example of medical and other social reformers in criticizing the established elites who controlled their institutions. They developed a new epistemology grounded in the practical experience of veterinary practice, which emphasized veterinary knowledge of the differences between species and contrasted it with medical tendencies to reason by analogy across them. After a long battle, they dislodged medical men from their powerful positions in the schools, and went on to create, by an 1844 Royal Charter, the Royal College of Veterinary Surgeons, a new regulatory body which still exists today. This event marked the formal establishment of veterinary medicine as a profession in Britain (Woods 2017a). However, it did not dispel medical interest or authority over animals. Later in the century, some of the first veterinary schools to be founded in North America forged close relationships with medical schools and were supported by significant medical figures, most famously William Osler at the Montreal Veterinary College (1874–84) and the School of Veterinary Medicine in Philadelphia (1884–9) (Smithcors 1959; Teigan 1983).

Veterinary schools were not the only institutions that fostered medical engagement with animals in the early age of empire. Zoological gardens were also significant. The most important at the turn of the nineteenth century was the menagerie of the Museum d'Histoire Naturelle in Paris run by Frederick Cuvier (Burkhardt 1999). Over the next few decades, other zoos were founded throughout Western Europe. A number of medical men built formal and informal relationships with them, and used their animal inhabitants to construct knowledge and professional reputations. They were attracted by the zoos' institutional commitments to studying comparative anatomy, the diversity of their animal holdings and the high rates of animal sickness and death – which produced plentiful opportunities for medical intervention in life and dissection after death. Other advantages included the absence of ethical concerns that surrounded human dissections, and the known conditions of animal existence which aided investigations into the identities and causes of their diseases (Hochadel n.d.; Baratay and Hardouin-Fugier 2002; Woods 2017d). As centres of animal population, farms offered similar advantages to zoos but, as they were not scientific institutions, it could be harder for medical men to win access and pursue their objectives. However, some doctors established their own farms, used those of friends or relatives, or built relationships with veterinary surgeons who facilitated their attendance (*Transactions of the Pathological Society of London* 1846–81). Another site for medical engagement with livestock opened up with the mid-century appointment in London of dedicated public health doctors, the Medical Officers of Health. Responsible for the sanitary condition of cities, they inspected urban dairies, slaughterhouses and butchers' shops in which live and dead animals were held. In France and Germany such activities were more commonly performed by veterinarians (Lee 2008; Atkins 2012; Mitsuda 2017).

Medical museums were also very important to the development of 'animal medicine'. In the late eighteenth and early nineteenth centuries, it was not unusual for wealthy doctors to amass very large, private collections of human and animal specimens which they used for research purposes and to teach comparative anatomy. Probably the most famous belonged to London surgeon John Hunter, whose comparative practices inspired future generations of medical men. When he died in 1799, his collection contained 13,682 specimens obtained from 500 different species, and was taken over by the Museum of the Royal College of Surgeons (Dobson 1962; Jacyna 1983). During the early to mid-nineteenth century, other private collections were acquired by medical schools for their expanding museums. As noted by Alberti, zoological specimens were well represented, because 'the boundaries between anatomist and naturalist, surgeon and veterinarian were permeable'. Later in the century, the emergence of pathology, biology and zoology as distinctive disciplines encouraged the removal of comparative anatomy specimens from medical museums. However, as shown below, pathological animal specimens continued to play a role (Alberti 2010: 57).

Outside of these institutions, much medical engagement with animals occurred in private spaces, where interested individuals conducted largely unpaid enquiries. These did not require specialist facilities or staff, and in a world full of animals there was no shortage of material. Doctors, their friends and families often owned horses, pets and livestock. Animals could also be obtained from zoos, farms and museums, while hunting, in serendipitous encounters on city streets, via veterinary surgeons and from patients and others who sought medical advice about sick animals. Doctors shared their findings via the meetings and publications of medical and zoological societies. Each year, several displayed specimens of diseased animals to members of the popular Pathological Society of London (PSL, est. 1846, which promoted the study of pathological anatomy) and published clinical case notes, post-mortem reports and lengthy expositions in its annual *Transactions*. These men came from all ranks of the mid-nineteenth-century British medical profession: elite London consultants, museum curators, grass roots general practitioners and corresponding members from the colonies. Some developed a special interest in animals, exhibiting them on numerous occasions and writing prolifically about their pathology. Many more presented animals just once or twice, but as the PSL permitted the exhibition of only interesting or unusual specimens, it seems likely that medical engagement with animal bodies was a widely distributed, if occasional practice. The records of other mid-nineteenth-century medical societies (for example, the Dublin, Birmingham, Sheffield and Reading Pathological Societies and the Odontological Society) indicate that they, too, discussed animals from time to time, and sometimes passed specimens on to medical museums for display. Vets were often mentioned as having supported these activities – in person, through the specimens contained in veterinary museums, or in their writings – but they rarely appeared in person at society meetings. Their involvement reveals the continuing overlap between medical and veterinary interests in diseased animals (*Transactions of the Odontological Society* 1856–89; Murray 1909).

WORKING ACROSS SPECIES

In their encounters with zoo animals, wildlife and domesticated animals, doctors applied knowledge of human health to the health of animals, used the study of animals to shed light on humans and compared and extrapolated across species to work out the relationships between them or the fundamental principles of life, death and disease. These activities drew strength from successive, overlapping scientific traditions that informed ideas about the relationships between humans and animals, God and his subjects, and the optimal organization of society. At the turn of the nineteenth century, natural theological ideas held sway. They were soon challenged by Lamarck's transformism, German naturphilosophie and the cell theory as developed by Schwann and elaborated by Virchow (who is widely quoted as stating that 'between humans and animal there is no dividing line', but the source of this quotation has not been identified). Subsequently, Charles Darwin's theory of evolution as expounded in *Origin of Species* (1859), *The Descent of Man* (1871) and *The Expression of the Emotions in Man and Animals* (1872) proved influential, as did Ernest Haeckel's evolutionary morphology and debates between Virchow and Weismann on the inheritance of acquired (pathological) characteristics (Churchill 1976; Jacyna 1984a, 1984b; Nyhart, 1995).

These traditions inspired some doctors to think about animal diseases in explicitly evolutionary terms. The notion that all species developed out of the same basic plan gave rise to suggestions in the 1830s and 1840s that malformations resulted from arrested development (Long 1841: 23–9), or that diseases themselves evolved along with the species affected by them. When signs of tuberculosis – then the biggest killer of humans – were reported in the bodies of various zoo animals, the *Lancet* editor asked, 'Is there a certain order in the series of diseases through which the human form passes, bearing some analogy with the gradual evolution of its organization? Do its morbid processes and productions, at various periods of its existence, correspond with those of a permanent and lower organization in the animal series?' (Editorial 1834: 147; Houston 1834: 285–6). Commenting upon the frequent deaths from tuberculosis of monkeys in captivity, John Simon, the Medical Officer of Health for London, observed in 1850 that with 'the dignity of standing next to man' came the 'inconvenience of this very human liability' (Simon 1850: 138). In such discussions, animals were not perceived as the threats to human health that they later became, but as fellow victims of disease.

Later in the century, this evolutionary perspective was updated and expanded by London surgeon John Bland Sutton, amongst others (for other iterations, see Williams 1888; Hutchinson 1892). As a prolific dissector of animals and humans, he believed that conditions regarded as pathological in one species might be natural in another (Bland Sutton 1890: 4), and that disease might actually be a product of evolutionary forces: 'The same laws which regulate physiology rule pathology . . . therefore the laws of evolution apply to pathology as well as to the ordinary events of animal life' (Bland Sutton 1886: 376). Bland Sutton's adherence to the widely held belief in the inheritance of acquired characteristics led him to conclude that disease could potentially drive evolution as pathologies passed on to the next generation could contribute to the differentiation of species (Bland Sutton 1885). He described the study of such matters as 'evolutionary pathology', 'zoological pathology' and 'general pathology in its fullest sense'. It was a branch of biology that could only be advanced by looking at disease in non-human species (Bland Sutton 1890: 12). Bland Sutton was influenced by Russian scientist Eli Metchnikoff, who applied a similarly comparative, evolutionary perspective to the study of embryos and subsequently, working under Louis Pasteur in Paris, to inflammation, resulting in his famous 'phagocytosis theory' of immunity (Tauber 1994). A different strand of evolutionary thinking can be detected in concurrent medical discussions on whether germs were similarly susceptible to the laws of evolution (Bynum 2002).

In emphasizing the proximity between humans and other animals, evolutionary theories reinforced existing medical tendencies to draw analogies between their bodies and diseases, and facilitated the application to animals of existing and emerging modes of medical practice, notably 'bedside medicine', 'hospital medicine', 'laboratory medicine', and 'public health' (Bynum 1994). In mid-nineteenth-century Britain it was not unusual for surgeons and occasionally physicians to treat animals as patients. Medical members of zoological societies performed surgical interventions on sick animals and instructed zookeepers on the treatment of their diseases (Woods 2017d). In rural areas where general practitioners were the main learned authorities on health, they were often consulted by animal owners, while in cities, the availability of vets did not stop animal owners from seeking medical advice. Reportedly, in 1830s London, doctors advertised openly for animal patients and interfered regularly with veterinarians' cases (Woods 2017a). They did not refer to this activity as 'veterinary medicine' or call themselves 'veterinary surgeons'. Consequently they were untroubled by the 1881 Veterinary Surgeons Act, which reserved this title for those with a veterinary qualification. Complaints about their treatment of sick animals continued to appear in British veterinary periodicals right up to the end of the age of empire.

The tendency to reason by analogy also informed medical investigations into animal diseases. The Pathological Society of London did not distinguish this activity from the study of human diseases. It was simply 'pathology', illustrated using 'specimens of the lower animals' (*Transactions of the Pathological Society of London* 1846–81). Some such specimens were incorporated into the 'general pathology' collections of medical museums and used to illustrate processes such as arthritis or fracture repair that occurred also in humans. Other attempts to shed light on human health through observing diseased animals in life and dissecting their bodies after death were referred to as 'comparative pathology'. During the later nineteenth century, this term was also used to describe the experimental investigation of infectious diseases using animals (Wilkinson 1992). To confuse matters further, vets sometimes applied it to their own investigations into animal diseases, which often involved no comparison and had no bearing on human health. For example, see the case reports published under the heading 'Comparative Pathology' by Youatt in 1836, or the contents of the *Journal of Comparative Pathology and Therapeutics* (est. 1888). Other forms of comparative enquiry were also posited. For example, during the 1870s, British asylum doctor Walter Lauder Lindsay used observations on animals to draw conclusions about diseases of the human mind, including suicide, while simultaneously studying asylum patients to understand the behaviour of animals (Ramsden and Wilson 2013). He documented his extensive observations in a 1,000-page work, *Mind in the Lower Animals: In Health and Disease* (1879), in which he called for the establishment of 'comparative psychology' as a scientific field (Finnegan 2008).

In focusing their attention upon the rise of experimental comparative pathology and the human health benefits that derived from it, historians have rather overlooked its pursuit through observation and dissection, which when applied to large numbers of animals began to resemble the 'hospital medicine' of humans. As noted above, this method was popular, easily accessible and widely distributed. It persisted alongside experimental comparative pathology and made its own significant contributions to human health through the study of spontaneously occurring diseases that were perceived to be analogous but not identical to those of humans. For example, in 1870s China, Patrick Manson – later known as the founder of tropical medicine – performed post-mortem examinations on dogs infected with the filarial worm in the hope of casting light on the parasite and its relationship to elephantiasis in humans. (He noted out that sudden death was not uncommon among dogs in China, and that medical practitioners were sometimes invited to examine them to determine whether they had been poisoned.) His findings led him to draw analogies between the worm and the malaria parasite, which informed his 1894 theory that the human-to-human transmission of malaria occurred via mosquito bites (Farley 1992; Li 2002). Another important advance derived from research into the nature and causes of rickets, performed by surgeon John Bland Sutton at London Zoo. Studying the disease in monkeys and carnivores led him to suspect a dietary cause, which he tested by adding cod liver oil to the diets of lion cubs. Its proven therapeutic and preventive benefits led the senior physician to the Great Ormond Street Hospital for Sick Children to declare the intervention 'a crucial one, and . . . conclusive as to the chief points in the aetiology of rickets' (Cheadle 1882). It informed the belief that rickets was caused by dietary deficiencies in fat and bone salts. This provided the jumping off point for Edward Mellanby's subsequent discovery that the key anti-rachitic component was a substance found in animal fat, later named fat-soluble vitamin D (Cassidy et al. 2017).

Reasoning by analogy was also embedded in the sanitary work of doctors, as pursued in the developing field of public health. In 1837, Dr Robert Harrison, Professor of Anatomy and Physiology at the Royal College of Surgeons in Ireland, stated that tuberculosis in captive monkeys was 'a sort of analogous experiment' that could extend and confirm knowledge of disease in humans. His investigations suggested that poor food and lack of exercise were to blame (Harrison 1837). Asylum doctor William Lauder Lindsay saw clear parallels between the disease in captive monkeys and in humans living in overcrowded dwellings, workhouses, barracks and asylums. Elsewhere, the zoo was compared to a factory whose lack of light and air rebounded on the health of its inhabitants (Lindsay 1878; Alexander 1879). Urban dairies were perceived in a similar light. Prior to their decimation by the 1865–7 cattle plague epidemic, these establishments supplied the majority of London's milk. Conditions were reportedly very poor, leading public health doctors to repeatedly highlight their capacity to undermine the health of animal inhabitants, neighbouring humans and milk consumers. According to Dr George Buchanan (1857),

> . . . cows live from one year's end to another with very insufficient exercise, and under artificial conditions of atmosphere and food . . . Never breathing the open atmosphere . . . but confined under densely-populated rooms, or even under-ground, without light, air, or drainage, fed on sour and decaying food, drinking water impregnated with their own excretions, the poor animals are a source of disease to the neighbourhood, they themselves lose their health, and cannot by possibility furnish a healthy milk.

Such views drove ongoing medical attempts to regulate and improve the dairies, which together with the growth of a railway trade in milk resulted in their almost complete removal from urban settings by the end of our period (Atkins 2012).

Until the later nineteenth century, outbreaks of animal epidemics (known as epizootics) were often attributed, like epidemic diseases in humans, to an 'epidemic constitution' of the atmosphere. Medical journals reported incidents in Britain and European nations where one followed the other, and suggested that by studying the rise and fall of epizootics, it was possible to learn something about epidemics in general and potentially predict their appearance in humans (Addison 1854; Lindsay 1854). The appearance of new epizootics during the 1840s and 1850s, such as foot and mouth disease and bovine pleuro-pneumonia, therefore attracted considerable medical attention. Later attributed to the spread of contagion via the rapidly expanding livestock trade, these diseases were suspected at the time to have arisen spontaneously due to atmospheric conditions. In 1851, the newly founded Epidemiological Society of London established an 'epizootic committee' jointly populated by vets and doctors who would work to investigate their causes for the benefit of human and animal health (Babington 1851).

The medical tendency to think zoologically about disease was evident also in their attempts to make sense of diseases that appeared to spread across the human–animal divide. Long before the development of germ theory, diseases such as rabies, glanders and smallpox were known to transmit in this way. In documenting the history of Edward Jenner's experiments, which showed that vaccination with cowpox lymph protected humans from smallpox infection, historians tend to omit the fact that Jenner (an enthusiast of natural history whose observations on the cuckoo won him the Fellowship of the Royal Society) believed that affected cows had originally been infected by horses. He also presented evidence to show that humans could be protected by the direct transfer of infection from horses (Baxby 1981). In 1847, when a pox-like disease appeared in newly imported sheep, two doctors followed Jenner's lead by using them to vaccinate 250 children against smallpox. Simultaneously, vets transferred infection between sheep in an attempt to generate immunity. All experiments failed (Simonds 1848; Budd 1863). Later in the century, in the context of discussions over the future of compulsory smallpox vaccination, the relationships between the various pox viruses provoked intense debate. While experimental evidence and reasoning by analogy led doctors to conclude that these were essentially the same virus that had been modified by the animal host, vets asserted that viruses were species specific (Baxby 1891), an argument that elevated their own professional knowledge of particular species over doctors' universalizing assumptions (Woods 2017a).

These myriad modes of medical engagement with animal diseases came together in responses to the 1865 outbreak of cattle plague in the London dairies. Already au fait with these institutions, public health doctors were among the first to raise the alarm, study the course of the disease, attribute it to insanitary conditions and query its implications for humans who consumed meat and milk from infected animals. The fact that cholera had appeared in humans just months before cattle plague broke out encouraged some doctors to cite atmospheric conditions as the causes of both. Working independently or on behalf of urban councils and farmers organizations, others turned to clinical practice to test out preventive or therapeutic medicines on cows (United Kingdom, Parliament 1866a, 1866b; Fisher 1993:61–9; Worboys 1991; Romano 1997). They also reported on the pathology of cattle plague. No fewer than eight accounts of the disease featured in the 1866 *Transactions of the Pathological Society of London* (*Transactions* 1866). William Budd, a Bristol doctor and early exponent of the theory that diseases were caused by specific, self-propagating agents, proposed that its pathological effects and contagious properties made it an 'exact counterpart' of human typhoid. He argued for its further investigation on account of 'the brilliant light which the demonstrable laws of this disease throw on the laws which govern the analogous diseases of our own species' (Budd 1865: 179; Pelling 1978). Further analogies were drawn between cattle plague and smallpox, which stimulated organized, high-profile but ultimately unsuccessful efforts to protect cows by vaccinating them against smallpox (Murchison 1865, 1866). Meanwhile, under the direction of a Royal Commission, some doctors performed experimental investigations into the nature and propagation of cattle plague which led them to suggest that living germs were the cause (United Kingdom, Parliament 1866c).

Eventually, cattle plague was eliminated from Britain through a policy of compulsory slaughter, quarantine and movement restrictions, as supported and effected by veterinarians. The success of this method confirmed rising suspicions that it was not generated spontaneously but spread through contagion. It established a new paradigm for the control of contagious animal diseases in Britain (Worboys 1991) and inspired influential doctors like James Young Simpson and Edgar Crookshank to make similar proposals (with quarantine in place of slaughter) for controlling human smallpox, in place of the government's unpopular policy of compulsory vaccination (Simpson 1868; Crookshank 1889). In their accounts of cattle plague, historians have tended to ignore or dismiss as misguided all medical responses to the disease except their experiments, which reportedly effected a 'sea change in British medical science' (Fisher 1993: 652). While in retrospect these experiments did contribute to the rise of germ theories and practices in Britain, it is important to remember that at the time they represented only one of many highly reputable modes of 'animal medicine'.

EXPERIMENTAL ANIMAL MEDICINE

Later in the nineteenth century, the long-standing zoological tradition within medicine and its interpenetration with veterinary medicine exerted important yet historically overlooked influences on the development of experimental pathology, research into zoonotic and other animal diseases, and the relationship between the medical and veterinary professions. During the 1880s, British public health and other doctors issued a host of reports of diphtheria-like illnesses in pigeons, fowls, pheasants, swine, horses and cats, which appeared to coincide with outbreaks of the disease in humans. It was suggested that the same bacterium might be responsible. After performing feeding and inoculation experiments, bacteriologist Emmanuel Klein claimed (mistakenly) to have isolated it, and proved that the disease in cats and cows was identical. Meanwhile, Medical Officers of Health presented evidence to show that scarlet fever and possibly typhoid could spread to humans via cow's milk. They suggested that the cows responsible for transmitting these diseases exhibited a mild ailment characterized by eruptions on the teats and udder, patchy hair loss and poor bodily condition. These findings provoked intense, wide-ranging concern amongst doctors and a robust denial from vets, who argued that the disease of cows was inconsequential and had no implications for human health (Local Government Board 1887; Brown 1888; Local Government Board 1889; Eyler 1986; Steere-Williams 2010). While in time, doctors abandoned their suspicions, this history shows that their late nineteenth-century conceptions of zoonotic diseases extended far beyond the handful of conditions (tuberculosis, anthrax and rabies) and species (cows, sheep and dogs) that feature in existing historical accounts.

The influence of zoological medicine can also be detected in how medical scientists engaged with animals within the laboratory. Historians tend to assume that their activities were oriented towards the production of animal models of human diseases which could be experimented upon as proxies for human bodies. In certain contexts this was the case, for example Haffkine's attempt's to devise a cholera vaccine (Löwy 1992). Elsewhere, however, scientists drew on elements of the older observational tradition of comparative pathology in approaching animals as subjects of naturally occurring diseases whose study could shed light on analogous diseases in humans, or the fundamental nature and laws of disease. For example, Pasteur worked out his ideas about germs through investigations into chicken cholera and swine erysipelas, which had no direct implications for human health. So, too, did the medical scientists who experimented on cattle plague in Britain (Bynum 1990; Worboys 1991). From the 1880s, British bacteriologist Edward Klein made extensive studies of sheep pox, swine fever and foot and mouth disease on behalf of the British government's Medical Department (Bulloch 1925). In colonial contexts, Robert Koch performed research on the tropical diseases of livestock which went on to inform his conception of the carrier state (Gradmann 2010).

The productiveness of such enquiries inspired national and colonial authorities, agricultural societies and leading landowners to seek medical aid when faced with animal diseases that threatened farming, international trade and colonial economies. In Britain, men like John Burdon Sanderson (Director of the Brown Institute of Comparative Pathology, London, who had performed experiments on the cattle plague (Romano 2002)), Thomas Cobbold (one of the most eminent parasitologists of the nineteenth century (Foster 1961)), Emmanuel Klein and David Hamilton (who held the first British university chair in pathology, at Aberdeen University (Obituary 1909)) were commissioned to investigate and ideally recommend ways of preventing diseases like contagious bovine pleuro-pneumonia, 'grouse disease' and the sheep diseases Louping Ill and braxy (Woods 2013, 2017e). In India, the devastating effects of cattle plague led the colonial authorities to summon Robert Koch (Mishra 2011), whose lack of success did not prevent his advice being sought again, with similar results, when the new cattle disease, East Coast Fever, broke out in South Africa in 1903 (Cranefield 1991). In 1884, the newly formed Bureau of Animal Industry in the USA appointed a doctor, Theobald Smith, to investigate livestock diseases. His work with the veterinarian, F. L. Kilbourne, established the principal of tick-borne infection, which was subsequently applied to human diseases (Méthot 2012). In fact many of the above diseases were suspected of having parasitic causes. Their investigation by men who were simultaneously engaged in the study of bacteria reveals (*contra* Farley 1992) considerable overlap in methods and concepts.

While Smith rejected any distinction between human and animal medicine, many vets were working actively to establish them. As shown above, in earlier years, vets had often quietly supported medical enquiries. However, as research gained more resources, and disease control became more embedded in the work of government, they became increasingly resentful of medical activities that overlapped with their own. Although professional confidence was rising, vets still possessed a lower status and scientific reputation than doctors, and consequently sometimes found themselves passed over or ignored in efforts to understand and manage animal diseases. One way in which British vets sought to counteract this situation was through echoing arguments made in the 1830s about the inadequacy of reasoning by analogy. Portraying medical men as theoretical and out of touch, they argued that animal diseases could only be understood through a deep familiarity with animals and their conditions of existence, which was the exclusive preserve of veterinarians (Woods 2013, 2017e).

CONCLUSION

This brief survey of 'animal medicine' reveals that although the identities and institutions of human and veterinary medicine began to follow separate trajectories from the 1830s, by the end of the century their boundaries remained highly permeable. Human doctors continued to intervene clinically in the health of animals and to study their diseases, not simply to shed light on human diseases, but also to advance animal health and understand the fundamental nature of disease. Early in the century, doctors worked *as* veterinarians, then in collaboration and subsequently in conflict with them. Although in practice this was not a linear transition but involved multilayered, overlapping ways of working, the overall direction of travel is sufficient to demonstrate the inadequacy of historians' tripartite framing of 'animal medicine', as described in this chapter's introduction. Contrary to the impression conveyed by existing literature, in this period there was no straightforward distinction between the *medicine of animals* and *animals in medicine*. Medical men pursued multiple activities that historians have tended to regard as 'veterinary' in character.

Moreover, this chapter has revealed that the history of *animals in medicine* is not what historians have taken it to be. While at times it did involve the much-documented practice of laboratory experiments upon animals that acted as stand-ins for human bodies, it was much more than that. There were many ways and many places in which doctors engaged with animals. Comparative, observation-based studies performed in sites ranging from zoos to museums to farms, private homes and urban dairies, were widely distributed and highly influential. Evolving over the century in line with changing understandings of disease and human–animal relationships, they established intimate associations between human and animal bodies that went on to inform the practice of experimental medicine and public health. Of course not all doctors participated in 'animal medicine', and of those that did, many (especially in the first half of the nineteenth century) were amateurs who acted without remuneration and in their spare time. Nevertheless, their activities are important in demonstrating the ways and extent to which human medicine was constituted by animals.

While originating from the study of embodied traces that historical animals left on the medical historical record, the account presented here is still a largely human story. It seeks to provide a broad overview of the shifting practices and parameters of animal medicine, rather than an in-depth consideration of how animals experienced, shaped and were shaped by it. However, their story is important, and is only just beginning to be told (Kirk and Pemberton 2013; Woods et al. 2017). Hopefully, by convincing scholars of the significance of animals to medicine, this chapter will encourage the development of more animal-centred histories of it. Future studies should also explore other national and transnational contexts, to show how the history of zoological medicine was shaped by different attitudes towards animals and ways of living with them, and by diverse intellectual and institutional medical trajectories.

The question of what happened to the zoological form of medicine described in this chapter also needs to be addressed. Certainly in Britain, its influence was waning by the end of the age of empire. The specialization, professionalization and institutional separation of medical from veterinary and agricultural research played a role, as did veterinary defensiveness and territoriality (Woods 2017e). Changes in human–animal relationships were key. The rich animal encounters that had characterized nineteenth-century life diminished as horses were replaced by mechanized transport, livestock disappeared from cities, natural history professionalized, urbanization progressed and hunted species were placed under protection. The disappearance of everyday animals made investigators more reliant on new types of animals that were materializing within laboratories. Drawn from a narrow range of species, these animals were selected, shaped and managed so as to produce model humans. No longer analogous but homologous to humans, their very animality became irrelevant to medicine, contributing to the rise of a more anthropocentric outlook which persists to this day (Churchill 1997; Logan 2002).

CHAPTER FIVE

Objects

ANNA MAERKER

INTRODUCTION

Objects took on new roles in the age of empire. In fantastical scenes imagined by artists such as George Cruikshank and J. J. Grandville, things came to life in ways both playful and uncanny, from anthropomorphic medicines and spools of thread metamorphosing into twirling ballerinas to the din of a mechanized steam orchestra and an animated gathering of empty clothes and hats (see Figure 5.1).

The advent of mass production made a new range of commodities available to ever larger communities of consumers; the expansion of global trade facilitated by imperial rule and expansions in infrastructure brought novel wares and materials to Europe. New materials, products and production processes were celebrated at industrial exhibitions. The flood of commodities was reflected in popular culture and communicated widely through the emerging mass media. In literary fiction, 'object biographies' told stories from the point of view of the thing itself. The genre began with early examples such as Charles Johnstone's *Chrysal; or, The Adventures of a Guinea* (1760), but came truly into its own in the long nineteenth century with works such as James Fennimore Cooper's serialized novel *Autobiography of a Pocket Handkerchief* (1843), which satirized the foibles of New York's high society. Charles Dickens's journal *Household Words*, in particular, celebrated and castigated the world of things with numerous articles on commodities, and their production, use and circulation (Waters 2008). The journal frequently made use of object biographical narratives. Harriet Martineau used the example of the humble button to reveal a world of sculptors, factory workers and child labourers, a

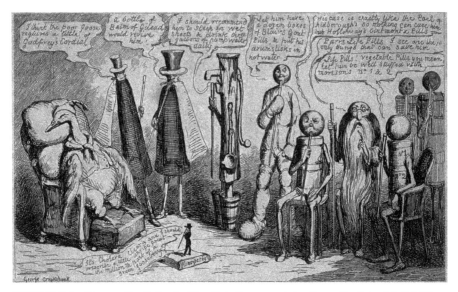

FIGURE 5.1: George Cruikshank, *The Sick Goose and the Council of Health* (1847). Wellcome Collection.

network of trades from Birmingham steel workers to Spitalfields silk weavers and Coventry fringe makers, and the shell divers of Singapore, Hawaii and Tahiti, on the other side of the world, snatching their livelihood from the jaws of circling sharks (Martineau 1852). Cheap print brought ever more stories and images of things into households; doctors and patients could now peruse the expanding range of available tools, instruments and prostheses through the emergent genre of the medical catalogue (Jones 2013; Sweet 2017). Thing stories were used by the medical profession to celebrate its exalted lineage. William MacMichael's *The Gold-Headed Cane* (1827) used the trope of the speaking object to tell the stories of eminent physicians – Radcliffe, Mead, Askew, Pitcairn, Baillie – who were the successive owners of the eponymous cane. In his narrative, the cane, fully conscious of its role as a 'relique' of the medical discipline, recalls its trajectory through the hands of celebrated practitioners as an opportunity to highlight medicine's progress and rising status (MacMichael 1827/1915: 1). Often dismissed as hagiographies, such texts may offer new interpretations for cultural histories of medicine.

The nineteenth-century fascination with objects did not just express itself in the creation of object-centred fictions. Increasingly, objects were theorized in their role for society, economy and education. Theorists of learning such as the influential Swiss reformer Johann Heinrich Pestalozzi advocated 'learning by head, hand and heart', stressing active physical engagement with objects as a central element of the learning process (Stadler 1988, 1993). In the nineteenth century, the medical museum became central to medical teaching, and the

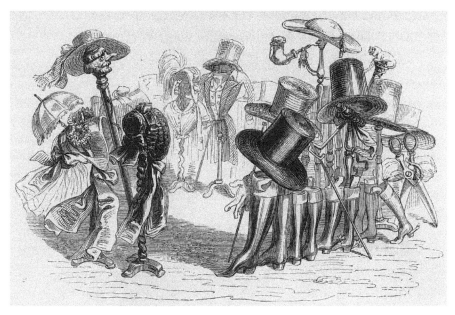

FIGURE 5.2: Grandville's animated garments. From J. J. Grandville, *Un autre monde* (Paris: Fournier, 1844), p. 71. Heidelberg University Library.

'object lesson' was a popular didactic approach for teaching children about natural and social worlds (Alberti 2011; Keene 2014). Just as Adam Smith had used pin-making as a paradigmatic case in his analysis of the market and its invisible laws, so influential didactic works like Elizabeth Mayo's *Lessons on Objects* (1863) used needles, whalebone and other household items to teach the children of the age of empire to perceive, describe and order the world (Mayo 1863). The role of things in society was addressed in an entertaining but no less serious way in Thomas Carlyle's satirical *Sartor Resartus* (1836), in which fictional scholar Diogenes Teufelsdröckh, professor of 'Things in General' at Weissnichtwo (Don'tKnowWhere) University, developed an imaginary philosophy of clothing which echoed Grandville's animated garments: 'Nay, is it not to Clothes that most men do reverence: to the fine frogged broadcloth, nowise to the "straddling animal with bandy legs" which it holds, and makes a Dignitary of?' (Carlyle 1833–4/1918: 172). In a more serious vein, Karl Marx built his philosophy of historical materialism around new articulations of things in society, especially his consequential concept of the commodity as 'an object outside us, a thing that by its properties satisfies human wants of some sort or another' (Appadurai 1986: 7). Such concepts brought things and technologies to the fore of social analysis, but also opened the path for technological determinism at the expense of human agency in ways which continue to be controversial in historical scholarship (Marx and Smith 1995).

Medical practitioners and their patients were part and parcel of this wider culture of things. The history of medicine in the age of empire is bound by emblematic objects: at the beginning, in the time of European upheaval and reform following the French Revolution, Laennec invented the stethoscope, while towards the end of the period, amidst fin-de-siècle anxieties about degeneracy and European scrambles for global supremacy, Röntgen discovered the x-rays which would quickly be taken up by the medical community as a means to make visible hitherto unseen elements of the human body. By sight and sound, objects of the age of empire such as the stethoscope and the x-ray machine afforded unprecedented access to the body's interior, while new instruments and assistive technologies afforded new forms of bodily intervention and alteration.

OBJECTS AND THE HISTORY OF MEDICINE: THE STETHOSCOPE

What can objects tell us about the history of medicine in the age of empire? A focus on 'things' has become prominent in popular and academic histories. In history books for general audiences, readers are eager to discover the object biographies of all manner of things from cod to potatoes (and how they changed the world), while Neil McGregor's ambitious blockbuster book promises to tell the *History of the World in 100 Objects* (Kurlansky 1997; Reader 2008; McGregor 2010). Meanwhile, academic historians have declared the advent of the 'material turn' in their discipline. This recent 'turn' encompasses a wide range of approaches, from a focus on the material culture of the past to theories of objects' agency.[1] Recent textbooks on the history of medicine do not always take this new turn to visual and material culture into account (Jackson 2011), and yet, in the history of medicine an interest in objects arguably predates the 'material turn' by several decades. Thus Henry Sigerist, one of the founding fathers of the discipline and an early advocate of attention to the culture of medicine, already pronounced in 1951 that the history of medicine was 'to a large extent the history of its tools' (Sigerist 1951; see also Davis 1978; Lawrence 1992).

It may therefore be useful to begin with a brief account of one specific type of object to generate overarching questions for research and interpretation. One invention which roughly coincides with the beginning of the period covered in this volume is the stethoscope, developed in 1816 by the French physician René Laennec. Worn around the practitioner's neck, the instrument would become one of the most emblematic objects of the medical profession. Before the development of modern methods of visualization, healers had few options when attempting to figure out what was going on inside a patient. Much was made of what came out of the patient's body: urinoscopy (the viewing of the patient's urine), in particular, was a popular diagnostic method as the bodily fluid's coloration and consistency could offer valuable clues to the patient's internal constitution. Physical interaction with the body was often restricted, both due to matters of practicality and considerations of politeness. Doctors could feel the patient's pulse on the wrist, but even this contact was morally dubious, and frequently lampooned in caricatures of male doctors attending to female patients (see Figure 5.3).

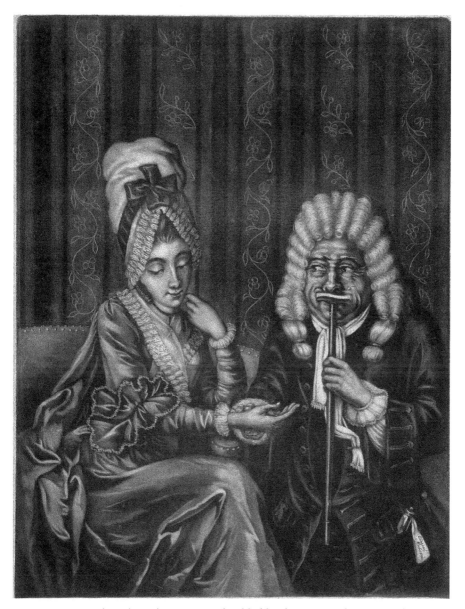

FIGURE 5.3: Feeling the pulse: *Doctor Blowbladder discovering the perpetual motion* (1772). Wellcome Collection.

Even more questionable was the practice of listening to the patient's heartbeat, which required direct physical contact with the patient's chest. Manual labour was rejected by university-trained physicians who desired a clear demarcation of their own profession from 'artisans of the body', such as barber-surgeons (Cavallo 2007). Above all, then, visual inspection and the patient's oral or written testimony, their own description of their symptoms and the progress of their disease, had formed the main basis of doctors' diagnosis since antiquity. By the end of the eighteenth century, physicians saw this reliance on patients' own words as increasingly problematic.

Among the diagnostic tools available to doctors around 1800 was the art of listening to the sounds of the patient's body: their heartbeat and breathing. In 1761, the Austrian physician Josef Leopold Auenbrugger improved on the simple method of passive listening. A hotelier's son, Auenbrugger knew that tapping wine barrels could be used to determine the levels of liquid in the vessel, and he applied this technique to patients' chests to examine the state of the patient's lungs. However, this new diagnostic tool of percussion still required the diagnostician to put his ear to the patient's chest. This practice was seen as problematic by many contemporary doctors for practical and moral reasons, but also as a threat to professional dignity. French physician René Laennec observed that the technique was 'not only indelicate but often impracticable' in the case of female patients, and 'disgusting' in 'that class of persons found in hospitals'. Confronted with a female patient with a suspected heart defect and a 'great degree of fatness', Laennec found a solution to the problem: by rolling up sheets of paper into a cylinder and listening through the resulting tube, the sounds of the patient's heartbeat were amplified, and the practitioner could simultaneously avoid direct physical contact with the patient's body (Laennec 1829: 5–6). The positive result led him to experiment with a range of materials, shapes and dimensions, until Laennec arrived at a model of a straight wooden tube which could be taken apart to enhance portability (see Figure 5.4).

Its interior was shaped like a trumpet to further improve the amplifying qualities of the device. Laennec called his new tool the stethoscope (from the Greek words for 'chest' and 'viewing'), and it would go on to become a key emblem of the medical profession, as well as profoundly reconfiguring the relationship between doctor and patient (Reiser 2009). Physicians could now link sounds of the living body to the subsequent observation of lesions in post-mortem examination. However, the introduction of an object into the diagnostic process created its own problems such as the reliance on the doctor's own sensory capacities. Did he have a 'good ear' for subtle differences in tone and tempo? Did the use of instruments put doctors' status as scholars into question, rendering them mere artisans of the body after all? Despite such early qualms, the stethoscope was adopted widely, in a period that witnessed an increasing

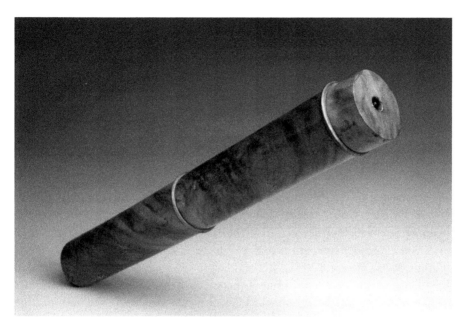

FIGURE 5.4: Laennec-style stethoscope, nineteenth century. Wellcome Collection.

rapprochement of medicine and surgery. Within two decades of the instrument's introduction, doctors reckoned that it would be 'positively suicidal' not to employ the stethoscope, as patients came to expect its use as a sign of cutting-edge medical practice: 'The public has proclaimed its fiat; the public *will have* auscultation' (Reiser 2009: 11). Thus, the stethoscope replaced the cane-and-wig of early modern medical men as a key marker of the profession. As Erwin Ackerknecht put it in his influential monograph *Medicine at the Paris Hospital* (1967), 'The symbol of the modern doctor is the stethoscope' (Ackerknecht 1967: vii). George Eliot exploited this association of the instrument when she introduced the character of the progressively-minded Dr Lydgate in her 1871 novel, *Middlemarch*, highlighting his use of the cutting-edge new instrument (Eliot 1871–2/2007).[2] The stethoscope's introduction into general practice also contributed to changing the relationship between patient and practitioner, the 'beginnings of modern therapeutic distancing' (Reiser 2009: 12; Furst 1998). This brief example opens up a range of questions through which objects contribute to an understanding of medicine in the age of empire. How did objects contribute to the development of ideas about health, the body and disease? How did they shape the identities of patients, practitioners and institutions?

Scholars have turned to objects in part in an effort to reject traditional histories of great men and great ideas, hagiographic celebrations of supposedly isolated individuals, or whiggish histories of progress (Huisman and Warner

2004). Read against the grain, object-centred sources such as the *Gold-Headed Cane* may be used to challenge such narratives. However, the turn to objects is not by itself an unproblematic remedy for such celebratory stories, as a linear account of new inventions may merely shift narratives of progress onto a slightly different plane if we replace histories of great men with histories of great objects ('the fish that changed the world'). Developments in the historiography of medicine, and in the related fields of the histories of science and technology, suggest that a successful 'history of medicine in 100 objects' would require a more nuanced approach which takes into account important phenomena such as the persistence of older technologies, the perspectives of users as well as inventors, and the networked nature of innovation, production, distribution and consumption.[3] It would also require attention to processes of maintenance, repair, reuse and loss: the fate of objects, not just as they come into being through invention and production, but during, and after, their lifetime of use (Werrett 2013). Beyond history-writing, anthropology has been helpful in articulating such alternative perspectives on objects beyond narratives of heroic innovation. Thus Daniel Miller, for instance, urges us to consider the 'humility of things'. In his view, 'objects are important, not because they are evident and physically constrain or enable, but often precisely because we do not "see" them' (Miller 2005: 5). Much of the current scholarship on objects in the humanities and social sciences is in broad agreement with the fundamental assumption expressed by Arjun Appadurai in the introduction to his influential edited volume on the *Social Life of Things* that 'things have no meanings apart from those that human transactions, attributions, and motivations endow them with'. Methodologically, these human actions and attitudes are made visible if we 'follow the things themselves, for their meanings are inscribed in their forms, their uses, their trajectories' (Appadurai 1986: 5).

OBJECTS AND THE SHAPING OF IDEAS ABOUT HEALTH, THE BODY AND DISEASE

The invention of the stethoscope heralded a quest for the development of new diagnostic tools which would allow unprecedented access to the inside of the body. The creation of new instruments fed into (and was fed by) the rise of physiology and pathology as central disciplines for the formation of medical knowledge and the emergence of new concepts of health, disease and the body. These technological developments also fuelled the development of medical specialization (Davis 1981). By the end of the nineteenth century, new fields such as ophthalmology, cardiology and gynaecology defined themselves not just with reference to a particular field of study, but also through a shared set of dedicated instruments (Rosen 1944; Weisz 2005). At the same time, many new instruments were also adopted by general practitioners – beyond the stethoscope, the ophthalmometer, the laryngoscope and the thermometer among others (Davis 1981: 124). Such devices could not only separate the diagnostic process from the testimony of the patient, but also make diagnosis increasingly independent from the sensory perception of the practitioner. Self-recording tools, such as the sphygmometer, turned the minute mechanical actions of the body itself – such as the pulse – into graphic curves which (supposedly) rendered personal judgement obsolete, thus turning medicine into a truly objective science at last (de Chadarevian 1993). The nineteenth-century ideal of 'mechanical objectivity', as described by Lorraine Daston and Peter Galison, held that mechanized observation and representation – in the form of devices including cameras, self-recording instruments and casts – would do away with the problematic interference of the human observer's subjectivity (Daston and Galison 1992). At the same time, however, the increasing importance of instruments prompted concerns among medical practitioners who worried that the patient might get lost in the process. Thus pioneering cardiologist James Mackenzie, a prolific user and developer of new measuring devices, expressed his fear that 'the day may come when a heart specialist will no longer be a physician looking at the body as a whole, but one with more and more complicated instruments working in a narrow and restricted area of the body' (Bound Alberti 2010).

Quantifying devices and other new technologies also played a key role in articulating the emerging concept of 'normality', adopted from the statistical works of Belgian astronomer Adolphe Quetelet, as well as new definitions and classifications of diseases. The thermometer, pioneered by the German physician Carl Wunderlich in the mid-nineteenth century, enabled the determination of normal body temperatures for humans and other species. Wunderlich also used his measurements to establish characteristic fever curves for different diseases (see Figure 5.5).

Beyond quantification, scientists such as Francis Galton and Cesare Lombroso used the newly emerging technology of photography to create 'composite portraits' of disease and criminality, superimposed photographs of sick or criminal individuals, in the hope that they would discover the features of the disease or the 'criminal type' (Cryle and Stephens 2017). Disappointingly, however, such composites, rather than bringing out distinct types, only managed to create the most average-looking faces. Thus, the introduction of new technologies did not always lead to success. In the case of photography, early medical adopters hoped it would allow for the creation of perfectly objective images of diseases and lesions, and thus put diagnosis and research on a firmer foundation. However, the question of the photographer's agency remained problematic throughout, and photographic atlases of anatomy and pathology often failed to deliver in capturing the relevant detail in a useful way (Curtis 2012). Thus many medical authors eventually returned to older, well-established

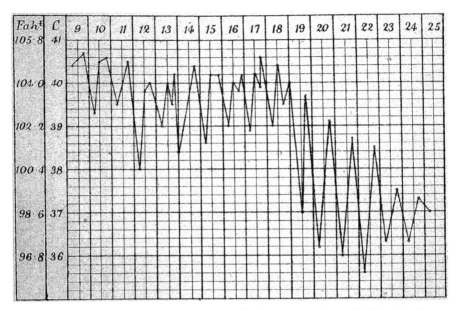

FIGURE 5.5: 'Intense, rapidly recovering typhoid'. From Carl Wunderlich, *On the Temperature in Diseases: A Manual of Medical Thermometry* (1871). Wellcome Collection.

techniques of illustration into the twentieth century (de Rijke 2008). Similar developments apply to the representation of normal and pathological anatomy in three dimensions as well. Rather than work with novel technologies, it was often the adaptation of older techniques which facilitated the creation of new material repositories of the body in health and illness. Thus the French anatomist Felix Thibert used coloured plaster casts of pathological lesions to create a 'living encyclopedia' (*encyclopédie vivante*) of diseases, while the Swiss anatomist Wilhelm His drew on the well-established tradition of wax modelling to document the early stages of fetal development (Thibert 1844; Hopwood 2004).

Such adaptations of older materials and methods also enabled the circulation of new images of the body beyond the medical community. Life-sized anatomical models in affordable, sturdy materials such as plaster and papier-mâché were introduced in institutions ranging from secondary schools to military training facilities, and they became a staple prop of itinerant medical lecturers. Thus, artificial bodies made knowledge of the body's interior available to a wide range of audiences. Such objects also enabled the circulation of European ideas and ideals of health and the body across the globe in projects which were frequently framed as 'civilizing missions' and justified further imperial conquest. Both objects and people involved in such missions were cast as 'agents of civilization', as for instance in the case of African slaves who trained as midwives

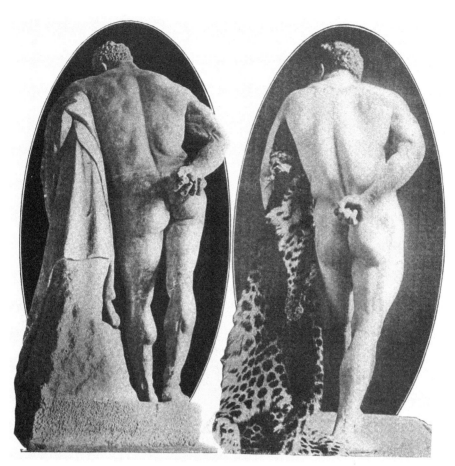

FIGURE 5.6: The Farnese Hercules and Eugen Sandow. From Eugen Sandow, *Life Is Movement: The Physical Reconstruction and Regeneration of the People* (n.d.). Wellcome Collection.

in Egypt with the help of French anatomical models and instructors (Maerker 2013).

Models and other popular representations of the body idealized the muscular, working body, especially with the advent of the public health movement which advocated self-knowledge and self-improvement as the path to individual perfection and social progress (Callen 1995; Callen 2018). Meanwhile, other proponents of healthy body initiatives looked not to the new artificial anatomies produced by model factories, but back to the material remains of Greco-Roman antiquity. The nineteenth-century revival of ancient ideals led to the beginnings of bodybuilding: showman-educators such as the Prussian-born Eugen Sandow presented ancient sculptures of muscular gods and heroes as ideals to be emulated, side by side with his own well-developed physique (see Figure 5.6). Others developed suitable training tools which would allow customers to achieve these ideals through suitable exercise, thus turning the body itself into an object of improvement, and stemming the tide of degeneration (Budd 1997).

OBJECTS AND IDENTITIES

If material culture is the 'mirror' which tells us who we are (Miller 2005: 2), then nineteenth-century medical communities could see themselves in a wide range of objects: in diagnostic tools and laboratory instruments, in professional clothing and paraphernalia, as well as in the very spaces of medicine, such as laboratories, hospitals and asylums. Dress, in particular, was a key marker of professional identity in the age of empire. In her classic study, *Adorned in Dreams: Fashion and*

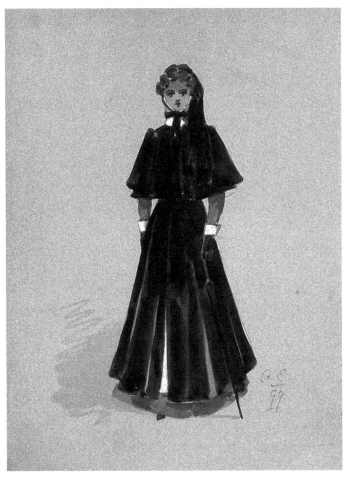

FIGURE 5.7: C.C., *An army hospital nurse in her outdoor uniform* (1899). Wellcome Collection.

Modernity, fashion historian Elizabeth Wilson has highlighted the ways in which 'dress . . . links the biological body to the social being, and public to private' (Wilson 1985). This was especially evident in the development of nurses' uniforms in this period. The uniform was an important part of the professionalization of nursing, and the entry of female nurses into the hitherto male dominated sphere of the hospital. According to Christina Bates, 'the uniform created patterns of behavior, values and identities that defined generations of nurses' (Bates 2012: 2; see also Brooks and Rafferty 2007). The garment incorporated elements from a wide range of other professional spheres including 'fashionable, occupational, academic, ecclesiastical, military and scientific wear' (Bates 2012: 10).

Nursing uniforms were introduced by the pioneering Protestant female nursing orders of the nineteenth century, beginning in 1833 with the Kaiserswerth Deaconess Institute's Nursing Training School, which would become a key influence for Florence Nightingale and other reformers of nursing. The uniform was modelled on traditional married women's clothing to accord moral standing and authority to nurses. Following the religious framework of the order, early nursing outfits called for simplicity and lack of ornamentation, such as silk accessories. Nightingale adopted similar guidelines for her Crimean nurses, insisting on plain grey tweed for winter outfits and printed cotton for the summer. Practical considerations shaped the outfits she requested for the Nightingale School of Nursing at St Thomas's Hospital, which opened in 1860. There, Nightingale insisted that 'crinolines, polonaises, hair-pads' not be worn, as 'the fidget of silk and of crinoline, the rattling of stays and of shoes' obstructed free movement and disrupted patients' rest (Bates 2012: 22). Unlike the earlier Protestant orders, she refrained from overt religious connotations in the design of uniforms in her quest to enhance the standing of nurses as professionals.

The dress of the male physician similarly underwent a change in the period: out went the wig and cane of the early modern doctor, in came the lab coat – in public representations, if not always in practice. With the emergence of laboratory medicine in the nineteenth century, the white lab coat came to signify modern, 'scientific' medical practice (Jardine 1992: 309–10; see also Jewson 1976). Conventions of dress were geographically specific as well. As one American physician observed, 'in England . . . the country in which the bedside manner has attained its finest development, convention prescribes the top-hat and frock-coat. A physician would as soon venture to call upon his patient without these appurtenances as without his collar.' In contrast, the American doctor praised his own country's more relaxed expectations: 'We ought to be glad that we are not shackled with purposeless conventions, and that the restoration of health does not depend on a return to the use of the full-bottomed wig, the robe, and the cane which were necessary in the time of Radcliffe and Sydenham' (Collins 1911: 307).

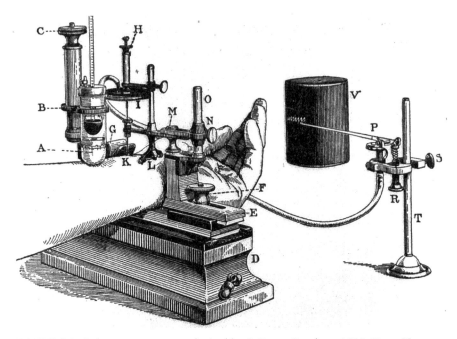

FIGURE 5.8: Sphygmomanometer devised by S. S. von Basch, *c.* 1881. From T. Lauder Brunton, *Therapeutics of the Circulation: Eight Lectures delivered in the Spring of 1905 in the Physiological Laboratory of the University of London* (1908), p. 62. Wellcome Collection.

Beyond dress itself, the materiality of laboratory medicine helped enhance the professional status of medical practitioners. Like the lab coat, new scientific instruments such as the stethoscope and the electrocardiograph functioned as 'tokens of medical practitioners' commitment to a precise, quantitative, cause-seeking medicine, and as emblems of the enhanced professional status and authority of the 'scientific' medic' (Jardine 1992: 310). Complex specialized instruments such as the early sphygmomanometer embodied the changing professional image of the medical practitioner as a man of science, as well as the global network which sustained it, from its French drums to its India rubber parts (see Figure 5.8).

However, the materiality of laboratory medicine had to be framed carefully to avoid threatening the status of its practitioners. The history of the laboratory was inseparable from domestic working spaces. Nineteenth-century physiologist Claude Bernard famously described the laboratory as a 'long and ghastly kitchen' (Latour 1992: 295; see also Gooday 2008). However, where common domestic items and techniques were adopted in the laboratory to solve practical problems in the process of growing germ cultures and for keeping the laboratory environment clean, items such as the humble potato had to be reframed carefully when they were used as a germ substrate in order to maintain the male practitioner's distance from feminine domesticity. Similar preoccupations with status frequently meant that innovation was prized above maintenance, which was usually left in the care of auxiliary practitioners. Thus, for instance, theatre nurses were in charge of the maintenance of surgical gloves (Newman 2017). It should be noted that not all medical practitioners readily embraced the new laboratory medicine and its material trappings. As John Harley Warner has emphasized, well into the twentieth century physicians rallied around Luke Fildes's painting *The Doctor* (1891), a sentimental scene of a practitioner attending to a sick child in a humble cottage, to articulate an alternative image of the caring doctor who drew on his empathy and experience rather than on new technologies, and who did not lose sight of the humanity of his patients (Warner 2014).

Objects could thus be used to articulate hierarchies among medical practitioners and competing images of the profession, but also to demarcate the boundary between experts and laypeople. For claims to medical authority in the age of empire it was important not just to use objects, but to use the right kinds of objects, and to use them in the right manner. Anatomical models, for instance, could be praised as innovative records of medical research, as for instance in the case of Wilhelm His, but also disparaged by medical professionals when used by popular lecturers such as Frederick Hollick, who controversially aimed to 'liberate the public from the oppressive monopoly of physicians' by educating the public in matters of health and reproduction (Haynes 2003). The meaning of medical objects was thus highly context-dependent: where Hollick used anatomical models to emancipate citizens from doctors' monopolies, the American women's rights activist Paulina Wright Davis employed the same objects to support her claim that women could and should learn about their own bodies, especially in matters of sexuality and reproduction (Maerker 2013).

The object culture of industrial capitalism also encouraged patients to act as consumers and connoisseurs of medical things, especially with the development of new kinds of assistive devices such as limb prostheses and hearing aids. Produced at large scales and marketed widely, these products were shaped by contemporary gender norms, beauty standards and expectations of productivity. They supported, and sometimes challenged, dominant concepts of 'normality'. Consumers' choices were shaped by complex constellations of shared and conflicting values, economic constraints and individual experience (Jones 2017; Virdi 2020).

HUMANITY IN MIND AND BODY

The tools of the new sciences of the body were used not just to articulate the identities of medical practitioners, but also figured prominently in attempts to identify humanity itself. Skulls, calipers, goniometers, photography and the very act of tool use itself were used to define what makes us human. Objects also contributed centrally to efforts to capture the nature of the human mind. In his influential 1801 treatise on insanity, Philippe Pinel asked whether insanity 'depend[ed] upon organic lesion of the brain', and proceeded to collect and analyse the skulls of 'maniacs and ideots' in an attempt to establish the relationship between mind and body (Pinel 1801: vii, 110).

However, unlike the phrenologists who postulated clear relationships between character and skull shape, Pinel remained cautious in his methods and conclusions. The human skull, he cautioned, was a recalcitrant object which defied easy geometrical description: 'Nothing, indeed, appears less capable of precise admeasurement than the cavity of the cranium' as it contained 'many irregular eminences and depressions' as well as resemblance to an ellipsoid 'whose convexity differs at different parts' (Pinel 1801: 119). Pinel was thus reduced to mechanical measurements of skulls, which he performed using a specially designed instrument, a 'parallelopipedon'. Overall, he concluded, there was 'no evident relation [of the shape of the skull] to the extent of the intellectual faculties' (Pinel 1801: 120–1).

Pinel's scepticism notwithstanding, the quest for material markers of human characteristics continued throughout the age of empire. Just as Galton and Lombroso used modern technologies such as photography to try to discern criminal types and types of disease, so others used a range of instruments to capture markers of race and 'civilization'. Craniometry, the measurement of the skull, became a defining practice of the emerging discipline of anthropology against the humanities' claim to authority in interpreting the human condition (Zimmerman 2001). Pioneering anatomist and anthropologist Paul Broca, in particular, was a prolific developer of new anthropometric instruments – among others, the craniograph (1860), a new goniometer (1864), the stereograph (1867), the *cadre à maxima* and the micrometric compass (1869), and the occipital goniometer (1870) – in his ongoing quest 'to detect the primitive type in a deformed cranium' (Broca 1863: 287). However, these instruments were more successful in defining the boundaries of the new discipline of anthropology, and in reifying the concept of 'race', than they were in generating consensus on the nature of humanity.

Equally elusive was the relationship between mental illness and its physical locus and expressions, a question which continued to occupy researchers in the nineteenth century. Such projects frequently involved heterogeneous assemblages of old and new techniques and technologies. Historians have made much of Charcot's attempts to use the new technology of photography to capture the essence of hysteria and other physical and mental afflictions, to capture typologies of paroxysms, postures and behaviours on camera (Didi-Huberman 1982/2003; Gilman 1982/1996). However, Natasha Ruiz-Gómez

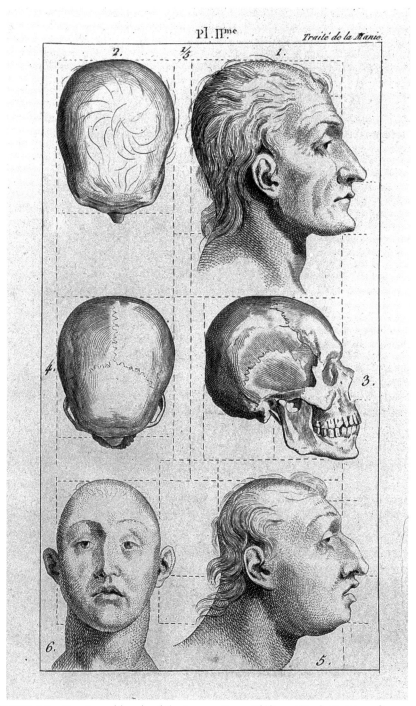

FIGURE 5.9: Crania and heads of the insane. From Philippe Pinel, *Traité medico-philosophique sur l'aliénation mentale, ou la manie* (1801). Wellcome Collection.

has shown that beyond photography, Charcot and his researchers established a much broader collection of artefacts in their quest for a better understanding of disease. The 'Musée Charcot' at the Salpêtrière Hospital in Paris contained a heterogeneous collection of pathological objects and made frequent use of the skills of artists, painters and sculptors in creating portraits of patients which went beyond the mechanical reproduction afforded by photography and casts (Ruiz-Gómez 2013). Contemporaries marvelled at the diverse and abundant collection. Thus, the Belgian philosopher and psychologist Joseph Delboeuf described Charcot's collection in the 1880s as

> . . . a large room, a kind of museum, whose walls, even the ceiling, are decorated with a considerable number of drawings, paintings, engravings, photographs sometimes showing scenes with various individuals, sometimes a single patient naked or clothed, standing, sitting or lying down, sometimes one or two legs, a hand, a torso, or another part of the body altogether. All around, cupboards with skulls, spines, tibias, humeri showing this or that anatomical feature; everywhere, on tables, in vitrines, a pell-mell of jars, instruments, machines; the image in wax, not yet completed, of an old woman, nude and lying on a kind of bed; busts, including that of [Franz] Gall, painted green.

Thus, he concluded, the collection presented 'a true specimen of a living laboratory' (Ruiz-Gómez 2013: 4). The institution circulated its growing collection widely in its own publication, the *Nouvelle Iconographie de la Salpêtrière* (published from 1888 to 1918).

Even the least embodied theories of the mind continued to rely heavily on objects, both as tools of therapeutic practice and as elements of conceptual development. As John Forrester has shown, Freud's ambition to act as an 'archaeologist of the mind' was supported by his collection of ancient (Roman, Greek and Egyptian) artefacts, and he had collected more than 3,000 pieces by the time of his death in 1939. Already in the 1890s, Freud's conceptualizations of the human mind had drawn extensively on the imagery of prehistoric excavation: 'our psychic mechanism', he contended, 'has come into being by a process of stratification'. In Freud's analytical work, everyday objects became meaningful, especially when they figured in the dream world of his patients. Through this exercise, Forrester contends, 'Freud's psychoanalysis did transform despised and neglected objects into precious things' (Forrester 1994: 241).

THE BODY AS OBJECT

The relationship between the body and its afflictions was never straightforward. Practices of turning bodies into objects in dedicated spaces such as museums and laboratories were central to nineteenth-century medical research and teaching. This process of transformation was often problematic for legal, cultural and practical reasons. Private anatomy teachers, in particular, had already begun to amass substantial collections of images, skeletons, wet and dry specimens and models in the eighteenth century as part of their teaching armamentarium (Chaplin 2009; Berkowitz 2015). But the nineteenth century was the heyday of medical museums: pathological collections were established in medical schools, hospitals and asylums, and became important markers of institutional and professional identity (Alberti 2011). As Edinburgh anatomist Frederick Knox put it, 'Without museums the profession would be in the state of man without a language' (Knox 1836: 3).

The ability to open up dead bodies had long been a privilege which distinguished physicians from other healers. In the early modern period this medical privilege was articulated in public dissections and embodied in miniaturized models of the human body for display by physicians (Klestinec 2010). As the supply of executed criminals was not sufficient to satisfy medical teachers' demand for dissection material, those in need of bodies – from anatomy instructors to articulators who prepared skeletons for teaching purposes – resorted to body-snatching, usually by digging up corpses recently buried in cemeteries. Jewish corpses were especially popular due to the Jewish custom of burying the dead quickly (Richardson 1988/2001: 62–3). In the early nineteenth century, gangs of professional 'resurrectionists' operated in centres of medical teaching such as London and Edinburgh (Richardson 1988/2001: 57). With this practice, the body was turned into a commodity. This development was facilitated by the fact that legally, the dead body was not considered property in Great Britain, and thus its appropriation was not theft, as long as it was stripped of all other objects a person might have been buried with. This 'horrid traffic in human flesh' caused public outrage and became a sufficiently urgent problem to warrant the creation of a Parliamentary Select Committee (*The Lancet* (1829), quoted in Richardson 1988/2001: 52). In 1828, high-profile medical practitioners, policemen and even a few anonymous body snatchers were invited to be interviewed before the Committee. President of the Royal College of Surgeons Sir Astley Cooper suggested the average price for a corpse to be eight guineas, though others claimed they had at times paid as much as sixteen or twenty. According to one body snatcher interviewed by the Committee, there was 'a good living' to be made in the trade (House of Commons 1828: 71). Responding to the findings of the Committee, the British Parliament in 1832 passed the Anatomy Act, which enabled licensed medical teachers to use unclaimed bodies for dissection. Similar provisions had already been in place in France since the Revolution, and had enabled Paris to become the world capital of anatomical instruction in the early nineteenth century. It should be noted, however, that both in France and Great Britain those laws merely improved medical schools' supplies of bodies, but did not fully extinguish the illicit trade in dead bodies. British and French newspapers continued to report on the scourge of body snatching, and as late as 1858, the writer (and former medical student) Henry Morley reported in *Household Words* on the continuing 'Use and abuse of the dead': 'the price of a subject to the student in this country is now four pounds, instead of ten. The Act, however, does not put an end to the villainous jobbing in corpses which is still within the power of an undertaker who can get the master of a workhouse to assist his views' (Morley 1858: 364).

Regardless of the legal framework regulating the use of dead bodies, the practice of dissection in itself articulated the object-like nature of the body in ways which were central to the identity of the medical profession. As John Harley Warner and James Edmondson have argued, the act of dissection and the custom of posing with the dead body were crucial markers of identity formation for medical students in the nineteenth and early twentieth centuries. The body itself was objectified, and the act memorialized in a photograph (see Figure 5.10).

These photos 'recount the rite of passage to a new identity . . . [and] present a professional coming-of-age narrative' (Warner and Edmondson 2009: 15).

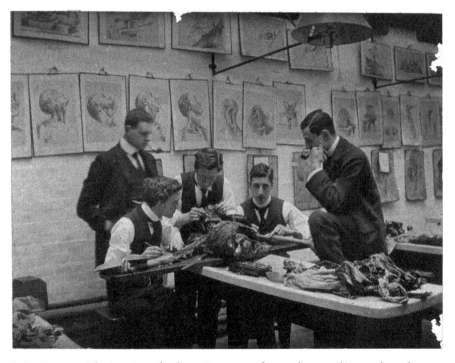

FIGURE 5.10: The interior of a dissecting room: five students and/or teachers dissect a cadaver. Photograph (*c.* 1900). Wellcome Collection.

Similarly ritualized processes of objectification also characterized the use of live animals as objects of medical study. As Nancy Anderson has shown, textbooks of medicine and the life sciences in the nineteenth century created images of 'faceless' animals to facilitate the perspective of the research animal as object (Anderson 2012; see also Guerrini 2003). The preparation of the 'sacrificial animal' as a transition from individual animal to object of study continues to be a crucial rite of passage for lab novices (Lynch 1988: 279).

However, turning animals and humans into research objects was always an incomplete process. While industrial exhibitions celebrated technological innovation, exoticizing shows of 'primitive' peoples aimed to demonstrate European superiority and thus to justify imperial domination. Such displays were highly popular with the general public, and gave researchers opportunities to study living examples of different races (Anderson 2008). Despite efforts to frame and police these encounters, human subjects frequently behaved in ways which did not conform to their expected roles, and spectators did not necessarily see what they were expected to see – rather than perceive 'primitives' to be inferior, observing those human groups and their interactions with each other and with visitors, a subversive sense of shared humanity could come to the fore (Qureshi 2011).

And even in death, bodies were frequently recalcitrant objects of observation. The preservation of body parts required a sophisticated array of techniques and materials to keep specimens looking and feeling like flesh. Just as the meanings of objects changed as they travelled in time and across communities, the very materiality of anatomical preparation was subject to change as well. Under preservation, colours faded, shapes distorted, tissues hardened or softened. Preparators highlighted these issues and developed different strategies for dealing with them. Thus, for instance, the brothers Robert and Frederick Knox, who produced pathological specimens for the Royal College of Surgeons in Edinburgh, diagnosed that the use of specimens, while of key importance for anatomy and pathology, was also highly problematic due to the inevitable distortions and users' lack of familiarity with preservation techniques. The two brothers arrived at radically different conclusions on how to make collections of preserved body parts useful, and their strategies involved two contrasting conceptualizations of users' agency. Robert Knox maintained that the creation of perfect representations would solve the problem of misinterpretation – and thus the main objective of the maker of such objects was to develop better techniques and materials. Frederick on the other hand suggested that only the education of the user could enable proper use and understanding of specimens. Good technique, in his view, was never enough – simultaneously owners and makers of collections always had to consider and reconfigure the perceptions and skills of collection users. 'My observations,' Frederick highlighted, 'will . . . enable the student at once to perceive whether the preparations have really had labour bestowed on them, or are merely preserved from decomposition; and will at all times put him on his guard with respect to the inevitable changes on the colour and delicate textures caused by the modes adopted for preservation' (Knox 1836: viii).

Towards the end of the period covered by this volume, the Great War prompted a new way of monetizing parts of living bodies. New weapons such as the machine gun had caused a wide range of bodily damage to soldiers, while combinations of old and new battlefield technologies such as ambulant x-ray units drawn by horse carts allowed ever higher percentages of wounded soldiers to survive a loss of limb or other severe disfigurement. While in the past, loss of limb as a result of workplace accidents had been compensated on the basis of loss of earning capacity, such calculations could no longer be justified in the face of increasing pressure to provide for veterans. In its stead, payments compensating for 'loss of amenity' were introduced, which calculated the precise value of every human limb. The loss of two fingers warranted a payment of 20% of the full military pension (Bourke 1996: 63–6). Those financial calculations were shaped by cultural assumptions about bodily perfection and its role for social integration, and the classical ideals of ancient Greece and Rome which fuelled the efforts of bodybuilders like Sandow also shaped efforts at rehabilitation, from the aesthetics of pioneering plastic surgery to the development of prosthetic devices (Carden-Coyne 2009).

CONCLUSION

Reconstructing the material culture of health and healing in the age of empire shows how medicine was inextricably embedded in the fabric of historical developments of the era: imperialism and global trade, the development of mass media and the modern professions, industrialization and mass production. Access to a new range of materials and the development of new industrial processes enabled the construction of new ranges of instruments for medical treatment, diagnosis and research, from stethoscopes to sphygmometers, as well as new assistive devices for patients. Adopting such tools as signs of progressivism and professionalism, doctors participated in consumer culture through journals, trade shows and catalogues. The mass-marketing of prostheses created new consumer choices for laypeople while simultaneously increasing pressure to conform to standards of beauty, productivity and normalcy. Objects influenced nineteenth-century medicine in many ways: things such as the stethoscope profoundly reshaped the relationship between patients and practitioners by replacing the patient's testimony with the doctor's own, technically enhanced observations of the patient's body, or even the results of self-recording devices and test kits. The use of new instruments simultaneously signalled the medical practitioner's allegiance to a new, scientific medicine, based on laboratory research in foundational disciplines such as physiology and pathology. By the end of the period, popular journals imagined that 'the modern physician deprived of the tools he familiarly uses to diagnose the conditions of a part' would be 'utterly lost' ('Progress' 1872: 252). Such rearticulations of healers' social and professional roles could be supported by auxiliary items such as clothing: the doctor's lab coat, the nurse's uniform. The 'proper' relationship with objects was turned into a marker of professional identity, especially the professional interaction with the dead body, the artificial body and the body of the laboratory animal. The use of objects also profoundly reshaped core concepts of medical knowledge itself: 'new instruments are leading to new trains of thought' ('Progress' 1872: 252). Self-registering and quantifying devices articulated new conceptions of the body as an 'elaborately constructed machine' amenable to optimization, and the concept of the 'normal' body as an ideal to be achieved through self-monitoring and self-improvement as well as specialist care and submission to expert authority ('Present state' 1883: 495). Humanity was defined in relation to its objects, especially the brain and its archaeology of strata of (repressed) memory. Throughout, however, the body remained a recalcitrant object; it defied easy 'reading', visibility optimization, and conservation.

Much more could be said about the role which objects played in the development of medicine in the age of empire. However, one might also reverse the perspective: how did modern medicine shape the culture of objects? Especially in debates about dissection and vivisection, medicine raised questions about the object-nature of things. The use of quantifying and self-registering instruments frequently encouraged the objectification of the body as a machine which required optimization (Rabinbach 1990). Medicine also shaped the emerging culture of mass consumption. Much of the thing culture of the early modern period had focused on practices of maintenance, adaptation and reuse (Werrett 2019). Indeed, despite the celebration of innovation and progress, much of nineteenth-century medical material culture still continued this tradition. Suppliers of medical and surgical instruments offered repairs as well as selling new commodities: catalogues listed services such as the sharpening of knives and syringe needles, the polishing of forceps, nickel-plating, replacing old springs, valves and rubber parts (Noyes Brothers and Cutler 1888: 71–2). This began to change towards the end of the nineteenth century, as the development of disposable medical supplies and new sterilizing devices was motivated by the advent of the germ theory of diseases. A range of competing, conflicting and complementary strategies were developed to keep medical objects and spaces clean, especially diverse forms of asepsis and antisepsis. In addition to those strategies, the development of throwaway items improved cleanliness. In 1912, army surgeon James T. Greeley filed a patent for a single-use hypodermic needle, designed for 'asepsis and celerity', which was adopted soon afterwards on the battlefields of the First World War (United States Patent and Trademark Office 1912). The development of a fully-fledged culture of disposables would, however, have to wait until the period after the First World War (Busch 1983).

NOTES

1. See, e.g., Green 2012; Alder 2007; and Daston 2008. For a useful summary of influential developments in archaeology and anthropology, see, e.g., Hicks 2010. For an overview of debates in history and related disciplines, see also Bennett and Joyce 2010. For material culture in the history of science, see, e.g., Werrett 2014.
2. The novel was set in 1829–32, when use of the stethoscope 'had not become a matter of course in practice at that time' (Eliot 1871–2/2007: 288).
3. For key historiographical developments focusing on users, maintenance and networks, the history of technology is especially valuable. See, e.g., Kline and Pinch 1996; Edgerton 2006; and Oudshoorn and Pinch 2003. For useful starting points in the historiography of medical objects, including instruments, technologies and materials, see, e.g., Timmermann and Anderson 2006; Klein and Spary 2010; and Lawrence 1992.

CHAPTER SIX

Experiences

ROB BODDICE

EXPERIENTIAL LANDSCAPE

To chart experiential change over time is a challenge when dealing with a single topic, such as one of the senses, or of pain, but becomes all the more daunting when faced with the cultural history of medicine as a whole.[1] Is it even possible, in a broad sense, to indicate the general tenor of experiential change over the long nineteenth century?[2] And whose experiences should we be looking at in any case – those who administer medicine or those who receive it?[3] My general sense of the answer to the first question is that there was, over this period, a growing sense of separation of patients from doctors, and with this came new fears, new anxieties and new hopes about the possibilities of avoiding disease or, if already sick, of getting better. To answer the second question we must examine the history of experience as the product of dynamic encounters.[4]

The history of experience is a fairly new field of inquiry, presenting its own peculiar challenges.[5] The question of medical experience presents these challenges acutely, for the meaning of the dynamic encounter between physician and patient was understood differently by the respective parties, yet the historical record privileges the point of view of medical personnel. Finding a history of experience in the history of medicine depends on the extent to which not only patient voices, but also patient gestures and senses can be recovered and reintegrated into medical narratives of what was happening.[6] This is often mitigated by the nature of patient testimony, which is contained within and framed by a structure of understanding and interpretation imposed by medical knowledge, institutions, procedures and practices. Nevertheless, there is scope to take such testimony 'out of the frame', as it were, and to listen to it anew. Equally, there is potential to recover the patient's body.[7]

Recent developments in neuroscience, in the study of the experience of emotion and pain and in understandings of the way in which placebo works have refocused the attention of neurobiologists and historians alike on the reliability and reality of subjectivity.[8] What had long been thought to be universal and hard-wired processes, such as pain sensitivity, for example, transpire to be highly subjective, heavily influenced by cultural context, so that we can point to no certain relationship between stimulus and response that exists outside of a cultural frame. The reality of experience as perceived by an individual is a construct of that individual's brain, a neuroplastic device, the neurological development of which is strongly tied to the world in which it is situated. We can, perhaps for the first time, add biological substance to the cultural history project and say that the social construction of reality is, in the most fundamental way, embodied.[9] There is no objective experience beyond the subjective apprehension of it. This insight allows us to approach the historical record afresh, to hear patient voices, see their gestures, and document their bodies. By the same token, we can better understand the political dynamics that make those things so difficult to discover.

The meeting of doctors and patients, of state-led medicine and the public in this period was often a meeting of acute tensions and incommensurabilities. The nineteenth century witnessed the active appropriation by surgeons and medical researchers of a doctrine of equanimity, afforded to them by the wonders of chloroform. They portrayed a supreme confidence in their ability to cure or prevent the most terrible scourges, and moved towards a notion that medicine should be administered by the state for the general good of the health of the commonwealth. This was a cool humanity, looking to distant goods, in contrast to the 'necessary inhumanity', in William Hunter's (1784: 67) terms, that had characterized the eighteenth-century surgeon (and from which Hunter had turned in disgust).[10]

On the other side, while patients benefited from the securities offered them by vaccination, of painless surgery, of new drugs (from morphine, first sold as pain relief in 1817, to Aspirin, mass-marketed by 1899) to heal them, they often met the equanimity, confidence and conceit of established medicine with fear, contempt and distrust. The encroachment of the state into the health of private citizens seems at times to have threatened the feeling of liberty of the citizen (compulsory vaccination is notable in this respect, from mid-century), and whereas medical experimentation promised great leaps forward for public health, the spectre of callousness ran through the population as the death knell of civilization. Medicine, especially toward the end of the nineteenth century and into the twentieth, was at once civilization's greatest hope and exemplary of the decline of morals in modern society. The rise of the medical professional and the medical specialist was suspicious enough to those who clung to gentlemanly independence and the ideals of amateurism. Combined with what was perceived to be an unbounded experimental curiosity that, to some, looked like the free reign of cruelty in physiological and toxicological laboratories, these new medical professionals took on an air of the monstrous.[11]

This chapter is organized around experiential categories, exemplified by a series of voyages that stress the encounters between medicine – its personnel, its institutions, its politics – and a variety of individuals, publics, patients and populations. There is a passage to another world beneath consciousness; a global excursion of smallpox vaccination; and an hysterical voyage to Australia. I begin with pain and sympathy, and specifically the question of what happens to patients in pain and the physicians who treat them after anaesthesia is introduced. Is the patient whose pain is benumbed still a pained subject, or merely a medical object? What was the physician or surgeon to feel about such an insensitive entity? And what was it like to 'go under'? This is followed by a medical narrative of fear – of disease and its prevention – where clear change over time can be marked according either to changes in medical knowledge or in the way in which medicine was administered or presented to the public. From fear I move to what I tentatively call 'performance'. The term will be readily understood as an adequate description of the ways in which the sick altered their behaviour and experience according to perceived changes in the scripts of illness over the course of the nineteenth century. Yet this 'performance' was not conscious or theatrical. These are instances of patients meeting the expectations of their doctors and deriving some medical benefit from it – a kind of gestural placebo effect – that can be precisely located in historical time. Thus, the presentation of hysteria in particular can be revisited as an 'authentic' experience of disease, in an emotive dynamic between patient community, medical community and society.

PAIN AND SYMPATHY

I began to be terrified to such a wonderful extent as I would never before have guessed possible. I made an involuntary effort to get out of the chair, and then – suddenly became aware that I was looking at nothing: while taken up by the confusion in my lungs, the outward things in the room had gone, and I was 'alone in the dark.'

—Spencer 1878: 575

So recorded a correspondent of the famous Victorian polymath Herbert Spencer, beginning a lengthy account of a trip to the dentist. The administration of chloroform, designed to render the procedure painless and the patient unconscious, seemed in this case to achieve neither in the fullest sense of those terms, yet the experience of the patient nevertheless took place as if somewhere else. The memory of the dentist's room vanished, replaced by an ethereal space were cruelty, pain and fear were anthropomorphized, looming from the darkness as embodied presences that had their way with the patient, who bore their torments because although they worked their terrible ways on 'him', the patient had no direct identification with the subject of his ethereal wakefulness. 'I' was not 'me'.

As the world 'outside my own body' disappeared, the patient was 'seized and overwhelmed by the panic inside', with 'every air-cell struggling spasmodically against an awful pressure', ripping each other apart until 'there was universal racking torture'. Consciousness was reduced to this: 'an isolated sense of torture, pervaded by a hitherto unknown sense of terror'. The ego, Spencer observes of his correspondent, was stripped away until such a point that the 'I' related only to the beating of the heart, with all other sensory and spatial components of consciousness stripped away. The patient put it more graphically:

> [A]ll of a sudden my heart sprang out with a more vivid flash of sensation than any of those previous ones. The force of an express-engine was straining there, and like a burning ball it leaped from side to side, faster and faster, hitting me with such a superhuman earnestness that I felt as if the iron had entered my soul, and it was all over with me forever. (Not that 'I' was now any more than this burning-hot heart and the walled space in which it was making its strokes: the rest of 'me' had gone unobserved out of focus).
>
> —Spencer 1878: 576

Nevertheless, this identity reduced to a heartbeat conceived of a 'profoundly cruel presence', 'unutterably monstrous in its nature', which suddenly became a 'pulsating *pain*, and I was all over one tender wound' (577). As the effects of the chloroform lifted, so the world flooded back into the patient's subjectivity, until he recognized that a '*tooth* was being slowly twisted out of my jaw' (578).

The account published by Spencer, which has been remarkably overlooked by scholars, gets to the core of the question of experience in the clinical encounter. In an age of high utilitarianism, the diminution of pain and the maximization of pleasure were not mere philosophies, but rules by which to live.[12] Spencer was trying to understand the nature of consciousness and the limits of the ego, but this nightmarish 'failure' of chloroform cut at the heart of modern medicine's greatest practical claim: pain was supposed to be a thing of the past. Indeed, the account strikes a familiar tone to that of Fanny Burney's (1810) graphic account of her (pre-anaesthetic) mastectomy. When 'the dreadful steel was plunged into the breast – cutting through veins – arteries – flesh – nerves', she 'needed no injunctions not to restrain my cries. I began a scream that lasted unintermittingly during the whole time of the incision' (442).

Indeed, for decades after the advent of anaesthesia, many surgical and dental operations, on working-class and non-white patients in particular, took place without it.[13] Nevertheless, despite doubts about the unknown dangers of anaesthesia, the painless era was feted for the change it would bring to the nature of (some) patients' fear of doctors, of medicine in general and of surgery in particular. Pain management had become the direct remit of medical practice, not ancillary to the treatment of disease, but central to that project. The comfort of the patient became, in the nineteenth century, part of the medical ideal.

The magnitude of this change can hardly be overstated. Painlessness promised practical experiential change on both sides of the clinical encounter. Until the advent of chloroform and ether at mid-century, most surgical and dental procedures involved a measure of resolve from both patient and surgeon, the callousness of the latter being a long held colloquialism. Though it is clear that the relationship between medical personnel and their pained patients did not lack a dynamic of sympathy, the age of anaesthesia seemed to usher in new possibilities for the emotional control of the surgeon or physician, making possible a great extension of techniques that would have been inconceivable if faced with a wracked and writhing body.[14] The fragile emotional dynamic between doctor and patient had long been understood. In matters of surgery, the mere sight of the instruments that caused pain could be enough to arouse terror in patient and observer alike.[15] Aesthetic responses to the signs of pain or discomfort involved doctor and patient in a reciprocity of sympathy, where resolve on the face of the surgeon might be key to the surgical subject getting through the operation. Anaesthetics promised to break this cycle of reciprocity by decisively removing the experience of pain in the patient.[16] The surgical subject was no longer a writhing individual, but a physiological *object*. While the promise of painless surgery was of great moment for those who were to go under the knife, this consequence for the surgeons themselves has been largely overlooked. By taking away the sympathetic concern for the body in pain, surgeons could operate without sympathy, with less fear or anxiety. Attention could be refocused on technique. Anaesthetics introduced an air of *procedure* to what had often previously been an atmosphere of alarm. The shift in atmosphere was marked by Thomas Eakins' famous 1875 depiction of the *Gross Clinic*, which captured the coolness of surgical procedure, the equanimity of the surgical student, the passivity of the surgical subject and the failure to understand the shift in register of pain, fear and disgust among the public, as here represented by the patient's mother (see Figure 6.1). As Spencer's correspondent would have attested, and as many others experienced, this new surgical ideal was not always met. Nonetheless, it was sufficiently powerful as an ideal as to change practices and to fundamentally alter the experiential disposition of both doctor and patient by the early twentieth century, especially in Europe and North America.

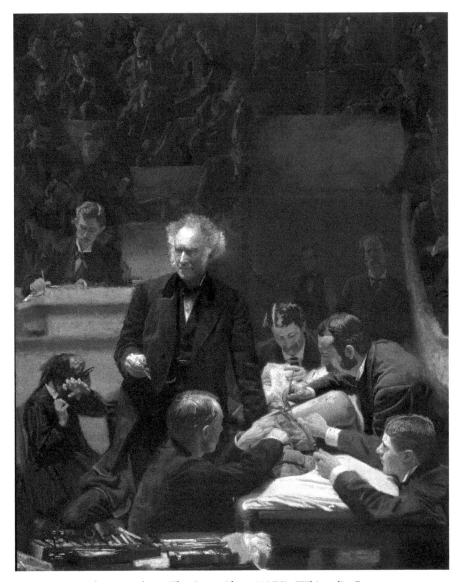

FIGURE 6.1: Thomas Eakins, *The Gross Clinic* (1875). Wikimedia Commons.

The high-point of the anaesthetic gaze came in 1889 when, before a graduating class of medical students at the University of Pennsylvania, William Osler (1925) gave his celebrated speech 'Aequanimitas'. As one of the leading physicians in North America, whose influence would thereafter spread to Britain, Osler's word was a kind of law among doctors. When he told these new doctors that the key to a successful career was 'equanimity', a form of bodily self-control that suppressed sympathy for the patient, he was certainly marking a notable recent shift in the experiential life of doctors, surgeons and physiologists. Osler professed a medical creed in which a theory of affective practice could be reified, so that the central idea of working for a higher good, aligned with the confidence derived from anaesthesia, resulted in an 'imperturbable' surgeon. Not only was such conscious self-command possible – it was essential. For if the surgeon did not have his 'nerves well in hand', or if he betrayed the slightest anxiety or fear, no matter if faced with the 'most serious of circumstances', then disaster beckoned. Osler reached for the experience of the patient and implicitly understood that patient confidence and comfort depended in large part on the extent to which they could willingly trust the expertise, authority and skill of the practitioner. And while such things were the product of a serious training, they were for nothing if they were not carried on with the correct bodily and emotional disposition. Hence, he demanded that his young colleagues put their 'medullary centres under the highest control', to retain a 'coolness', 'calmness' and 'clearness of judgment in moments of grave peril'. This phlegmatic physician or surgeon would be necessarily 'insensible', a quality that was essential for the 'exercise of calm judgment, and in carrying out delicate operations'. Osler knew that, as a social value, a 'keen sensibility' was virtuous, but felt compelled to go against the grain when it came to the experiential qualities of practising medicine, which required 'a callousness which thinks only of the good to be effected . . . a judicious measure of obtuseness' that met 'the exigencies of practice with firmness and courage, without, at the same time, hardening "the human heart by which we live"' (Osler 1925: 3–6).

There is sufficient reason to assume that, by and large, Osler's generation had already adopted such a practical callousness, within certain limits, though they did not label it as such.[17] A key indicator of this was in the medical establishment's growing association with the administration of public health at the level of the state.[18] Medical progress depended on new refinements of specialist knowledge and such feats of administration that it was as if it ceased to be within the ken of the general public, which was asked to trust that the establishment had its interests at heart. Public health policy and medical research took place at a distance from the critical scrutiny of the public eye, especially in the last quarter of the nineteenth century, arousing suspicion at medical and governmental motives. For those practitioners working in such fields, the public became a sort of nuisance to be condescended to lest it check the important work being done in its name. Controversies over vivisection and vaccination, for example, ran uninterrupted across the West from at least the 1870s until after the First World War, focusing in particular on public concerns about medical overreach and the establishment of callousness in the governing class. I will say more about such fears presently, but seldom are the experiences of medical personnel during this time highlighted.[19]

The testimony of individual members of the medical establishment about such thorny issues as medical research by vivisection or the legitimacy of compulsory vaccination, for example, show a certain bewilderment that the public had been allowed to raise such a pitch of objection. While senior figures in the medical establishment in the US, Germany, France and Britain all made careful noises about their tender sensibilities, their gentlemanly qualities and their moral compasses, they nevertheless averred a kind of banal procedural quality to medical research, perceived as a deep sense of satisfaction in the prospect of progress being made, knowledge being advanced.[20] Individual research questions, such as the search for diphtheria serum or a rabies vaccine, to take two prominent examples, took place with a keen sense of the damage done by those diseases, to the extent that the plight of the experimental animals who were sacrificed for medical progress was considered as of little consequence in the balance. Public objections were considered to be not merely ignorant, but sentimental, and with little direct knowledge of the implications for human society of the work being done. Much of the opposition was written off as womanish, and the debate was clearly gendered.[21] The satisfaction derived from doing such work was therefore tinged with a clear air of defiance of the public will, of service to a higher good, and of a vision of fealty to society that most of society could scarcely understand.

In Germany, the more acute development of state-run medical research led to the claim that medical research was a (satisfying) job, and that addressing the ethical concerns of an ill-informed public was simply beyond the remit of an employee.[22] Elsewhere, a more delicate line was drawn, but the mask occasionally slipped. When the German physiologist Edward Klein famously testified to the Royal Commission on Vivisection in 1876 that he really had no regard for the sufferings of animals used in his research, and that he only used anaesthetics to keep the animals still, not to prevent them suffering pain, he was faced with a barrage of criticism, not least from his own peers. On the back foot, Klein tried to amend his testimony, to bring it into line with English sensibilities. But, he noted sourly, the English public would do well to behave more like those in Europe, not 'to take care of other people's consciences in matters they do not clearly understand' (UK Parliament 1876: 183–5, 328).

All of this notwithstanding, we should be mistaken to think that the utilitarian war on pain in the nineteenth century did anything to diminish the more quotidian pains of illnesses and diseases. The agonies caused by cancer or gout – a pain described by Sydney Smith as like 'walking on my eyeballs' – for example, were almost at the level of colloquial knowledge (Porter and Rousseau 2000: 166), and those without access to medical care would have had to undergo toothache and anaesthesia-free extractions well into the twentieth century. Everyday pain, and the pain caused by protracted illness, still had to be borne as an expected part of the sufferings of life, which many still saw as divinely instilled. Indeed, the word 'patient' still resonated with its original meaning of virtuous suffering, alive with distant cultural memories of the notion that worldly pains would offset any suffering to come in the afterlife.[23] Despite the best intentions of those in political and medical authority to diminish the aggregate of suffering, it is likely that the continued processes of urban migration, industrialization and increasing population density in the 'age of empire' made the everyday sufferings of most people worse over time.

One might view the increasing advertisement and ready availability of nostrums and cures throughout the nineteenth century to be evidence of novel possibilities for the killing of pain (and indeed, we find such things as Aspirin among the snake oil), but it is perhaps more fitting to view the popularity of such self-cures as evidence of a rising tide of pain. Much of this pain was specifically tied to modernity itself, some of the phenomena of which I will return to in the section on 'Performance'. Not all of it was newfangled or mysterious, however. The pain of labour – both work and parturition – was likely heightened by the acute sense of fear that stalked a failure to deliver: the industrial wage labourer stood to lose everything if injured; the pangs of birthing in an industrial age were heightened by the loss of common community wisdom and presence of disease in crowded centres. The labouring bodies of women were drawn further under the purview of (largely male) medical gazes and procedures; clinical knowledge of parturition gradually replaced folk knowledge; and the location of childbirth slowly began its shift from the home to the hospital in this era.[24] In a standard narrative of the history of parturition, we might look at evidence for the decrease in infant and mother mortality and the advantages of aseptic birthing environments. A counter narrative, which has begun to appear in the medical humanities, concerns the increase in both fear and pain as women gave up their bodies to medical authority. The flip side of progress in medical knowledge and technique is the simultaneous diminution of such knowledge among the population. Since the experience of any apparently painful or emotional ordeal is known to be contingent on the extent to which the person going through the ordeal feels a measure of control, reassurance and the ability to manage attention, we are left with the potential paradox of an increase in the perception of fear, pain and suffering, despite medical claims to the overall 'improvement' of the birthing process.

Then there are those pains wrought by the industrialization of warfare. Phantom limb pain, for example, had been known to a few philosophers for centuries, but seldom did those relieved of a limb in the field of battle survive before the mid-nineteenth century. Improvements in field surgery, especially in terms of the immediacy of aseptic treatment, meant that many more maimed military men survived their theatres of war and returned to civilian life with claims of suffering that mystified the medical establishment. Phantom limb pain had been observed in the American Civil War, but really emerged as a common phenomenon during and after the First World War.[25] Phantom pains are still not entirely understood, though most pain experts now understand the pain not to stem from the periphery or from the injury site itself, but from a problem in central signalling caused by the failure of the periphery to respond. Early twentieth-century neurologists responded to the problem of phantom limb by attending principally to the site of the injury, but this approach was also intertwined with a discursive trend that laid the blame on the character or moral fibre of the patient. Horrific injuries acquired in combat were compounded by feelings of emasculation. A generation of war-torn men lived in lifelong agony, made worse by being told that the pain was in their heads. Psychogenic pain was written off as malingering, or as a psychological flaw.[26] The resulting suffering is almost unimaginable. Not unlike Spencer's correspondent who was 'conscious under chloroform', there remained an experience gap between the doctors who said the pain was gone, or was never there, and the patients who knew the reality of their own pain.

FEAR

In 1803, Francis Xavier Balmis set out from La Coruna, Spain, on a grand voyage with the intention of vaccinating the Spanish Empire. He is celebrated as a global vaccination pioneer, taking the lymph to Central and South America, the Philippines and China (where it was administered by the British). His journey, which took nearly three years, saw him and his team vaccinate more than 100,000 people, setting up stations everywhere he went in order to ensure the continued process of vaccination of the population. This included the 'Vaccination Junta' in Mexico City, which would oversee the vaccination of the entire population, and a constant effort at local instruction, that the knowledge of this procedure would be preserved after the voyagers had moved on. Balmis sailed on the orders of King Charles IV, an early convert to vaccination, which had only been announced to the world by Edward Jenner in 1798. This global effort was truly monumental, perhaps the first centrally organized attempt to administer public health on a worldwide scale.[27]

Tales of Balmis's voyage usually focus on the importance of thwarting smallpox across the empire. The disease, after all, did not discriminate between colonizer and colonist, and whatever advantages the empire had gained from introducing smallpox to the indigenous populations in the first place,[28] by the beginning of the nineteenth century, epidemics threatened to shake the strength of the empire itself. To local colonial administrators and to the mixed population alike, the promise of safety from smallpox was doubtless a wonderful prospect.

There is something missing in the story, however, which should be recovered and unpacked. While it is well documented that Balmis used live vaccinifers (the people who supplied lymph) to transport the vaccine, seldom are the experiences of those vaccinifers dwelt upon. That these vessels tend to be called 'live carriers' or 'vaccinifers', instead of *children*, speaks to an acceptance of the fact that ethics then were not what ethics are today, and a certain resignation: after all, what choice did Balmis have if he wanted to keep the vaccine active while travelling such long distances?

I do not wish to gainsay such acceptances and resignations. They are, in many ways, apt. Nevertheless, there is an astonishing history of experience to be reconstructed of the people who, without choosing it, brought vaccination to a large portion of the globe. They were the unwitting instrumental objects of grand public-health visions and their subjectivity has been essentially lost. They were on the front line of a new politics of medicine, for vaccination was not simply a means of protecting the health of the population, but an instrument of colonial power. The child carriers of the vaccine were powerless in the extreme in being compelled to embody this medico-political ambition, and one can only assume that they met the task with a great deal of reservation, if not outright terror.

The first cohort of twenty-five children, all orphans aged eight to ten, were pulled from orphanages in Madrid and La Coruna. Five orphans from Madrid carried the original vaccination to the port, where twenty more were placed aboard, bound first for the Canaries and then on to Puerto Rico. One need not look too far for a rationale for the selection of orphaned children. The vaccinifers had to be free from any encounter with smallpox, which ruled out most adults. And they had to have no ties to parental authority that would have doubtless blenched at the prospect of the voyage ahead. The selected orphans set sail on 30 November 1803, reaching San Juan on 9 February 1804. They were eventually sent back to Spain from Mexico City, without the nurse who had accompanied them on the outward voyage, after more than a year abroad. The nurse remained because, wherever Balmis and his team went, new children had to be taken up and shipped to the next location. The vaccination mission was a great chain of forced orphan transplantation. Their fates are generally unrecorded. Twenty more children were found to sail from Mexico to the East. We know something of their journey. They left Acapulco on 1 February 1805, destination Manila: 'The children slept on the floor in crowded quarters and accidentally came in contact with each other, with their arms producing unexpected skin lesions, which caused them to have elevated and prolonged fevers' (Aldrete 2004: 377). The voyage took two and a half months and, while all the children survived, they must have been in poor health and low spirits. Having been the battery for the vaccination of 20,000 people in the Philippines, the children were sent back to Mexico by Balmis, who took a fresh batch on to Macao and Canton. These instruments of the imperial state did not seem to be accorded any of the courtesies that might be afforded to *persons*, but were simply objectified vessels. Care for their survival was, primarily, care for the survival of the vaccine. Few have reflected on the paradox of such dehumanization, in the name of disease prophylaxis. Then again, the saving of life was perhaps only an ancillary care to the preservation of power and trade. This first great humanitarian mission was, in its tone, coldly calculated. Balmis's return was met with great praise, not least from Edward Jenner (1807), who announced, in the midst of Napoleonic warfare, to have made his own private peace with Spain.

The lost experiences of these children are the more surprising when one considers the general air of fear and loathing that dogged the first century of vaccination, much of which centred on the risk of corrupting children with animal and venereal diseases. A child born in 1800 was, on the whole, likely to get smallpox, one way or another. Vaccination – a safe and, so far as its proponents could tell at the time, effective prophylactic – was met with great resistance in England, its country of origin, not least because a great many doctors derived an important part of their income from inoculating children with smallpox. Indeed, the medical establishment preserved smallpox among the population in the hope that purposeful infection would lead to a mild case, followed by lifelong immunity. It was by no means a certain outcome, and had the distinct disadvantage of making the child fully contagious after inoculation. Still, elaborate procedures and performances were established in a bid to make the inoculation process seem as safe and as medically specialized as possible. By contrast, Jenner offered both the vaccine and instructions on how to use it to anybody who cared for it, without charge. It was a simple procedure, without ritual elaboration, and it directly challenged the medical status quo.

The storm that broke around the nature and morality of vaccination introduced new strains of fear among the population, and a distinctly novel sense of anxiety about the motives of both the institutions of medicine and the state. Existential concerns about catching smallpox were rivalled in some communities by concerns about the consequences of vaccination. The perceived evils of the vaccine very quickly became a kind of urban folklore, where evidence-based studies of its positive effects were rivalled by a well organized slew of alternative facts, pushed forward by medical doyens who had something to lose if vaccination were to succeed.[29] The case is particularly telling because it demonstrates the difficulty with which anybody could legitimately establish medical authority in an era where medicine was beginning to be organized on a national basis. Then, much like now, authority was supplanted by force of personality and rhetorical flourish. Medical truth became a flimsy concept for some. From an experiential point of view, it gets to the heart of what it was like for the lay public to weigh medical information and risk among competing narratives of danger.

The initial vaccine debate centred on the risks of inadvertent sexual deviance and the profane comingling of the divinely-conceived human with animal matter. A prominent inoculator (Moseley 1800: 183) classified cowpox as bovine syphilis and publicly wondered whether vaccination was not a form of bestiality, risking an era of bovine chimeras. This was the background to Gillray's famous satirical print of 1803, depicting a community of hybrids transformed by the vaccine (see Figure 6.2). There were elaborate attempts by anti-vaccine doctors (Rowley 1805) to reify Gillray's print, bringing forth the 'cowpoxed ox-faced boy' and the 'mange girl' in order to demonstrate the tangible dangers of the new procedure. It is difficult to gauge the popular reaction to all of this in the short term, but it is easy to see the extent of such fears over the longer run.

Rumours of syphilis dogged vaccination throughout the nineteenth century, and were particularly frequently cited after the introduction of compulsion in England and Wales in 1853. While it is most common to judge the vaccination protests as illegal conscientious objections, and open defiance of the vaccination laws by certain radical city Guardians (notably in Leicester) as manifestations of a deep resentment of government intrusions into the liberty of private citizens, an examination of anti-vaccination sentiment shows that opposition lay chiefly in the fact that vaccination was perceived to be dangerous. This is borne out by anti-compulsion protests in Rio de Janeiro (1904) and Toronto (1919).[30] In the

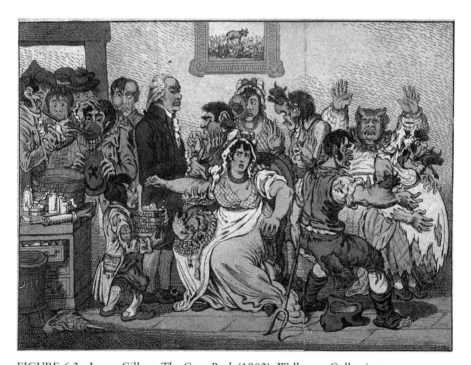

FIGURE 6.2: James Gillray, *The Cow-Pock* (1802). Wellcome Collection.

compulsory law's first incarnation, resistors could be sent to prison with hard labour for failing to vaccinate their children, and some endured multiple prosecutions for failure to comply. In most cases, the stubbornness of these vaccine martyrs was borne on a deeply held conviction that vaccination killed children, or else maimed them, or tainted them with other diseases.[31] There were enough outlying cases – a result of the vicissitudes of arm-to-arm vaccination – to fuel concerns that vaccination caused syphilis, erysipelas, fever and so on. While the liberty argument circulated among philosophers such as Herbert Spencer and the evolutionist Alfred Russel Wallace (1898), the case against vaccination lay in the raft of statistics that could be brought forward that apparently proved either its inefficacy as protection against smallpox, or else its clear correlation with outbreaks of other diseases. Yet a general lack of statistical sophistication meant that exactly the same statistics were employed, by key figures such as John Simon, the first Chief Medical Officer, to make the opposite argument in favour of vaccination's efficacy. Such was the revolt against compulsory vaccination that, for the duration of the Royal Commission into the matter, between 1889 and 1896, enforcement of the law was held in abeyance. On an unprecedented scale, the population had declared itself more afraid of the state's handling of measures against the spread of smallpox than of smallpox itself. This despite a devastating epidemic in 1870–1.

Domestic difficulties aside, the British undertook their own colonial vaccination voyages, notably around the Indian subcontinent, a country where Jenner was lauded for having reined in an angry God. As with the voyages of Balmis, there are unspoken stories of mistrust, suffering and the dynamics of colonial power. While the vaccination of large swathes of the British Empire was generally greeted among medical and governmental establishments as a positive force, doubtless the vaccine itself was often administered to populations who feared what it might do, as well as the authority of those delivering it.[32] Those Indian vaccination voyages depended, in large part, on the use of subaltern orphan children as vaccinifers in order to keep the vaccine alive in tropical conditions.[33] Accorded less attention than the experimental animals of the physiological laboratory, or the animal batteries in which vaccines were first generated before being distributed among the population, their experiences have to be reclaimed from what was never said or recorded.

The story of vaccination in the long nineteenth century serves as a useful lens for scrutinizing how new public-health politics and the nuts and bolts of public-health administration were received by a public which, by and large, was meant passively to receive what the state had deemed fit for it. In the case of those without power, there was little choice but to comply, irrespective of the world of uncertainty in which they found themselves. Others complained loudly, and long, and to some extent succeeded in pushing back against checks on the liberty and authority of private citizens. Those victories, which saw the relaxation of laws concerning compulsory vaccination, for example, might have been experienced not so much as triumphs for the principle of liberty as they were a release from a great existential fear: fear of the medical state.

PERFORMANCE

Between Christmas and New Year 1874, John Hudson, the Staff Surgeon of the emigrant ship *Earl Dalhousie*, on its way to Adelaide from London via Plymouth, found himself dealing with sixteen cases of hysterical tetanus. It was not so much a ship of fools, according to his report in *The Lancet* (1875), as it was a vessel of sexual deviance, fraudulent posturing and feminine nervousness. The epidemic was precipitated by one Susan Bickford, a twenty-two-year old who betrayed 'signs of good and evil training, such as bad language and pretty hymns'. She had spent time in the workhouse, given birth at fifteen (though her child was not with her) and was a 'victim of nymphomania'. Lest that phrase mislead, the nymphomania was her own. Her problems, according to Hudson, stemmed from compulsive masturbation. At the peak of her hysteria, Bickford would fall into convulsions that would eventually result in 'complete and general rigidity [opisthotonos], the body being arched backwards, so as to rest on the head and heels'. The presentation was of tetanus, a disease known by its posture, not by a specific pathogen (the tetanus bacillus was only discovered in 1884, and the transmissibility of the disease worked out only in 1890). Yet the surgeon looked upon it as malingering, attention-seeking and deceit. Nevertheless, this hysterical tetanus was remarkably contagious – a function of 'sympathy' rather than any more modern notion of contagion – quickly affecting others among the female passengers, with twelve cases occurring on a single day. The medical perception of these manifestations of tetanus can be summed up by their characterization as 'delusions and vagaries . . . feigning and deception', in individuals marked by 'uterine weakness' and sexual depravity. Hudson summed up the cause of all the cases as 'probably emotional, and the nature of each apparently a reflex action of the nervous centres'. That these postures might have signalled a genuine illness, or an authentic expression of pain, was not entertained. Nevertheless, the women all recovered once they had been diagnosed and treated with a range of methods and materials, including chloral hydrate, potassium bromide, henbane, valerian, aperients, bleeding, cold compresses and isolation. In Bickford's case, the moral exhortation to cease masturbating roused her from her symptoms.

To understand why, we have to go back to the beginning of the nineteenth century. The Scottish surgeon Charles Bell published his *Essays on the Anatomy of Expression in Painting* in 1806, the implications of which went far beyond the world of art. This is perhaps implicit in the republication of the work, in

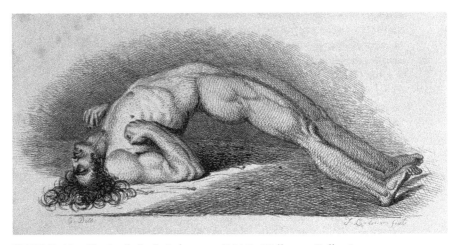

FIGURE 6.3: Charles Bell, *Opisthotonos* (1844). Wellcome Collection

1824, as *The Anatomy and Philosophy of Expression*. Central to Bell's treatise was a critique of the deficiencies of artists throughout history, but in equal measure he used the art-historical record to spot cases of fraudulent illness and disease, as if providing a guide for differential diagnosis. The classic case in this regard was of the arched form indicative of tetanus (see Figure 6.3).

The tetanic arch was, in earlier times, a signifier of demonic possession rather than a worldly pathology. Bell examined the depictions of such arched postures in various artistic representations, finding that, in most examples, the body was in an unnatural position, indicating fraud on the part of the afflicted. True tetanus, he observed, was uniform and unmistakeable. This was long before the tetanus bacillus was discovered. Tetanus literally described the bodily posture, rather than a specific pathogen, leaving it open for sufferers of all descriptions to exploit. With Bell's help, the imposters were supposed to be easy to spot. The trouble was that such arched contortions were steadily on the rise throughout the nineteenth century, coming to represent a classic sign, not of possession, but of hysteria. For physicians, telling the difference between tetanus and hysterical tetanus was a diagnostic challenge.

The historian of experience asks how it is that a distinct sign of illness can suddenly become widespread, when the illness itself does not directly cause such a sign. The cause of hysteria was still debated throughout the nineteenth century, with some still pointing to uterine mobility, others to nymphomania, and others still to psychological disorders. In general, however, it was understood that hysteria was not a somatic disease so much as a problem that inhered in the female constitution. There was nothing in it, however, to suggest that it should manifest as tetanus. Yet throughout the period in question, more and more women were identified as hysterics precisely because they fell into arched postures that were, in appearance, extremely painful.

While historical research has shown that the hysterical arch was effectively coached into hysterical patients by doctors who specifically sought out its appearance – in particular the noted neurologist Jean-Martin Charcot at the Salpêtrière hospital in Paris – this has tended to lead to analyses of medical authority and the vagaries of transference.[34] On the patient side, however, there remains more to say. The arch of hysteria may not have been directly connected to a medical cause, but its appearance nevertheless did often signal the beginnings of recovery. I have theorized elsewhere (2017a) that such physical gestures were unconscious efforts to match an expression of an inward feeling – of despair, depression, grief and so on – to a readily understandable prescribed gestural script. Extending William Reddy's (2001: 128) formulation of the 'emotive' as a process whereby an individual tries to match a feeling to an acceptable expression of emotion, I have proposed that similar work is done in the clinical setting matching a sense of ill feeling to an acceptable appearance of disease. Hysterical patients, especially in the third quarter of the nineteenth century, found succour in correctly achieving the posture sought by their physicians. Far from the fraudulence imputed by Bell, these patients found comfort for their genuine distress by conforming to a diagnosable representation that was assented to by the medical establishment. This convergence of illness feeling and disease rule had a positive effect on the initial feeling, for the simple recognition of a problem was often sufficient to begin to be able to alleviate it.

How did the women aboard *Earl Dalhousie* know the script? I suspect Bickford herself had direct knowledge of the hysterical arch, having spent time in the workhouse asylum in her youth. Her situation was personally and financially perilous, and doubtless the voyage itself was a significant additional source of anxiety. She was alone, escaping a life of difficulty, but heading to another of great uncertainty, and loaded with baggage of past trauma of giving birth as a child and then having to give up that child. She broke down on board and gave expression to her illness in a way that was likely to garner her medical attention. The diagnosis of nymphomania supplied her with a recovery plan that, having nothing really to do with the cause of her initial distress, nevertheless ushered her condition into a medical-moral category that could be treated. The simple fact of diagnosis and treatment was doubtless sufficient attention to begin a successful recovery. This emotive process, completed through bodily 'performance', brought the experience of the medical personnel and the experiences of the patient into accord. Such was the dynamic (and entirely unwitting) process of placebo at work. The other women, seeing both the drama of the tetanus posture and the attention it received from the medical authorities on board, quickly succumbed to its power. This is not to say that they consciously performed their hysterical arches, but rather that their emotional problems found succour in a script that a ship's surgeon could interpret.

Contemporary medicine understands the beneficial power of diagnosis as part of a broader and growing understanding of the science of placebo.[35] The invention of an hysterical script on the front lines of alienist and proto-psychiatric medicine helped frame the experience of hysteria for the hysteric. For a brief period, great hopes were raised for the treatment of hysteria as a readily recognized form of faux tetanus. The benefits were short lived. Once the tetanus bacillus was discovered, the disease ceased to be defined by its posture and became distinctly associated with its pathological cause. With real tetanus now clinically distinct, hysterical tetanus was taken less seriously as a manifestation of disease. As the medical script changed, and as physicians no longer looked for the arch as a sign of hysteria, so hysteric patients looked for other ways to find purchase with the institutions of medicine.

The gendering of this particular script should not be overlooked, the well-known presence of a cohort of hysterical men under Charcot's gaze notwithstanding.[36] Women presenting with tetanus were much more likely to be written off as hysterics than men, who would in many cases be treated for tetanus itself. Even long after tetanus had become a distinct disease caused by an identified bacterium, men presenting with cases of hysterical tetanus were generally more likely to be believed. Arthur Hurst (1918: 581) pointed out that war surgeons were troubled by mysterious cases of localized tetanus (in the hand, for example) in patients who had been vaccinated. Medical researchers wasted time looking for new forms of tetanus to explain these presentations, when they should have been 'curable at a single sitting by psychotherapy'.

These stories of hysteria and tetanus, of finding a posture to fit a pathology, are indicative of wider trends in the long nineteenth century for psychological disorders. Similar narratives could be constructed for the sufferers of 'railway spine' and their doctors, for the nostalgic (literally, those suffering from home pain), for the neurasthenics who were affected by the electricity and energy of the modern city, and for the victims of 'shell shock', whose nervous conditions were causally connected to material circumstances rather than to an authentic trauma of the mind.[37] The 'discontents' of civilization, as Freud (2002) would style them, strove to find scripts they could perform that they might find an audience in the medical establishment, and that they might find a course of treatment to help them out of their own ongoing traumatic experience. That the audience they found fell largely outside of the medical establishment, and within the rapidly expanding world of psychiatry, suggests the very limited extent to which medical authorities sought to understand and to treat emotional trauma as a medical condition in its own right.

KNOWING HOW TO FEEL

This brief account homes in on the quality of experience in an era in which imperial nationhood and medicine were becoming much more closely intertwined, both in terms of the administration of public health and in terms of new medical politics and philosophies. I characterize this period as one where the institutions of medicine became much more present in the lives of the public, but where the public viewed that increasing presence with suspicion, even outright fear. An era defined by the quest to defeat pain and disease was also marked by new kinds of suffering and novel methods of objectifying and instrumentalizing individuals. In the nitty gritty of these medical encounters, the experiences of medical personnel often obfuscate those of patients and subjects of medical research. That does not mean, however, that the latter cannot be reclaimed.

It is impossible to characterize the experience of medicine, even when delimited to the dynamic encounter and the journey, for all people and for every case. What I have sketched here leaves out far more than it contains. Nevertheless, there is here an outline for the way in which the history of experience might be approached as a central part of the cultural history of medicine in the long nineteenth century. It depends on an ability to hear the silences in the medical archival record, or else to find testimony in non-traditional places. It depends on a willingness to take at face value, or at least to try to understand the face value, of subjective accounts of pain and fear, and to interpret novel embodiments of illness as authentic statements about subjective experiences of illness. It depends on a willingness to try to capture the sensory experience of the encounter, the distances between touching and being felt, listening and being heard, seeing and being seen. And it depends on an acceptance that (emotional) experience is itself contingent on the 'context of possibilities', subject to the available repertoire of knowledge and expression of a given time and place.[38] Perhaps the most fruitful way to open up those possibilities is to challenge, in historical context, one of the most basic health-related questions. The question 'How are you?', or more tellingly, 'How do you feel?' seems straightforward enough. Anybody might readily give an answer. But if how one feels is intrinsically tied to the cultural context in which one is embedded, to the available scripts one has to guide expression, then it becomes a legitimate task to try to discover how one knows how one feels. When historians carry out this task for past actors, we open up a rich experiential seam to mine in the cultural history of medicine.

NOTES

1. The pathfinding studies in the history of the senses were Classen 1993 and Corbin 1995. A sense of the scale of the undertaking of a history of experience was realized in Classen 2014.

2. For an appraisal of this challenge, in even broader terms, see Condrau 2007.
3. The latter question goes beyond the human, the experience of the medical-experimental animal being one of the chief challenges of the post-human turn in the humanities and social sciences. See Boddice 2012, 2016; Gray 2014; Kirk 2016.
4. An approach encouraged initially by Porter 1985, and picked up latterly by Condrau 2007.
5. It is decidedly different from previous strands of historiography that were conducted under the umbrella of the 'history of experience' and should be thought of as a new historiographical departure. See Boddice and Smith 2020.
6. See Rees 2014 and Willenfelt 2014 for two entirely different approaches to this problem. The connection between the history of emotions and the history of experience has recently been elaborated. See Moscoso and Zaragoza 2014; Moscoso 2016; Boddice and Smith 2020.
7. For an appraisal of the 'somatic turn' and the implications of finding the history of the body, see Cooter 2010.
8. On neuroscience and emotion, see Feldman Barrett 2006, 2006a; on neuroscience and pain, see Eisenberger 2003; on placebo, see Mogil et al. 2015 and Hall et al. 2015. For an historical theorization of how to apply all of this, see Smail 2008.
9. See Boddice 2017, ch. 7; Boddice and Smail 2018.
10. See Moore 2005: 136.
11. The best account of specialization is Weisz 2006; for examples of fear of experimental medicine and the medical professional, see Lansbury 1985; Willis 2006; Boddice 2016: 56–71; Boddice, 2021.
12. For a much broader context of utilitarianism and medical ethics, see Gere 2017.
13. For a careful review of the class and race implications of the ethics of anaesthetic usage around mid-century, see Wall 2006.
14. For the emotions of surgeons before the age of anaesthesia, see Brown 2017; for the post-anaesthetic era, see Boddice 2016: 49–52, 72–92; Schlich 2007; White 2006.
15. The famous passage of David Hume is quoted in Mercer 1972: 31. Adam Smith's version is in Smith 2009: 45.
16. Here, the worlds of surgery and physiology were drawing on aesthetic theories of emotional projection, particularly in the consumption of art. See Burdett 2011, 2011a.
17. See the extended discussion of this in Boddice 2016: 49–52, 72–92.
18. See, for example, Lambert 1962.
19. For a general overview, see French 1975 (vivisection) and Porter and Porter 1988 (vaccination). For an approach to the feelings of medical researchers in this context, see Boddice 2016, 2021; White 2006, 2009.
20. Boddice 2012, 2014a; Lederer 1995.
21. For an overview of the literature here, see Boddice 2011, 2021
22. For a general overview of the distinct relation of German doctors to the state, the law and the public, see Weindling 1991; Maehle 2009.
23. For an introduction that particularly focuses on experience, see Moscoso 2012. See also Bourke 2014a; Boddice 2017.
24. See Wood 2012; Marland 2006; Wolf 2009; Leavitt and Walton 1984.
25. Devine 2014: 314, n. 134; Bourke 2014.

26. See also Goldberg 2012 for a general appraisal of the historical attitude towards pain without lesion.
27. For accounts of Balmis's voyage, see Aldrete 2004; Tuells 2002; Tuells and Martin 2011; Franco-Paredes and Lammoglia 2005.
28. Cook and Lovell 2001.
29. The long-durée story is told by Kitta 2011.
30. For Rio, see Sevcenko 2010; for Toronto see Arnup 1992.
31. For Leicester, see Fraser 1980. For a general account of working-class resistance to compulsory vaccination, see Durbach 2004. For the account of maimed and killed children, see Murdoch 2015a.
32. See Arnold 1993; Brimnes 2004; Bhattacharya 1998; Bhattacharya et al. 2005.
33. See Murdoch 2015.
34. See Charcot 1877; Gilman 1993; Furst 2008; Scull 2009; Micale 1995.
35. The potential for historians to revisit this subject are vast, if we consider the recent findings of Hall et al. 2015 and Mogil et al. 2015, about the cultural and genetic plasticity of placebo response.
36. See Micale 2008; Showalter 1985; Stirling 2010.
37. On railway spine, see Erichsen 1867; Goldberg 2017; on neurasthenia, see Kenny 2015; Killen 2005; on shell shock, see Bourke 1996: 107–22.
38. The phrase is a coinage of Hernández Brotons 2017: 20, in turn drawing on Koselleck. See Boddice and Smith 2020 for a full elaboration.

CHAPTER SEVEN

Mind/Brain

REBECCA WYNTER AND STEPHEN T. CASPER

In 1865, T. Fenton wrote to *The American Phrenological Journal and Life Illustrated* to take issue with J. McM., an earlier correspondent to the periodical. The nature of mind and brain was at the centre of Fenton's complaint. McM. had argued, '"The musician cannot play if his instrument is broken." True, not on *that* instrument,' responded Fenton as he began to draw on metaphors that would become familiar between 1800 and 1920, 'yet recollect the instrument may be broken, yet *not the musician* ... Phrenologists and physiologists compare the brain with a galvanic battery ... a very good comparison; but a battery has an operator, and cannot act without his positive will.' Even so, Fenton complimented McM.: 'he makes us think, and very few writers do that; they take the softer food that saves chewing; but the chewing saves the teeth, and the teeth help the digestive system, and the system makes the man' (Fenton 1865).

The separation of 'Mind/Brain' reflected in this exchange carries with it the baggage of centuries of the Western philosophy of mind. Of course the intellectual tensions between the two – articulated by René Descartes (1596–1650) and later Immanuel Kant (1724–1804) – shaped culture. However, in this chapter we will go beyond these traditional philosophies. Fenton's analogies point to more variegated and time-specific cultural meanings for mind and brain. We will here consider how the two were conveyed, understood and manifested in culture, from institutions, medical treatises and poems, to ideas surrounding race, class, disability and gender. In doing so, like McM., we hope to offer food for thought.

Since the 1960s the historiography of mind and brain medicine and science has been dominated by key figures who emphasized the mind in the modern world. Located close to the Annales school and channelling the anti-psychiatry movement, the French philosopher-historian Michel Foucault asserted that 'madness' was a social construct, built through discourse and dialectically thrown into sharp relief by Enlightenment reason. It was caught, like a fly, by the web of power and surveillance apparatus of the modern state in a so-called 'Great Confinement' (Foucault 1961/1995). Andrew Scull rejected Foucault's thesis in 1979: there was no social control, no determined, unilateral and organized move to shut away the 'mad'. Instead, a land grab by professionalizing 'alienists' (proto-psychiatrists) created a novel nineteenth-century empire – asylumdom (Scull, 1979).

Employing in response a politically-aware social history, Roy Porter and Elaine Showalter excavated patient experience. Porter (1985, 1987/1990, 1987/1996) called for the 'patient's view', and enthusiastically employed an array of sources to retrieve it. Feminist historian Showalter (1987), taking hysteria as her object, demonstrated the construction of a diagnostic category through cultural material. Some, like Patrick McDonagh (2008), also embraced eclecticism. Others, such as Sander Gilman (1982) and Rick Rylance (2000), concentrated on specific source types to analyse cultural perceptions of mind. However, like the subjects of their work, many historians have stayed locked in the asylum. Nevertheless, institutional studies continue to inform our understanding of the mind in the long nineteenth century (see bibliography).

Within the historiography of mind medicine, the brain has been sidelined, though the influence of the history of the body is beginning to change that (for example, Wallis 2017). In comparison to the history of psychiatry, the history of neurology has been only modestly investigated. L. Stephen Jacyna and others have charted the intellectual and professional development of neurology, neurosurgery and neuroscience. Jacyna and Casper (2012) also co-edited the first text to consider the neurological patient's perspective. Moreover, there has been a wider shift in scholarship that has enabled voices from outside the academy to intervene through politically-informed histories that challenge medical models of psychological and neurological difference (see Silberman 2015).

With the mainstreaming of medical humanities, there has also been a deeper willingness to engage with other cultural histories of mind and brain in the 'Age of Empire', with mixed success. *Neurology and Modernity*, edited by Laura Salisbury and Andrew Shail (2010), captured major themes, including railway spine and shell shock. Andrew Scull (2015) published *Madness in Civilization: A Cultural History of Insanity*, which found an intersection between neurology and psychiatry. Considerations of literary, visual and material cultures have certainly gathered pace since 2000 (see Coleborne and McKinnon 2011; Guenther and Hess (eds) 2016; Kaes 2010; Rose 2004; Sirotkina 2002; Stiles, Finger and Boller (eds) 2013; Wynter 2011). Nonetheless, the cultural history of mind and brain together remains virtually untouched.

In what follows, we offer a tentative beginning. We first suggest familiar spaces in which cultures of mind and brain can be readily located (and localized). We then discuss less demarcated terrain, observing how histories have ignored reciprocally weighing meaning across colonial and colonized borderlands, treating routes shaping 'mind' and 'brain' as one-way streets. Such blind spots appear also in the treatment of the two as matters of high culture – low-brow constructions might well have exercised power in shaping mind and brain throughout the nineteenth century. In our final section, we shift in tone and emphasis to propose further avenues for historical research.

SITES AND LOCALIZATION

In 1800, in Aveyron, France, a boy walked out of the woods and into the nineteenth century. Previous attempts had been made to adopt him. The feral child, estimated to be around twelve, however, left the wild and entered civilization of his own accord. Victor, as he became known, embodied the collision of two principle themes of the European Enlightenment: nature/nurture and reason/unreason. As such, the partially-successful work of Dr Jean Marc Gaspard Itard to teach and socialize the developmentally-delayed 'Wild Boy of Aveyron' represented the murky borderlands of both Enlightenment dichotomies (for more on Victor's cultural impact, see McDonagh 2008). Underpinning them lay mind and brain.

The eighteenth century had witnessed a great interrogation of 'mind' and 'brain'. In Britain and France the zeitgeist manifested in a shift in the treatment of those labelled as 'lunatic': an ancient catch-all term for people considered to have had mental illness, neurological issues and developmental, learning disabilities, which carried into the modern period archaic notions of moon madness. Progressive practice was present elsewhere, from the seventeenth-century care and 'musical therapy' of Ottoman hospitals in Turkey (Narter 2006), to St Luke's Hospital, London, opened in 1751 (Smith 2007). But it was The Retreat at York, in northern England, and Paris's Bicêtre and Salpêtrière hospitals at the cusp of the nineteenth century that have come to represent the change (see Digby 1985). Indeed, the Paris sites acquired the story that revolutionary inspiration had persuaded senior physician Philippe Pinel to break the manacles of the insane (see Foucault 1961/1995, Weiner 1994).

In Portugal and Britain the subject of a distracted mind acquired political significance through the illnesses of Maria I (1734–1816) and George III (1738–1820). The angst surrounding the king's ill health seeped into press coverage, cartoons, poems, material culture and religious services (Macalpine and Hunter 1969; Agland 2009). If the monarch was appointed by God, and something of God was present in everyone, including those who had lost their reason (as the Tukes, Quaker founders of the Retreat, believed), then a 'crack'd brain' did not mean an irrevocably broken mind. Thus – and following the much wider pattern of specialization – the 1800s initiated the Western emergences of psychiatry, neurology and psychology, all fields which emerged as autonomous areas of expertise in the early twentieth century.

In post-revolutionary France, educated people remained suspicious of pronouncements about mind and brain that hinted at revolutionary ideologies, particularly the sensationalist psychology that had coincided with Jacobin excesses. They were equally cautious of welcoming mechanistic or deterministic discoveries. Romantic French culture envisaged a free-willed body. Such elite efforts, as described by historian Jan Goldstein (1987), indicated that the psyche was a contested subject in nineteenth-century Europe.

In such circumstances, legal cultures stepped in and helped shape the meanings of mind and brain. Clemency for 'the mad' and recognition that free will could be compromised had been built into religious and legal codes around the world, including the Jewish Talmud and traditional Chinese tenets. Enlightenment legal systems posited that courts should take into account the state of mind at the time of the offence. Many nations followed Britain's lead, especially after the 1800 ruling that one of George III's attempted regicides, James Hadfield, was not guilty by reason of insanity. The precedent was rigorously tested in court in 1843; the resultant M'Naghton Rule 'created a common law standard in many countries'. A defendant was not held accountable if 'labouring under such defect of reason, from disease of mind as not to know the nature and quality of the act he was doing; or if he did "know" it, that he did not know what he was doing was wrong' (Simon and Ahn-Redding 2006: 7). What these precedents, manifesting a 'lesion of the will', actually meant was controversial. As such, these trials and the refinement of how someone in or out of their 'right' mind behaved was determined by cultural factors, including emotion and physiological response (Dixon 2012; Bates 2016). Historian Joel Eigen (1995, 2003, 2016) has revealed the involvement of lay and medical witnesses, lawyers and judges in producing what constituted 'insanity' and the edges of consciousness through assessments of fugue states. However, such explorations of feelings and substantial studies of courtroom actors have been largely limited to Britain and North America (Moran, 2019; Rosenberg 1995).

Mind and emotion were rendered further visible by phrenologists, among them German-born Franz Joseph Gall (1758–1828), Johann Spurzheim (1776–1832) and Englishman George Combe (1788–1858). Their itinerant work and their supporters generated the collection of skulls and circulation of specialist journals in Africa and Asia, with ideas disseminated by penny post and translated into Bengali and Japanese. It has been argued that phrenology was a 'global scientific movement' (Poskett 2016), but while key phrenologists may well have had worldwide reach, the plasticity of the central theory meant there were

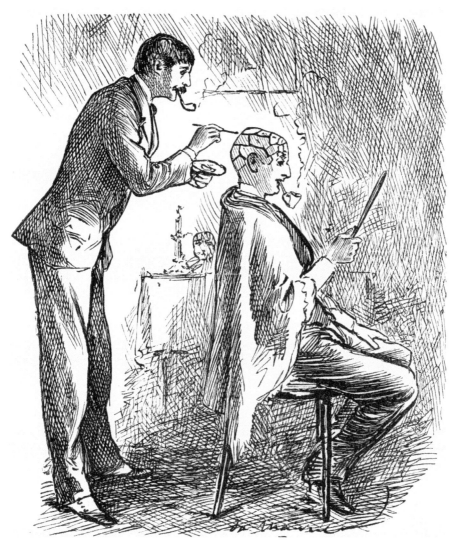

FIGURE 7.1: George du Maurier, 'New Idea for a Fancy Ball. Shave your head, and go as a phrenological bust', *Punch Magazine*, 22 June 1878. Private Collection / Look and Learn / George Collection / Bridgeman Images.

many phrenologies and dichotomous deployments (see Figure 7.1). In some sites, the doctrine fixed the nature and the constitution of human beings in the physiognomy of the body. Elsewhere, such as the north-eastern United States, the ability to localize human weakness and aptitudes promoted equality of opportunity. Phrenologies offered enlightened subjects self-improvement or social reform.

Mind and brain were also fixed in a particular Anglo-French political economy. Such Enlightenment philosophers as the Marquis de Condorcet (1743–94) and Erasmus Darwin (1731–1802) had imagined unchaining the downtrodden by enabling the cultivation of mind. Some industrialists and thinkers – Robert Owen (1771–1858), Charles Fourier's (1772–1837) or Étienne Cabet's (1788–1856) disciples – had followed, building new versions of social harmonies and novel, yet ephemeral, utopian cultures of mind (see Pitzner 1997; Claeys and Sargent (eds) 1999). Less transient was, for example, the work of Édouard Séguin, a pupil of Itard and influenced by Henri de Saint-Simon's utopian socialism. Establishing a school for children with learning disabilities in Paris in 1840, and publishing *Traitement Moral, Hygiène, et Education des Idiots* (1846), Seguin later emigrated to America, taking his practices and ideas about mind and brain with him.

Such cooperative ideologies clashed with laissez-faire, Liberal-Whig, and Malthusian counterweights that emerged contemporaneously. These invited questions about natural order and predicted, not social improvement, but demographic miseries following benevolence (Hale 2014). The mind's natural sympathy was made suspect by its rationality (Musselman 2012). The brain, observed German philosopher Georg Hegel in 1807, was a source of an 'existential form of self-conscious individuality' (Hegel 1939/2003: 189). Its emotions had to be checked by cultural mores that later defined Victorian sensibility (Oppenheim 1991).

The sites and localizations of mind and brain appear to have flowed from the broader political, legal, industrial and economic context that made the modern European world. Nineteenth-century metaphors connected machines to the natural forces of the nervous system, particularly supply and demand (Lawrence 1979; Oppenheim 1991: 74). Market forces were also evident in the expansion of facilities for the treatment of the minds and brains for which the modern world had become too much. Across Europe had existed public facilities for people considered 'unmanageable' or dangerous due to their mental states, including the archetypal Bethlem, London, whose bowdlerized name ('Bedlam') embedded a grimy, sensational image of institutionalized mental health care in modern culture.

From the eighteenth century, these public sites began to be supplemented more determinedly, and not only by those alms- or workhouses whose authorities found it necessary, cheaper or more convenient to retain 'the mad' poor. As the corpulent Scottish doctor George Cheyne was postulating that 'Riot, Luxury . . . [and] Excess' had stimulated 'Nervous Diseases', including his own (Cheyne 1733: 49), in England the so-called 'trade in lunacy' responded to a new wave of fragile minds. While Germany maintained public sites, France also began to witness the increase of private *maisons de santé* to support public facilities like Salpêtrière.

With little regulation and the lure of profit, the comparative number of private madhouses in England outstripped elsewhere. Alarm about the detention of sane people proliferated as swiftly, and eventually legislation enabled public alternatives inspired by a charitable institution. The York Retreat was noticeably different from general hospitals in this period. It was established by Quakers for Quakers. Its entire design and ethos was rooted in faith practices. Plainness in surroundings, connection to the natural world, nourishing food, non-violent intervention, useful activity and the sort of peacefulness that Friends employed to hear God and conscience were built into the site (for more, see Akehurst, 2020). This simplicity, which can be clearly discerned in the image of the Retreat (see Figures 7.2 and 7.3), refined as 'moral management', became the Western ideal for care, and was exported to the Americas, Australia, Africa and Asia.

It is ironic that the enlightened asylum was a hybrid of English nonconformist religious practice and French Revolutionary ideals, and went on to be a cultural form of modernity. Its pastoral image and location were often used to counteract both the picture conjured by 'Bedlam' and the life stresses and dislocation visited by industrialization and urbanization. Moreover, their physical presence in the landscape meant that asylums became cultural beacons for mind and

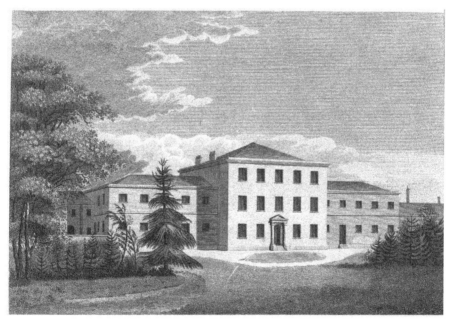

FIGURE 7.2: 'A View of the North Front of the Retreat near York', frontispiece, Samuel Tuke, *Description of the Retreat, an institution near York, for insane persons of the Society of Friends : containing an account of its origin and progress, the modes of treatment, and a statement of cases* (York, 1813). Wellcome Collection.

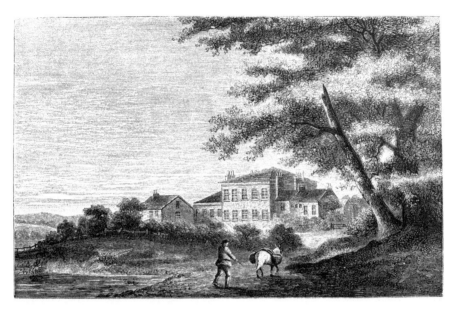

FIGURE 7.3: 'The original buildings. The Retreat', in Daniel Hack Tuke, *Chapters in the History of the Insane in the British Isles* (London: Kegan Paul, 1882). Wellcome Library, London.

brain medicine and science. Through specialist professional publications – including France's *Annales médico-psychologiques* (established 1843), *The American Journal of Insanity* (later *Psychiatry*, 1844), and Britain's *Asylum Journal* (1853, later renamed the *Journal of Mental Science*) – therapeutic ideas were disseminated and taxonomies of alienated minds and brains were established. Foundational textbooks or 'diagnostic bibles' began to take shape. The first of global importance was Britons John C. Bucknill and Daniel Hack Tuke's *Manual of Psychological Medicine* (1858), superseded after 1883 by German psychiatrist Emil Kraepelin's *Compendium der Psychiatrie*. Even so, the reception of such texts could be greeted by parochial cultures; the *Compendium* was 'designed for the German student in psychiatry, [but could not] fail to prove useful to the English medical psychologist', who '[found] it necessary to know the conclusions arrived at by a nation – or, at least, its psychologists – having such a singular aptitude for delicate psychological distinctions', presumably in comparison to 'the classification of the psychoses' arrived at by '"German Retrospect"' (Anon. 1886: 254). All the same, in their professional development those English psychologists would soon be known by the German word, psychiatrists.

Writings that developed professional cultures, understandings of mind and brain and cultures of treatment and containment were not the only literature to emerge from lunatic asylums. Some, like the early poetry of private madhouse keeper William Perfect (1737–1809) and the literary criticism of non-restraint pioneer John Conolly (1794–1866), was produced by physicians themselves. Patients also wrote, from John Clare's (1793–1864) poems to in-house magazines, such as the Royal Edinburgh Asylum's *Morningside Mirror* and *The Opal* of New York State's Utica. Indeed, institutions for 'lunatics' were both producers and consumers of culture in the long nineteenth century, as historian Benjamin Reiss (2008) also observed (see also Clark 2015; Harpin and Foster (eds) 2014). Painting and folk art emanated from the asylum; reading, music, dances and handicrafts took place there, in part as therapeutic occupations; theatre troupes, bands, amateur sports teams and fashions crossed into and actively contributed to institutional cultures and offered asylums a richer and even a more culturally-specific and locally-embedded identity.

The arts provided extensive illustrations of the mind and brain as cultural preoccupations well beyond asylum walls. American Emily Dickinson's poems (1830–86), for example, served up a relative anatomy of brain and mind (Baumgartner 2016; Sielke 2008) and in *c.* 1861 the loss of reason as 'a Funeral, in my Brain'. The worried, depicted by Dickinson, were middle class and Romantic – tragic individuals with brains of unlimited capacities grappling with the metaphoric and metonymic. Within thirty years of Dickinson's real funeral, Romantic struggles were long lost in the mud of the First World War. In 'Mental Cases' (1918), poet Wilfred Owen – himself invalided briefly to Scotland's Craiglockhart War Hospital for officers with 'mental' or 'nervous' issues, under anthropologist, neurologist and psychiatrist William Rivers – described 'men whose minds the Dead have ravished'. The poem has come to symbolize one great cultural marker of the 1914–18 war: shell shock, a condition partially constructed by the new psychoanalytical theories of Austrian Sigmund Freud.

Beyond a loss of reason lurked other horrors for the consumers of literature in the long nineteenth century. Mary Shelley's *Frankenstein* (1818) intimated at the use of electricity to reanimate what was construed in the post-Napoleonic world as the latent animal electricity of the body. Alexandre Dumas's *The Count of Monte Cristo*, published on the eve of the 1848 revolutions, caricatured the dissolution of volition after M. de Villefort's stroke. Paralysis appeared with similar terror in Émile Zola's *Thérèse Raquin* (1867). Indeed, the subject provoked such concern that some began to create hospitals serving their needs, including Johanna Chandler's foundation of London's National Hospital for the Paralysed and Epileptic in 1859.

Bram Stoker's *Dracula* (1897) developed further horror by constructing an agent without free will, the vampire, a materialization of the 1870s cortical localization theories of Gustav Fritsch, Eduard Hitzig and David Ferrier. Such animal behaviour also characterized the addict, a figure who appeared in the fiction of Samuel Coleridge (1772–1834), Thomas De Quincy (1785–1859) and Wilkie Collins (1824–89). Collins's *Woman in White* (1859) immortalized yet another persistent terror of the Enlightenment imagination that recurred frequently in the long nineteenth century: a sane person locked in a lunatic asylum. This trope – drawn directly from ex-patients' exposés (a distinct and persistent feature of Western mental health care), and from the pages of newspapers (see Reinarz and Wynter 2015; Scull 2015; Wynter 2015) – reveals that madness was a cultural concern and the subject of art throughout the century. Masterpieces devoted to madness – from Alexander Pushkin's *The Bronze Horseman* (1833) and Charlotte Brontë's *Jane Eyre* (1847) to Kate Chopin's *Awakening* (1899) – seemed to dominate European and North American readerships, and circulated anywhere a cosmopolitan readership could be found.

Perhaps the most inventive of these nineteenth-century literary endeavours was the shift from stimulating the mind to localizing visceral embodied experiences. As historian James Kennaway has described, these 'pathological dimensions' were evident in music and exercised medical opinion throughout the century (Kennaway 2012: 69). By 1900, musical audiences in cafés and salons turned to the melancholic music of Chopin or Debussy in order to reflect somewhat psychoanalytically upon their interior emotions, doubtlessly aided by narcotics, alcohol, nicotine, chocolate and caffeine. Yet the spine-tingling and hair-raising corporeal experience invented by the gothic authors was of a different order, and moved towards a modernist style that sought to elicit physically erotic reflexes, epitomized by, for example, the writings of D. H. Lawrence (1885–1930).

These currents were reflected in individual composers' own lives. Hector Berlioz, for example, in his 1830 *Symphonie fantastique*, used his gigantic orchestral arrangement as a self-styled confessional of his own *maladie morale* 'characterized by melancholy, nervous "exultation", black presentiments, and a malignant *idee fixe*' (Brittan 2006: 211). Rimsky-Korsakov during one of his droughts of production developed crippling neurasthenia (Abraham 1945: 30), which some critics later saw in the 'deep-rooted tendency to cover his inspiration and emotional traces' in his music (Walsh 2003: 68–9). Discord could even appear with literal force in musical composition as it did in the years before 1914 – for instance, Stravinsky's multi-tonal harmonies that defined much of his oeuvre and rang, in Adorno's words, with an abiding 'schizophrenia' (Weiztman 1974: 294).

Art was no less saturated by cultural references to mind and brain, and also moved from early nineteenth-century emotional studies towards multi-perspectivism on the eve of the First World War. J. M. W. Turner (1755–1851), the famous landscape painter, whose works conjured emotional textures in their subject matter, found patronage and friendship through Thomas Monro, chief physician at Bethlem (Abell 2009: 84). Turner inspired art for the rest of the century. Yet as the unromaticized truth of artistic Realism lost out to the fictitious realism of photography, the arguments of the Impressionists and Cubists began to resonate with a clearer vindication of the claim that reality came in bits and pieces (Novak 2003: 3). Through photographs and staining innovations, Santiago Ramón y Cajal (1899) demonstrated that the sensory central nervous system fragmented reality into components, then reconstructed from human perception. The point was made more clearly by Guirand de Scevola, who developed First World War camouflage paint by drawing inspiration from Pablo Picasso and others 'who, because of their very special vision, had an aptitude for denaturing any kind of form' (Kern 2003: 303).

The nineteenth-century cultural footprint of mind and brain far surpassed these artistic touchstones. Philosophical contemplations, medical and scientific investigations and banal conversation brought mind and nerves into everyday parlance. As historian Roger Smith has shown, Victorians' inhibited passions fashioned a theory of inhibition of the nervous system, which then reaffirmed the ideals of self-control and self-governance and cast their lack as evidence of a weakened nervous system (Smith 1992). Jean-Martin Charcot's (1825–93) hysterical women and Silas Weir Mitchell's (1829–1914) neurasthenic men became proof of these principles. Such constructions of nervousness came before lay audiences in numerous ways. *Good Housekeeping*, for instance, described in 1914 a bodily neurology in which a 'ganglia of the sympathetic system make a protest that is heard at the headquarters in the brain. Hence your headaches, your indigestion, your feelings of apprehension and depression, your wakefulness at night and lassitude by day, your irritability and "nervousness"' (Hirshbein 2009: 17–18).

Mind and brain as frames of reference and metaphors worked similarly on the industrial city. The creation of public spaces, for example, was meant to salve the minds of newly-urbanized peoples. The Paris Menagerie became a place for public and scientific encounters with animal intelligence (Jacyna 2017). For Honoré de Balzac (1799–1850), these encounters would subsequently frame other exotic and sensual encounters with non-Europeans (Kelly 2011). Conversely, Istanbul's Taksim Gardens (opened in 1869) was crafted in a Parisian style and was meant to showcase the modernizing Ottoman bureaucratic mind. Yet this public park, as other spaces, also asserted an orderly set of relations, between men and women, subjects and the state, and psychological theories of leisure and work (Çelik 1993: 68–9). These relations were mediated further by a growing statistical culture that viewed the average human as a predictable unit with measurable regularities in morality and behaviour. That view would underpin, for instance, Adolphe Quetelet's statistical studies in post-Napoleonic France. It would find outsized expression in Frederick Winslow

Taylor's efficient labour theory, promoted by *The Principles of Scientific Management* (1911) (see Porter 1986).

These images of mechanical-statistical humans shifted the aesthetic of the city, which was filling with the technologies of industrial modernity. Physicians began to highlight collisions upon the human senses. Some thought that the optical senses of the brain, for example, experienced compounded stresses while reading on a train (Schivelbusch 2014: 68). Railways, cables and eventually telephone exchanges contributed to the neuroses of modernity that so many believed sprang from the clatter and speed of late nineteenth-century modern life. Moreover, these technological systems lent themselves by the 1850s to metaphors for the human nervous system (Otis 2002).

Later in the century Fordism, built from Taylorist physiological principles, began altering the industrial aesthetic (Harvey 1989: ch. 2 passim, particularly 25–8). Environmental transformation wrought by electric lighting made the changes yet more complete, and for psychologist Hugo Munsterberg (1863–1916) redefined vision into a psychotechnical study of how public light altered attention, reaction times and motor coordination (Blatter 2014: 141). There were deeper changes in human neurobiology. In former times, sleep was discontinuous. The nerve physiology that produced eight uninterrupted hours of sleep was, quite literally, the product of modern lighting (Ekirch 2001, 2006: 6).

A salient backdrop for these sites and localizations of mind and brain was growing secularization, in which neurology and psychology played a significant role. In the early 1800s, anatomist Charles Bell complained that his examinations of the brain were viewed as a search for the soul (Casper 2014: 10). Yet, by 1900, the study of religion became an act of psychological anthropology. Thus, in 1902, US philosopher and psychologist William James observed that 'the attempt to demonstrate by purely intellectual processes the truth of deliverances of direct religious experience is absolutely hopeless' (James 1902/1982). In 1800, mind, brain and spirit came forged together. By 1900, the occult protested that the psyche fell within its purview while the divide between science and religion increasingly widened (Hayward 2004).

This splintering of ideas and practices was also apparent in the reshaping of psychiatric and neurological modes of care. In the mid-nineteenth century, the public institutional model had been accepted and rolled out across the Western world and from there increasingly its empires. With a broad cultural acceptance, but without the faith community underpinnings, Retreat-inspired asylums quickly found themselves overwhelmed with long-stay patients. So much so, that their scale (some built to accommodate over 2,000) at once redoubled institutional design to offer more specialized care for minds and brains and provided evidence of the degeneration of Western civilization. The expansion of neurology as a discipline in its own right spurred further developments. The creation of hospitals for nerve, paralysis and epilepsy patients did much to cater for acute and ongoing intervention, as did a new 1910 'wonder drug', Salvarsan, for some with General Paralysis of the Insane (tertiary syphilis). Biological psychiatry and psychoanalysis were, therefore, contemporaries; their adherents – broadly speaking, Germany and Britain on one side, America on the other – would sculpt different paths for nations and cultures, especially after 1920.

Other long-term neurological conditions proved a challenge. Another irony, then, that inspiration was again found in a new 1880s religious establishment: Bethel epileptic colony at Bielefeld, Westphalia, influenced by Pastor Friedrich von Bodelschwingh. Bethel's model – welfare to work in a small community atmosphere, where the anxieties of urban living and trying to find employment were removed and health stabilized – proved influential, particularly to care in Britain and North America. That is not to say alternatives to gargantuan institutions were not already evident. In Scotland, unwell minds and brains were 'boarded out' to family homes (Sturdy and Parry-Jones 1999). At Geel, in what is now Belgium, the ancient open community dedicated to St Dymphna, in many ways a precursor to 'boarding out' and Bethel, continued to provide care (Parry-Jones 1981). More strikingly, Japan and China only established their first lunatic asylums in the late 1800s, the latter by American medical missionaries in 1898 (Blum and Fee 2008; Hashimoto 2010; Messner 2009; Suzuki 2003). Eastern traditions had no sense of mind/brain duality, considering psyche and soma holistically, and treating them likewise, overwhelmingly in patients' own homes (Li Chiu 1986).

ROUTES AND BORDERLANDS

Western sites and localizations of mind and brain might appear benign and cosmopolitan. Literature, art, philosophy and science, constructed in an age of empire, equipped with the mentalities of industrial capitalism, were derived of and provided Europeans with a pompous self-confidence. It was self-evident to many nineteenth-century Europeans that their languages, religion, arts, textiles, science, industry and militaries had reached the apogee of human progress (Stocking 1991). Such views both constructed and were informed by medical and scientific theories of mind and brain, sometimes in direct comparison to imperial projects. 'Those who have had the opportunity of observing the restoration of reason,' wrote Samuel Tuke in 1813, 'will be aware, that she does not, in general, at once, resume her lost empire over the mind' (Tuke 1813: 180). That reason was perceived as colonial was no accident and would become a nineteenth-century cultural motif. Such metaphors provide insights into how Europeans saw the world, oversaw their colonial subjects, and materialized a ready-made geography for white supremacy masquerading as enlightened reason. This view arose from the wellspring that was the Metternichian consensus. However, it foreshadowed what would become for Westerners, particularly in the late 1800s, existential fears of cultural degeneration (Pick 1993). These fears reveal that there were distinct routes and borderlands that structured the cartographic European imaginary, not least those roads that connected imperial designs with the minds and brains of colonizers and the colonized.

Joseph Conrad's 1899 *Heart of Darkness* provides a late illustration of the ways that craniometry, madness and theories of mind collided in colonial projects. Since at least the Enlightenment, 'the savage' had prefigured the notion of civilized humanity. The places of savagery – the American West, Central Africa, the Andes mountains, the Pacific archipelagos – all presented, as the scholar Chinua Achebe observed specifically of Africa, a desire 'in Western psychology to set [such places] up as a foil in Europe, a place of negations at once remote and vaguely familiar in comparison with which Europe's own state of spiritual grace [would] manifest' (Achebe 1977). The excess and insanity in *Heart of Darkness* only showed white readers that the dark hearts of the Other were theirs to carry as well.

The themes of novellas like Conrad's could only have been possible culturally through nineteenth-century routes connecting madness, psychiatry, psychology, neurology and evolutionary theory to Enlightenment concerns about race, gender, politics and social progress. For some, theories of mind and brain bordered rhetorical justifications for the domination of non-white races and of women. They played a silent, but starring, role in the visual iconography of the Dreyfus affair in fin-de-siècle France, which depicted an anti-Semitic physiognomy meant to stir the masses against the accused (Hyman 1989). Even the modern, scientific cerebral localization theories and establishment of French anthropology of Paul Broca (1824–80) should be seen in the light of these European concerns about their place in a world they sought to rule (Porter 1996: 201; see also Schiller 1992).

Savagery, like Victor the feral child, resided within the borderlands of Enlightenment dichotomies and bordered the limits of mind and brain in the nineteenth century. Philosophe Jean-Jacques Rousseau (1712–78) constructed 'the savage' as in a state of nature more hopeful than that of the civilized. The savage also lent a particular force to Enlightenment natural history. The race theories, involving both physical and cognitive features, of Georges-Louis Leclerc, the Comte de Buffon (1708–88), for example, influenced nineteenth-century evolutionism. Deterministic race theories set the stage for liberal, Whig and conservative political arguments about the abolition of slavery. These theories also informed monogenic and polygenic debates about the races. They were central in the short-lived 1851 diagnostic elaboration of 'drapetomania', a supposed insanity seen in the American South that led enslaved people to desire to abscond from their masters (Bynum 2000).

Among the evolutionists who considered how European understandings of mind and brain were shaped by 'primitive' Others was Herbert Spencer (1820–1903), who observed, 'we err in supposing that the savage has feelings such as they would have in his place. Want of rational curiosity respecting these incomprehensible novelties is a trait remarked of the lower races wherever found; and the partially-civilized races are distinguished from them as exhibiting rational curiosity' (Spencer 1876: 16–17).

These ideas were serious and reverberated around scientific enterprise. Dr Andrew Halliday observed in an 1828 survey of British mental health care: 'We seldom meet with insanity among the savage tribes of men . . . Among the slaves of the West Indies it very rarely occurs; and . . . the contented peasantry of the Welsh mountains, and the Western Hebrides, and the wilds of Ireland are almost free from this complaint' (Halliday 1828: 79–80). Based on his observations at Earlswood Asylum for Idiots and Imbeciles, in 1866 superintendent John Langdon Down described 'an ethnic classification' of child patients that provided evidence for retrogressive monogenic inheritance: 'A very large number of congenital idiots are typical Mongols. So marked is this, that when placed side by side, it is difficult to believe that the specimens compared are not children of the same parents' (Langdon Down 1866: 259–60). Psychiatrist Henry Maudsley, in 1873, pronounced that developmental disability was evidence 'that certain human beings are born with such a native deficiency of mind that all the training and education in the world will not raise them to the level of brutes' (Maudsley 1871: 68). William Gowers, a British physician of nervous diseases drawn to imperial politics, wrote in 1888 that hysteria was 'almost unknown among barbarous races, and seems to be a product of the cerebral development that accompanies the process of civilisation' (quote in Scott, Eadie and Lees 2012: 199). French psychologist Alfred Binet in 1907 claimed that the philosophy of materialism originated 'in the beliefs of the savage tribes' as his way of showing that Karl Vogt's claim that the brain secreted thought as the kidney did urine was not as radical as it appeared (Binet 1907: 141, 143).

These ideas manifested in an extreme form in the writings of Italian criminologist Cesare Lombroso (1835–1909), who argued that criminality and anarchism derived from observable physical regression (Pick 1986). For Lombroso, the female criminal was a rare creature because primitive man 'refused to marry a deformed female, [and] ate her', eradicating this breeding stock (Lombroso and Ferrero 1895: 109). He added, with evident flourish, that 'the aboriginal Australian . . . in reply to an inquiry as to the absence of old women in his country, said, 'We eat them all!' (Lombroso and Ferrero 1895: 109–10). Lombroso's writings call attention to how evolutionary psychiatry and neurology grounded in race theory othered people beyond Europe *and* within it. While Lombroso was controversial, his writing influenced literary and scientific figures. His crudeness was not lost on US psychologist G. Stanley Hall, who nevertheless discussed the Lombrosian school in *Adolescence* (1904). The feeble-minded child, the lunatic pauper, the hysterical woman or the shell-shocked soldier was in a eugenic age a matter of grave public concern. Lombroso's determinism, if extreme, contributed to the debate.

Those concerns placed a fixed location on mind and brain and also found routes connecting temporalities, which constructed moral and neurological economies. The construction of both, of course, was European and cosmopolitan. Their chief disease, insanity, as Catharine Coleborne has noted, came to be 'viewed as an inherent feature of all new societies' (Coleborne 2015: 14). Shell shock, for instance, spoke to the way that civil life and war were 'woven into the fabric of modernity' (Barham 2004: 2). Shell shock also revealed a moral geography for mapping the decline of manly spirit in an age of machines; a theme that animated such utopian classics as Samuel Butler's *Erehwon* (1872) and E. M. Forster's *The Machine Stops* (1909) and jerked in the echo between patients' movements and the playback of the medical film *War Neuroses* (1917).

Although it would appear that European ideas about mind and brain radiated outwards from the metropole towards the colony, there was a direct reciprocal transfer of knowledge back from those peripheries (Coleborne 2015). Observations on mental illness among the supposedly inferior neurobiological structures of Australian aboriginals who were being forced through 'civilization processes', for instance, were further evidence for the claim that civilization helped shape white insanity. Whereas aboriginals were considered to experience simpler insanities, white madness was more complex because white brains were deemed more advanced. That the effect of civilization could be seen in both was a point legitimating a universalistic psychiatry (Murray 2007).

Yet, as historian Sally Swartz has commented of 1890s South African asylum care, the presumption of this universalistic psychiatry limited explorations of novel forms of mental illness that might have existed in colonial contexts. At a time when novel and endemic disease was a commonplace trope used to legitimate imperial control, the lack of interest in endemic insanity indicates colonial doctors' views of the mental life of indigenous peoples. In segregated asylums, as Swartz shows, their attitude 'was performed as authoritative knowledge' and justified both incarceration *and* deficient care and treatment (Swartz 1995: 415). Psychiatric and neurological thinking in colonial contexts exerted cultural force in other ways. Rebellious social movements in East Africa were described through psychological terms of reference (Mahone 2006). In Zululand, authorities struggled to determine the difference between witchcraft and madness among indigenous women who claimed to be possessed. Historian Julie Parle, reviewing this episode, has described it as a means for the sick to recover some state of mental health in a context of intense social and political 'disruption and conflict' (Parle 2003: 131).

Lost in all of this to us, tragically, are the ways in which indigenous peoples themselves constructed what Western science and medicine declared to be minds and brains, as well as their own experiences of 'normality' and 'abnormality'. Although it might be possible for a subaltern reading of colonial primary sources to recover these lost local and subjugated perspectives, such a project, which still awaits an historian, would require explicit awareness of the ways such sources function to validate European cosmopolitan, cultural binaries.

HIGH MINDED AND LOW BROW

While non-European Others offered numerous opportunities to construct cultural economies of mind and brain globally, European sources reveal complex class stratifications within European vernaculars of mind and brain. Such social distinctions were most evident in discussions of nervous conditions, perhaps originating with Cheyne's 1733 class-conscious treatise *The English Malady*. Whatever the origins, as historian Melville Logan has commented, 'The nervous body was a paradigm that the middle class used to explain itself to itself and differentiate itself from other classes' (Logan 1997: 4). Similarly to refined taste and etiquette, nervous conditions suggested that the wealthy and middling sort were not like the poor and working classes, and that class differences would translate into novel pathologies among the cultured as well as moral evaluations of the deprived.

The cultural manifestations of class took many forms. Early nineteenth-century industrialists, responding to the metaphors of political economy attached to the nerves, extolled their self-control in order to justify their social position (Musselman 2012; see also Lawrence 1979). In literature, characters followed real-world fashions, taking the waters or resting nerves in expensive spas, kurorts, resorts and sanatoria, often located in Alpine retreats (Guenther 2014). Thus scenes in Leo Tolstoy's *Anna Karenina* (1873–7) seem to resemble episodes in Charles Darwin's life (1809–82) (Browne 1995: see 493, for example). Similarly, some nineteenth-century circles in Germany and elsewhere hypothesized that homosexuality was marked among upper-class high achievers because it was an evolutionary altruism inherited by 'better types' (Greenberg 1988: 411). Emotive music caused similar apprehensions about middle-class sensitivities, particularly among young impressionable women. James Johnson, man of letters and physician to British king William IV, observed that 'young ladies of the elite were in serious danger from being "excited, stimulated, electrified" by music', but 'the vibrations of music fall inert' on mere '"factory girls"' (Kennaway 2012: 39–40). The Parisian bourgeoisie were as impressed by Joseph Babinski's discovery of his famous neurological sign as they were by the fact that his sibling was the culinary genius behind Ali-Bab's 1907

Gastronomie pratique (Philippon and Poirier 2008: 68–73). Esoteric religious experiences, such as mind cures, American psychologist William James reasoned in 1902, could give 'to some of us serenity, moral poise, and happiness' and prevent 'certain forms of disease as well as science does, or even better in a certain class of persons' (James, 1902/1982: 122).

Such high-minded conceits, which abounded across the long nineteenth century, were also inherited from a metaphoric anatomy of the nerves, which dominated cultural sensibilities in everything from pedagogy to politics. In a direct sense, a somatic theory underpinned these high-minded views. Metaphors of the body politic, going back to Thomas Hobbes (although the notion was older) had situated the head as sovereign over the body in a way that mirrored political organization. This pliable symbol aligned well with other nineteenth-century cultural tropes, especially the commonplace belief in the great chain of being. It also determined frameworks of comparative zoology, most provocatively Jean-Baptiste Lamarck's, who, now pilloried for his theories of the inheritance of acquired traits, is often forgotten to have introduced the great binary zoological division determined by backbone (Lamarck 1809/1963: 62). Lamarck's distinction between spinal regions and cortical processes ultimately constructed, according to Melville Logan, 'a body with two distinct stories' which 'helps to explain why the bodies that appear in Victorian novels function so differently from those of the earlier century' (Logan 1997: 168).

These attitudes were reflected throughout a range of emerging European cultural forms and contradictions. Clinicians in Britain, for instance, denigrated the emergence of specialties, seeing them as manifestations of divided minds, lowly Americanism or social dissolution. They preferred instead to extol classical education and the unity of knowledge (Casper 2014: 1–19). Likewise asylums throughout Europe routinely contrived a sociology within their internal organization that reflected the wider world – and that sociology had enormous influence on the attitudes neurologists and psychiatrists brought to the sick and healthy alike. In a comparatively late expression of these snobberies, British neurologist Henry Head (1861–1940) damned the anthropometric deficiencies of the working classes and enlisted military men. Indeed, Head once postulated that:

> As refinement increases, the intrusion of the body into the regions of the soul is disturbing and offensive. In a lower stage of development both body & soul can comfortably dwell together under one roof like the Irishman & his pig without offense to either tenant of the room.
>
> —Jacyna 2008: 196

Head's comments characterize the paternalistic views held by most physicians of their patients throughout the long nineteenth century. In his 1813 and his

1815 texts, Samuel Tuke explained in a much earlier example that class formed a dominant consideration for understanding his patients' states of mind as well as where they should be housed (Tuke 1813, 1815: 11). In this way, class operated throughout the century as an organizational philosophy for asylums and hospitals and as an epistemology of mind in health and illness.

Given the preponderance of such attitudes towards mind and brain it is easy to forget that they reflected elite philosophies applied within Victorian common knowledge. It seems unlikely that there were no contrary vernacular epistemologies or proverbial economies that challenged these values. Such a study has yet to be undertaken, but there are sources which might reveal them if consulted. Erotica, bawdy humour, lewd songs, rebellious ideas and unhealthy religious fervour were held contemptuously as low-brow cultural pursuits that played upon the lowest nerves and lowest common denominators, and thus also justified why some people dominated others through social status (Smith 1992).

Drunkenness provides a clear illustration. It was routinely instantiated within Victorian understandings of morality as a loss of reason, a libertine pursuit, a waste of potential amongst the upper classes and decried by middle-class reformers and medical practitioners. Nevertheless, as historian Matthew Warner Osborn has shown, the cultural construction of *delirium tremens* granted to 'individuals of cultivated minds, lofty sentiments and glittering prospects' a medical diagnosis which was otherwise described as intemperance in poor, Black or indigent people (Warner Osborn 2014: 79). However, for French socialist Flora Tristan in 1839 the material cultures of drunken orgies in London's 'finishes', replete with their spectacles of perverse wealthy appetites among 'those who . . . seem to be dedicated to the night', proved less striking than the brutal entertainments that accompanied their loss of reason, including the intentional provoking of convulsions in women who had lost consciousness to drink (quoted in Carey (ed.) 1987: 310–13). The apprehension that observations like these might signal more revolutionary aspirations in subjugated minds was not lost on attentive or compassionate onlookers. It was a time, after all, as historian E. P. Thompson noted, that 'working men formed a picture of the organization of society, out of their own experience and with the help of their hard-won and erratic education, which was above all a political picture' generative of a more 'clearly defined class consciousness' (Thompson 1966: 712).

Doubtlessly, however, revolution incarnate was but one vernacular expression among many. The manifestations of colloquial dualisms throughout a variety of sources was yet another. The brain, as historian Anne Harrington has described, was itself a dual organ (Harrington 1989). Dual personalities, as described in Robert Louis Stevenson's *Dr Jekyll and Mr Hyde* (1886), tapped into Victorian debates which were potentially shared and discussed across the social strata (Styles 2012: 29). James Hogg's *The Private Memoirs and Confessions of a*

Justified Sinner (1824) adopted the divided self as a literary conceit playing upon the tension between 'true' mental illness and the occult as reality. Mesmerists purported to tap into hidden selves and other worlds. Psychical practices, which so enamoured scientific men such as Alfred Russel Wallace (1823–1913) and Oliver Lodge (1851–1940), convinced many, educated or otherwise, of realities beyond the immediately tangible (Oppenheim 1988). Hypnotists – immortalized stereotypically in George du Maurier's *Trilby* (1894; serialized in *Harpers Magazine*) as the sinister Jewish Svengali – had been producing public spectacles since the 1700s, anticipating the more scientific Braidism in fashionable nineteenth-century circles (Otis 2000: 120). All of these pursuits indicated the ways that morality, spirituality, mind, brain and dualism manifested publicly, ideologically and commercially among lay publics.

A further conjuncture linking high-minded pursuits and low-brow interests emerged with moving pictures. There appears to have been a relentless focus on motion in animals and humans from 1870. These left marked material legacies in the archives of neurology, psychiatry and physiology. The innovations of Etienne-Jules Marey (1830–1904) and his exact contemporary Eadweard Muybridge on animal motion, represented in sequential pictures, came to symbolize greater truthfulness and offered the promise of mechanical objectivity (Braun 1994; Daston and Galison 2010: 133).

These photographers' staggered images are echoed in Marcel Duchamp's painting *Nude Descending a Staircase, No. 2* (1912). However, Duchamp's Cubist formulation conceals nudity, in contrast to Muybridge's technique of filming clearly naked subjects. In post-1890 pathographies, physicians interested in nervous and mental conditions aped these tendencies by filming often-naked patients in seizures or paralysis (Cartwright 1995: 48–75). Such film suggests more than mere clinical gaze now, though their study might yet benefit from the sort of attention found in John Harley Warner and James Edmonson's history of contemporaneous medical school dissections (Warner and Edmonson 2009). Whether the influence on cinematic pornography originated from such studies, or pornographic photography prefigured the gaze of clinical films remains an open question. However, the psychological laboratory constructed many of the special effects that would define cinema's melodrama, later decried by the high minded as low brow (Blatter 2015). At the same time, the answers to that open question might well offer lines of investigation revealing much about Victorian sexuality, patriarchy and the making of permissible, salacious imagery in a culture that we often pretend was above such things (Foucault 1976/1990).

SOURCES AND PRACTICES

We have hitherto sketched key features for a grand narrative of mind and brain in the cultural history of medicine during the long nineteenth century. We have sought simultaneously to reveal substantive lacunae that unsettle this history. In this section, we shift in tone to directly address some areas that we see as remaining unexplored in a landscape where historians often return to familiar institutional and professional habitations. There are numerous sources untapped or underexploited, shielding ways of seeing, voices and experiences that have not yet edged or fit into contemporary view. Moreover, the practices of different academic disciplines have still to be fully employed towards the enhancement of the history of mind and brain. Indeed, we argue that a more synthesized and holistic approach needs to be considered, particularly by historians of mind and brain, to avoid perpetuating false truths and divisions. To date, the historiography of the modern period, trained on Western experiences, has tracked back today's demarcations of specialized medicine, imposing a flawed and ahistoric narrative on the past. We contend that scholars need to rethink histories of modern neurology and psychiatry so that they commence, not from within current frameworks, but from the point where self-specializing generalists and the burgeoning number of alienists were the medical experts of the great unseen.

However, also frequently forgotten are the experts and professions that have influenced and organized mind and brain sciences and medicine beyond clinicians and the pre-1800 triad of 'medical statements . . . legal sentences [and] police action' outlined by Foucault (Foucault 1969/1972: 32). By neglecting these cultures of meaning, historians have inadvertently contributed to obscure negotiated or compromised readings of contemporary issues, potentially permitting warped approaches to current mental and neurological health and welfare. For example, the Great Depression of the 1870s in Britain shifted welfare strategies and discussions about 'deserving' and 'non-deserving' people, and the institutional and political response that grew out of this parsimonious atmosphere was complicated by Darwinian notions of dependency, degeneration and eugenics. The machinery needed to implement the English and Welsh legislation of 1913 that sought to identify, manage or detain 'mental defectives' provides a clear indicator of how many different local and/or working cultures shaped the meanings of mind/brain and outcomes. In Birmingham, England, a communiqué was sent out from the city authorities to ascertain 'what defectives are to be found within [the] area'. The intended recipients included Poor Law authorities; hospitals, dispensaries, sanatoria, medical practitioners; lodging houses, shelters, refuges, charities, charitable institutions; religious ministers, probation officers, district nurses; labour exchanges, friendly societies, 'working-class organisations' and a city insurance body (Mental Deficiency Sub-Committee Minutes 1914–17: 7–9). The trouble was, there was no definition of what constituted 'mental deficiency' locally, nationally or internationally, which meant each person or organization brought their own preoccupations to their own definition. Such diverse communities' understandings of mind and brain and how they functioned across society – as separate entities, as nodes, and as part of a multiagency nexus – are absent from our histories.

Though omitted from the list, links with the educational authorities were already established. Birmingham was at the vanguard of establishing special classes for 'Defective and Epileptic' children under permissive legislation of 1899. This in itself points to the role of distinctive local cultures, with specific and peculiar preoccupations and understandings of abilities and disabilities, behaviours and actions in the understanding of mental and neurological health and the practices drawn from this localized understanding: the terroir of mind and brain. With their new access to appointments in educational authorities under recently-established local councils – and aside from roles in private asylum businesses, institutional staff and visiting committees, and medical missionaries – this was the first time that women like Birmingham figure Ellen Pinsent had an official and wide-reaching influence on what the mind and brain were, and what people did and looked like when they were thought to have 'gone wrong' (see Wynter 2015). With the onset of the First World War, this territory increased for lay and medical women through the local administration of war pensions, voluntary involvement with nursing and organizations such as the Ex-Services (Mental) Welfare Society (established 1919) and via the opening of medical positions for female physicians and psychiatrists. This cultural shift – accompanied by women's suffrage as an international and a militant movement – in who was involved in shaping, understanding and conveying mind and brain was echoed at different rates throughout the Western world and its colonies. Still we really do not know how or in what way transnational comparisons, exchanges and debates shaped these experiences or how they were adapted or resisted locally.

Most of the community figures and organizations trusted to identify 'mental defectives' in Birmingham are largely missing from the broader (cultural) history of mind and brain. Care in the community, or lack thereof, has come into clearer focus since the 1980s/1990s Western deinstitutionalization process. Even so, beyond Weir Mitchell's 'rest cure', there is limited recent cohesive or comparative work about men and women with psychological and neurological issues living and/or cared for outside state institutions (see Bartlett and Wright (eds) 1999; Marland 2004: ch. 3, 65–94, 80–94; Suzuki 2006; Gatley 2012). Fresh pathways are being cut that utilize war pension records by new, as yet unpublished research in the UK (including by Jessica Meyer and by Rebecca Wynter), though these often skirt 1920. With some exceptions, notably Germany, the employment of such material is limited, given the date that pensions were introduced, but insurance records and the archives of friendly societies – and, indeed, other records where ordinary people can be 'heard' – have yet to be explored for understandings and approaches to mind and brain outside institutional medicine. Following so many former patients, this would push or resettle the meanings of mind and brain into the community, where medical framing may have seeped, but understandings were inflected through other professions and organizations, and lay, personal, localized and a host of other cultural lenses.

Malingering is another potential topic for which pension or insurance records might contribute to the cultural history of mind/brain (for malingering, see Bergen 1999/2004; Cooter 1988; Siritkina 2007; Wessley 2003). It is also just one of the connective tissues which sat within the broad anatomy of defined psychiatric and neurological responsibility, as the areas began to refine, in part through international congresses, from the later nineteenth century. Reflecting on one such meeting in Germany, an event in Newcastle in 1893 – a city on the North-East coast of England, associated with coal mining – brought together physicians to consider 'the legitimacy of concussion of the spine', which, it was argued, was a result of so-called 'railway spine', something rarely experienced by colliers, despite their supposed predisposition to back injury. A central theme of these international discussions was the role of the mind in traumatic physiological neuroses, and objectivity in evidencing their existence (Anon. 1993). A greater scrutiny of conference reports, contexts and discussions can enable an investigation of the production of 'mind' and 'brain' and their meaning at specific points in time. Even within medicine, then, there are significant nineteenth-century sources that remain largely untouched.

Beyond medicine and science, there are many more overlooked sources for the study of mind and brain between 1800 and 1920, including material culture, music, popular fiction and magic lantern shows. Yet numerous items with which we might genuinely access everyday understandings of mind and brain medicine and cultures remain undervalued – in oral traditions and in song, but mostly in print, including music hall material, penny dreadfuls, magazines and newspapers – though some should find great prominence with the employment of 'big data' and culturomics or corpus linguistics in historical research, and even the use of virtual reality. Since the appearance of Foucault's studies, the dialectic of madness and civilization has resulted in intense investigation of insanity in society. Strangely, however, we know almost nothing about the construction of sanity in civilization. It is, perhaps, no surprise that such an example, and many others, offer the promise for rich investigation through a popular lay-culture perspective. Indeed, to borrow historian Mathew Thomson's words,

> There has been a tendency to focus on an elite . . . or an 'educated reading public', leaving relatively little insight into more middlebrow, let alone working-class, attitudes. There is the problem that a focus on the downward diffusion of ideas, not only from the upper echelons of mind and brain medicine and science, but also from the great psychologists – Freud in particular – [tend] to leave out of the picture a more eclectic range of

intellectual influences, let alone the possibility that ideas and practices might emerge from below.

—Thomson 2006: 20

It is not simply fresh sources that will widen historical horizons. For all the noise about collaborative practice and interdisciplinary working, to date this has largely been achieved through personal determination. The digital and medical humanities have helped support individual initiatives, though pointedly these have often been facilitated by the visions of funding bodies. Even so, the visible successes mostly remain outposts, in part because scholarly publishing and discipline-specific ways of working and speaking are not responsive to ideas and articulations that do not fit; nor, it must be said, does the framework enable the integration of first-hand accounts by 'service users', patients or survivors, whose lives or conditions may not adhere to academic timetables or deadlines, often rendering the prime outlet as sensationalist media and helping tether mental healthcare reform to scandal. While there are clearly significant systemic issues and obstacles, scholars should ideally be aware of research happening in other disciplines and attempt to garner insights; this is, potentially, more important than ever with the emergence of the animal turn, and One Medicine and evidence-based medicine in health. There are significant questions remaining in the history (cultural and otherwise) of mind and brain medicine and science for which tools might reside in other disciplines.

*   *   *

We close then by returning to our own areas of expertise. Is there a cultural history that might incorporate both mind and brain? The answer we have found in writing this together is most certainly 'yes'. And there are many reasons to pursue such an endeavour. With the embrace of the cultural history of medicine comes a willingness to think across occupational divisions of medicine's past. In such work, we find promise that even the older approaches to exploring the intellectual and social history of medicine can find renewal beyond the history of the professions, the institutions and diseases. We understand that such intersectional approaches, and the openness and exchanges they necessitate intellectually, may sound naive or idealistic. But so what? There are many excellent reasons to foster collaborative work and double down on history as a way of knowing that is salient to being human. After all, it is history, not splendid isolation, that makes minds and brains.

CHAPTER EIGHT

Authority

MICHAEL BROWN AND CATHERINE KELLY

INTRODUCTION

In August 1855, in the English city of York, the Provincial Medical and Surgical Association met for the last time under that name. Founded in 1832, the Association encompassed some 2,000 medical practitioners from throughout the British Isles and beyond. What began as an organization promoting medical science and encouraging medical sociability had, during the intervening years, come to play host to widely divergent opinions concerning its culture, purpose and identity. Matters had come to a head at the previous year's meeting in Manchester when an argument broke out over the suggestion that the Association take a more active role in politics and change its name to the 'British Medical Association'. The fallout from this ensured that the York meeting attracted an 'unusually small' attendance ('Association Intelligence' 1855: 774). Nonetheless, 453 members of the Association, most of whom were pointedly absent, took the opportunity to submit a memorial to the meeting. It read:

> The profession of medicine in the British dominions is at present devoid of any recognised head or authoritative council possessed of powers and privileges, and invested with corresponding duties and responsibilities, which would constitute it a body politic.

The consequences of this state of affairs were numerous, the memorial suggested. For one thing, medicine and surgery, lacking adequate self-regulation, were open to 'imperfectly educated individuals, incompetent to the performance of the public and private duties they subsequently undertake' who thereby brought 'discredit on the whole profession'. Moreover, it meant 'the absence of any recognised medical authority to which the government and the public might appeal in cases of general or local sickness, the rise and progress of epidemics, the breaking out of war and pestilence, and in questions of public hygiene generally' ('Association Intelligence' 1855: 799).

This text made numerous references to the concept of 'authority', but what exactly was being invoked? On the one hand, 'authority' might refer, as in these quotations, to a legally-recognized and mandated body which regulated the practice of medicine and surgery and which might cooperate with government in matters of public health. As it stood, no such organization existed; in England, professional institutions such as the Royal College of Physicians and Royal College of Surgeons (founded 1518 and 1800 respectively), together with the Society of Apothecaries (founded 1617) had few powers outside of licensing and enjoyed a limited jurisdiction. On the other hand, 'authority' also suggested something more complex and amorphous: a recognition of medicine's value and knowledge system by those in government and by the public at large. This cultural authority, or what, to follow Pierre Bourdieu, we might term 'cultural capital', was as much the concern of the memorialists as the legal and administrative aspects of medical power (Bourdieu 1986). Thus, they claimed that another consequence of medicine's disorganization was 'the degradation of the social position of the medical profession below that of the other learned professions'. Even so, these memorialists saw their interests not as sectional or self-interested, but as commensurate with the public good. Hence, another negative outcome was:

> In the general community, an excess above that which is necessarily incidental to our actual state of civilization, of sickness and misery, and of mental and bodily deformities and incapacities; with a great increase of pauperism, and the premature severance by death, of the dearest ties of humanity.
> —'Association Intelligence' 1855: 799

Social historical scholarship on the 'rise' of the medical profession in the nineteenth century has generally focused on this first meaning of authority. Informed by a functionalist sociological model of professionalization, it has conceptualized the medical profession as a self-regulating, monopolistic and highly differentiated form of labour characteristic of modern industrial society and has largely focused on tracing the structural forms of this monopoly, through such measures as the establishment of colleges and institutions and the passage of legislation, such as Great Britain's Anatomy Act of 1832 or Medical Act of 1858.[1]

Since the 1990s, however, scholars have begun to conceive of medical authority in more complex and nuanced terms. Drawing from a diverse range of influences, including art history, literary and poststructuralist theory as well as the cultural interpretation and symbolic interactionist schools of anthropology and sociology, historians of medicine began to place increasing emphasis upon the ways in which medical practitioners claimed and asserted authority through such means as literary and visual self-representation, discursive and rhetorical elaboration as well as performance and social display. They have also become more sensitive to the political and ideological dimensions of medical authority and to the myriad ways in which medical authority was challenged, frustrated or negotiated.

This ideological contrast between institutions and ideas, between the concrete and the imaginative, and between established reality and reforming vision, was prominent at the 1855 meeting. For example, at one point in the discussion concerning the change of name to the British Medical Association, the London surgeon Henry Ancell predicted a 'great fight' between 'the profession – in our sense of the word "profession" – and the profession in the Government sense, viz. the Councils of the Colleges' ('Association Intelligence' 1855: 790).

For Ancell, this change of name therefore encapsulated a reformist vision of a democratic and unified medicine opposed to institutional oligarchy (see Figure 8.1). Moreover, it was indicative of another aspect of medical authority to which the cultural history of medicine has become increasingly sensitive, namely the associations between medicine and the national/imperial state. The word 'Provincial' may have had an alluring ring to it in 1832 in the Board Room of the Worcester Infirmary – a self-consciously parochial and anti-metropolitan statement of identity – but by 1855, at the height of the siege of Sebastopol, at a time of growing national self-belief and imperial reach, and when the railway network and the rise of mass society were beginning to elide the distinctions between metropolis and province, some thought it utterly redundant. 'I am sure I am only expressing the mind of the London members of the profession,' claimed the surgeon and naturalist Edwin Lankaster, 'when I say that they do not feel themselves in any position as a distinct body from the members of the profession in the provinces. They feel more than ever that there is but one profession in this country' ('Association Intelligence' 1855: 787). Meanwhile, Benjamin Ward Richardson, the pioneering anaesthetist, asked:

> There are sister kingdoms: there are colonies; there is the great empire of Hindostan; and why should not the Association have its branches there . . . Why should we not have branches at Berwick-upon-Tweed, Glasgow, Edinburgh, Aberdeen, Dublin, Montreal, Calcutta and Bombay? Why not extend the Association over the whole world and make it a British Association in every sense of the word?
>
> —'Association Intelligence' 1855: 788

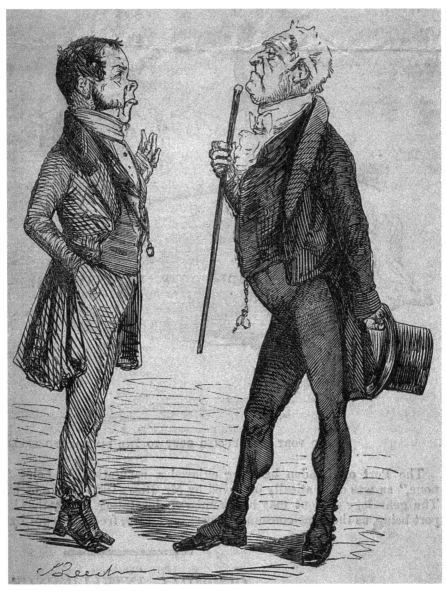

FIGURE 8.1: Competing visions: John Leech, 'When Doctors Disagree', Etc., Etc. (*c.* 1840s). Wellcome Collection.

Ultimately the memorialists were victorious and the motion to change the name to the British Medical Association was passed by 50 votes to 31, the name it retains to this day. This change of title might seem trivial, but it is indicative of so much more: of a medical profession with ambitions to exercise authority over the health of the population as a whole, and one which worked increasingly through the mechanisms of state and imperial governance. These ambitions were often negotiated as other groups such as nurses pursued their own professional projects occasionally, as discussed below, making knowledge system and authority claims in opposition to the medical profession. Neither was Britain alone in this transformation. While some countries, such as France and later Prussia/Germany took the lead in formalizing the social and political prerogatives of the medical profession and establishing the biopolitcal imperatives of 'medical police', even more decentralized and non-interventionist nations such as the United States witnessed attempts to secure and extend the social, political and intellectual authority of medicine and surgery. Indeed, the American Medical Association, founded in 1847, can be said to have been the first truly national medical and surgical organization of its kind, while, by the early twentieth century, the United States would be home to some of the most prestigious medical schools and research centres in the world.

This chapter explores developments in the cultural history of medical authority in the age of empire. While it focuses on new areas of analysis, it also demonstrates how new analytical frames have enabled historians to revisit established areas of study. It is true to say that historians of medicine have, for the most part, eschewed a radically culturalist agenda that dispenses with socio-political notions of power in favour of a postmodernist dissolution of such established analytical categories as class, gender and race. Rather, and like much of history as a whole, historians of medicine have assimilated some of the methodologies and sensibilities of the cultural turn, such as discourse, performance, embodiment, materiality and a sensitivity to the multivalent nature of power, into an established tradition of social history, creating a hybridized form of socio-cultural history which maintains its link with the past.[2] This chapter therefore seeks to analyse some of those continuities as well as demonstrating the ways in which cultural history has informed new directions and approaches. Needless to say, a chapter like this cannot cover every topic relevant to the broad field of medical authority. Instead, it focuses on the following key themes which address the most significant aspects of medical authority discussed by historians generally, which have attracted the most innovative and interesting work by cultural historians and which are closest to the authors' own areas of expertise: identity, performance and self-representation; knowledge, power and resistance; war, empire and the state.

IDENTITY, PERFORMANCE AND SELF-REPRESENTATION

As we have suggested, it is practically impossible, as well as intellectually limiting, to attempt to distinguish the earliest cultural historical accounts of medical authority from the broader field of the social history of medicine. Historians of medicine had, to an extent, long been interested in medical identity and self-representation and one can find articles on such professional signifiers as the gold-headed cane in early quasi-antiquarian publications like the *Annals of Medical History*. However, it is with the maturation of the social history of medicine in the 1980s that we begin to see more sophisticated and culturally-sensitive understandings of medical identity. Although slightly before our period, one of the earliest examples of this tendency is the collection edited by William F. Bynum and Roy Porter entitled *William Hunter and the Eighteenth-Century Medical World* (1985). Alongside chapters on Hunter's contributions to obstetrical knowledge and accounts of his income, the collection is notable for essays by Roy Porter and Chris Lawrence which seek to situate Hunter within a much broader social and cultural milieu, and to understand his public identity as a polite and learned gentleman of the Enlightenment (Porter 1985; Lawrence 1985).

Within the traditions of British medical history, at least as it concerns the nineteenth century, these gestures towards a culturally-sensitive history of medical identity often focused on the body of the practitioner and its visual representation. For example, in his 1998 essay 'Medical Minds, Surgical Bodies: corporeality and the doctors', Chris Lawrence draws attention to the varied visual representations of physicians and surgeons across the nineteenth century and to the ways in which these representations were linked, in both the public and the professional mind, to changing ideas about the relative value of mental and manual labour, or brain and brawn. Lawrence's essay is notable not simply for its engagement with visual representation, but for its links to an emergent scholarship on the history of masculinities and its acknowledgement of the role of gender in shaping professional identities.

This interest in medical bodies and their representation is especially evident in two books published around the turn of the millennium. The first of these is Ludmilla Jordanova's *Defining Features: Medical and Scientific Portraits, 1600–2000* (2000). Jordanova's sweep is as broad as the book is short, although, in reality, the objects of her analysis tend to cluster in the eighteenth century. Nevertheless, Jordanova's work brings an art historical sensibility to bear on the issue of medical self-presentation and is highly instructive on the cultural construction and public commemoration of medical heroism; like Lawrence, she is also sensitive to the gendering of professional identities. The other book is Roy Porter's swansong, *Bodies Politic: Disease, Death and the Doctors in Britain, 1650–1900* (2001). Porter was resolutely a social historian, but his last book suggested an openness to the interests of cultural history, if not necessarily to its methodologies. Like Jordanova, Porter is concerned with images, although he deals as much with patients as with practitioners. Also like Jordanova, his chronological sweep is broad, though his preference for the early modern period over the nineteenth century is similarly evident. Even so, the book draws attention to the role of corporeal and sartorial stereotypes in the representation and elaboration of medical professional identities, from the bewigged and corpulent figure of eighteenth-century satire to the sombre and upright Victorian idealist. Complementing this analysis, Lisa Rosner's *The Most Beautiful Man in Existence: The Scandalous Life of Alexander Lessassier* (1999) demonstrates through the surgeon Lessassier's own diaries how aware contemporary practitioners were of the importance of such outward signifiers of authority, and how strategically some could pursue philanthropy, the right address and an appropriate carriage to enhance their social position and ameliorate some of the socially undesirable aspects of surgery and anatomy in particular.

The title of Porter's book hints at the political dimensions of medical identity and authority, another key pathway from the social to the cultural history of medicine; Porter himself acknowledges the politically fraught nature of early nineteenth-century medicine and suggests that professional rivalries and antagonisms were often diffused by humour and satire. The origins of a politically sensitive and sophisticated approach to the history of medicine in the nineteenth century can be traced back, at least in part, to the influence of the 'Edinburgh School' of the sociology of scientific knowledge, to the early reception of Michel Foucault and to developments in critical theory and cultural anthropology. Perhaps because of the political, social and intellectual turbulence of the period, historians of this ilk found particularly rich pickings in the early nineteenth century. Roger Cooter's *The Cultural Meaning of Popular Science: Phrenology and the Organization of Consent in Nineteenth-Century Britain* (1984) was especially pioneering in its complex and careful mapping of medical knowledge onto the politics of the period and onto competing claims to social and cultural authority.[3] Adrian Desmond's *The Politics of Evolution: Morphology, Medicine, and Reform in Radical London* (1989) was similarly influential. As a comprehensive study of the politics of knowledge in an era of reform it remains unsurpassed. It demonstrates how revolutionary French anatomy and Lamarckian evolutionary theory found a receptive audience among the radical, non-conformist and materialist practitioners of the metropolis at a time of convulsive political upheaval. Another important work is Stephen Jacyna's *Philosophic Whigs: Medicine, Science, and Citizenship in Edinburgh, 1789–1848* (1994), which shows how the Thomson family in particular, and the Edinburgh medical community in general, were shaped by the reformist and progressive values of a politico-philosophic Whiggism, not simply in terms of their public and private identities, but in the very nature of the medicine they taught and practised. Together with the work of Cooter and Desmond, Jacyna's book convincingly argues for the 'inescapable presence of the political in the world of nineteenth-century medicine' (1994: 6).

Such interests in medicine's cultural and political identity were mirrored by developments in the United States. Here, the work of John Harley Warner has been particularly important. *The Therapeutic Perspective: Medical Practice, Knowledge and Identity in America, 1820–1885* (1986) and *Against the Spirit of System: The French Impulse in Nineteenth-Century American Medicine* (2003) explore the ways in which the professional identities of American medical practitioners were shaped by both theory and practice and by the importance ascribed to therapeutic intervention. Whereas many members of the Bostonian medical elite were influenced by French clinical practice to see disease in increasingly universalist terms and to practise relative therapeutic restraint, other less professionally secure practitioners recognized that their authority over patients depended less upon theoretical novelty than upon a therapeutic interventionism founded upon an individualistic model of illness. This emphasis upon the centrality of quotidian practice and public perception was subsequently developed by Steven Stowe. His book, *Doctoring the South: Southern Physicians and Everyday Medicine in the Mid-Nineteenth Century* (2004), draws upon a rich body of letters and casebooks to demonstrate the many ways in which medical identity and authority were mediated by local customs, cultures and expectations.

In the last decade and a half, cultural historians on both sides of the Atlantic have developed these themes to present a rich and complex picture of medical identity in the age of empire. They have combined a sensitivity to practice with an emphasis upon ideology, ideation and self-representation. Michael Brown's work, for example, has sought to nuance established understandings of medical professionalization in the nineteenth century by drawing attention to the political and cultural dimensions of medical discourse and performance. His book *Performing Medicine: Medical Culture and Identity in Provincial England, c. 1760–1850* (2011) traces the transformations in what it meant to be a medical practitioner from the polite, learned and sociable ideals of the Enlightenment through the turbulent age of reform to a vocational identity 'based upon expertise, professional self-identification and a political engagement with the care of the social body' (Brown 2001: 9). Like others before him, Brown is at pains to demonstrate the fundamentally political dimensions of this transformation, but is also alert to the ideational aspects of medical identity, arguing that the medical profession was as much an 'imagined community' as a structural reality.

In the United States, a cultural sensitivity to the issues of medical identity and self-representation have encouraged a particular engagement with the figure of the dissector. Michael Sappol's *A Traffic of Dead Bodies: Anatomy and Embodied Social Identity in Nineteenth-Century America* (2004) argues for the centrality of the corpse in the construction of American medical professional identity and authority. An otherwise taboo object, the anatomical body was also subject to theft, pranks and fantasy, a powerful symbol of medical acculturation. Moreover, its manipulation and mastery conferred the authority of medical science and the ability to heal, factors which enhanced the credibility of orthodox practitioners at a time of intense competition and heterodoxy. But, as Sappol demonstrates, the corpse was also a cultural object which moved from the dissection room into sensationalist fiction, dime museums and minstrel shows. John Harley Warner and James Edmondson's *Dissection: Photographs of a Rite of Passage in American Medicine 1880 – 1930* (2009) explores the visual dimensions of dissecting room culture, presenting an astonishing array of photographs of medical students variously posing and performing with their anatomical subjects. As the authors argue, this rite of passage formed a fundamental part of student culture, marking their transition from laymen to medical professionals. Both of these books are sensitive to the particular racial politics of dissection in the United States. The fact that it was the bodies of poor, disenfranchised blacks which so often provided the raw material for medical schools strengthened an association between dissection and racial violence that could sometimes become explicit (Warner and Edmondson 2009: 25). The capacity for medical authority and identity to be founded upon the bodies of the socially and racially marginalized is also evident in Helen MacDonald's study of anatomical dissection in Australia's Van Dieman's Land (2006).

If race has played an important role in recent literature on medical identity, then so, too, has gender. Brown has demonstrated how masculinity was central to the public identities of nineteenth-century medical practitioners, who sought to capitalize, albeit ambivalently, on the imaginative associations between medicine and war and to present themselves as heroic and self-sacrificing servants of the state (2010). Together with Chris Lawrence, he has elaborated similarly heroic imaginative associations between surgery and imperial exploration (2016). This new work on gender and medicine has also reshaped how we view the early history of women's entry into the medical profession, providing a more nuanced and complex picture than that of traditional hagiographies. For example, Laura Kelly's work on female medical graduates in Ireland, as well as her most recent work on Irish medical students, has provided a rich and intriguing insight into the gendered cultures of medical education. Kelly argues that while Irish institutions led the way in admitting and qualifying women to practice, men and women inhabited separate if parallel spaces at university. Women were trained in separate dissecting rooms and 'ladies rooms'. Significantly, she notes that women participated in this gendered division through their own cultivation of a distinct self-identifying cohort (Kelly 2013, 2017). Similarly, Claire Brock's study of female surgeons demonstrates the complex experiences and identities of women entering what was, by the mid-nineteenth century, perhaps the most swaggeringly masculine branch of the medical profession (2017).

The history of surgery also provides an indication of how cultural history is moving beyond words and images to consider the performative and affective dimensions of medical identity. For example, Thomas Schlich has demonstrated how the meaning and display of surgical skill shifted across the nineteenth century (2015), while Brown explores the role of the emotions in shaping practitioners' identities and in structuring relationships between them and their patients, suggesting that detachment was a less ubiquitous emotional state for nineteenth-century surgeons than has generally been assumed (2017, 2019). Such new avenues of inquiry promise to further our understanding of the multitudinous aspects of medical and surgical identity in the age of empire.

KNOWLEDGE, POWER AND RESISTANCE

The long nineteenth century was a period of increased parliamentary activity in most European and North American legislatures. Increasingly, and often at the behest of medical practitioners, public health and the practice of medicine became the focus of legislative and regulatory measures. Historians have given detailed accounts of how a regulated medical profession in Britain emerged from a confused early period described by John Pickstone as one of shifting and fragmented medical authority (1992: 140). Any discussion of the cultural authority of medicine across this century must necessarily be set against the background of key markers of the formal or legal authority bestowed on certain forms of medical practice by the Apothecaries Act 1815 and the Medical Act 1858.[4] The efforts of medical reformers to exclude the 'unqualified' from practice are the background noise against which, and under which, many other claims and challenges to medical authority must be understood. As M. J. D. Roberts reminds us in his nuanced study, 'The Politics of Professionalization: MPs, Medical Men, and the 1858 Medical Act', 'professional authority, however defined, rests on more than professional assertion . . . it requires some measure of cultural acceptance as well' (2009: 38).

Social historians have long been sensitive to the ways in which, during the nineteenth century, medicine came to assume an ever-closer relationship with the structures of state governance, especially through the medium of public health. Indeed, the narrative of the 'rise' of public health had been integral to established conceptualizations of medical professionalization and monopolization and changed relatively little from the 1950s until the 1990s.[5] However, since the turn of the century, socio-cultural historians have presented a more complex picture of public health and have explored the ways in which medical authority in the public sphere was mediated, challenged and even frustrated. Though not strictly speaking a work of cultural history, but rather a densely sophisticated social historical account, Christopher Hamlin's *Public Health and Social Justice in the Age of Chadwick: Britain 1800–1854* (1998) has been hugely influential in this regard. Hamlin's triumph is to transform our understanding of public health by situating it within a much more extensive political, economic and intellectual matrix. He thereby demonstrates that the aetiological correlation between filth and disease enshrined in the Public Health Act of 1848 owed more to the doctrines of political economy and utilitarianism and to solving the 'problem' of pauperism than to a simple and unproblematic desire to 'clean up' the streets. Moreover, Hamlin's work also charts the vagaries and limitations of public health practice, especially as it involved large infrastructural investment which required the active support of local authorities, many of whom were distinctly unenamoured with the centralizing impulse of the Act. Another work of this period which set the tone for subsequent research in the field is Michael Worboys' *Spreading Germs: Disease Theories and Medical Practice in Britain, 1865–1900* (2000). Worboys' work emphasizes the plurality and complexity of germ theory in the early decades of its elaboration and argues that germ theory 'on the streets' could take a markedly different form to that which has come down to us in the laboratory-based practices of Koch and his followers.

Hamlin's and Worboys' books were part of a raft of literature published in the late 1990s and early 2000s that revivified the study of public health and which increasingly brought to bear the concerns and approaches of cultural history. Some, such as Andrew Aisenberg's *Contagion: Disease, Government, and the Social Question in Nineteenth-Century France* (1999), take inspiration from Michel Foucault's theories, especially his ideas on 'governmentality', to situate public health debates within the complex balance between liberal individualism and state interventionism that characterized many nineteenth-century political contexts. Others, such as David Barnes's *The Great Stink of Paris and the Nineteenth-Century Struggle Against Filth and Germs* (2006), draw upon anthropological theories of disgust as well as the traditions of sensory history to develop more culturally sensitive models of public health. And others, such as Pamela Gilbert, explore the cultural practices of cartography as well as the political contours of the cholera epidemics that defined the image and experience of health in the nineteenth-century industrial city. In her *Imperial Hygiene: A Critical History of Colonialism, Nationalism and Public Health* (2004), Alison Bashford contributes to a growing and influential literature considering the relationship between public health and governance in colonial contexts. Using the Australasian colonies in particular, she draws out the importance of the rhetoric of hygiene and contamination to the control of those societies through various means including, importantly, 'spatial forms of governance' such as segregation and quarantine which sought to regulate the circulation of matter and people. Meanwhile, one of the most interesting developments, signalled by Nancy Tomes's *The Gospel of Germs: Men, Women, and the Microbe in American Life* (1999) and in evidence in Victoria Kelley's

Soap and Water: Cleanliness, Dirt and the Working Classes in Victorian and Edwardian Britain (2010), is the move towards understanding public health as an individualized and internalized set of social practices rooted in new forms of commercial consumption.

For our immediate purposes, however, perhaps the signal achievement of this recent work on public health has been the way it has emphasized the relative contingency of medical professional authority (see Figure 8.2). Far from being the principal drivers of public health, medical practitioners were often simply one of several stakeholders who were involved in the complex negotiation of sanitary practice. Two recent works have drawn particular attention to this aspect of historical experience. One is Graham Mooney's *Intrusive Interventions: Public Health, Domestic Space and Infectious Disease Surveillance in England, 1840–1914* (2015). Mooney's book is influenced both by Worboys on germ theory and by the work of Patrick Joyce and others on the nineteenth-century state, to demonstrate how the application of an intrusive system of medical surveillance was shaped by local political circumstances and mediated by the attitudes of the urban working classes, at whom it was principally targeted. The result was a system which oscillated between the

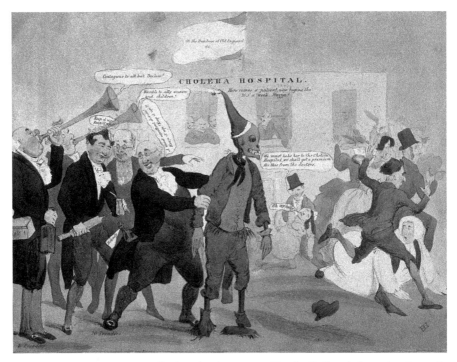

FIGURE 8.2: Contesting medical authority: Henry Heath, 'A Sketch from the Central Board of Health: The Real Ass-I-Antic Cholera!!' (1832). Wellcome Collection.

values of liberal voluntarism and a more coercive and compulsive regime, one which emphasized the citizen's duties as much as their rights. The other work is Tom Crook's *Governing Systems: Modernity and the Making of Public Health in England, 1830–1910* (2016), which is even more indebted to post-Joycean work on governmentality. Like Mooney, Crook is concerned to balance established accounts of medical professional expertise with a narrative that emphasizes the role played by numerous, overlapping and often highly localized systems of government in the creation, maintenance and extension of public health provision.

This same emphasis upon the limitations of medical authority and the ways in which medicine was shaped by public sentiment, including outright antagonism, informs much of the recent literature on other aspects of medicine's public presence in the age of empire. Just as the mid- to late nineteenth century saw the passage of legislation aimed at combating the generation and spread of epidemic disease, so, too, did states seek, in other respects, to secure the health of the 'social body' (Baldwin 1999). Perhaps one of the most notable instances of this, and one which has attracted a good deal of recent attention from historians, is the practice of vaccination, particularly compulsory vaccination. Like Crook and Mooney's work on public health, Deborah Brunton's *The Politics of Vaccination: Practice and Policy in England, Wales, Ireland, and Scotland, 1800–1874* (2008) downplays the importance traditionally ascribed to medical expertise in favour of a focus upon the operations of local power and the variations of regional and national experience. Whereas Brunton argues that resistance to vaccination has often been overstated, Nadja Durbach's work focuses almost exclusively on that side of the debate. Her *Bodily Matters: The Anti-Vaccination Movement in England, 1853–1907* (2004) explores the complex range of interests arraigned against compulsory vaccination for smallpox in later nineteenth-century Britain, as well as their rich and occasionally lurid rhetorical strategies. This campaign, she maintains, cut across class and gender boundaries but, as with opposition to other aspects of an interventionist public health, found its clearest and most cohesive expression in a discourse that set liberal individualism, with its associated values of freedom of action and of conscience, against the tyranny of statism and legislative compulsion.

The anti-vaccination movement was thus part of a broad challenge to medical authority which, emerging in the mid-nineteenth century, coincided precisely with the profession's social and legal establishment. This opposition drew its strength from a complex constellation of reformist beliefs that were prevalent in later nineteenth-century Britain and North America and which included new forms of religious and social heterodoxy such as Swedenborgism, spiritualism and vegetarianism as well as political ideologies such as Chartism, socialism and suffragism. As Katherine Gleadle has demonstrated, many political radicals were drawn to alternative therapies, such as homeopathy and medical botany, precisely because they were in opposition to what was quickly becoming a medical establishment. For female radicals in particular, such 'physiological reform' allowed them to turn the domestic sphere, and indeed their own bodies, into a space for political expression and resistance (Gleadle 2003).

Feminism and its political corollary, suffragism, played a particularly vital role in two of the most prominent anti-medical movements of the later nineteenth century, namely anti-vivisection and the campaign for the repeal of the Contagious Diseases Acts (CDAs). In both cases, the perceived cruelty and oppression of medical practitioners could be linked, both imaginatively and politically, with other instances of male violence and exploitation, such as that of the wife-beater or the proprietor of 'white slaves' (as prostitutes, particularly unwilling ones, were euphemistically known). Such associations were made as long ago as 1985, with Carol Lansbury's *The Old Brown Dog: Women, Workers and Vivisection in Edwardian England*, and they have been developed more recently by Ian Miller (2009). However, other recent work by Paul White (2006) and Rob Boddice (2016) has sought to understand the other side, especially the ways in which physiologists and vivisectors navigated the complex affective politics of the issue, positioning their own emotional restraint against what they presented as the emotional incontinence of their opponents.

The campaign against the CDs has seen the development of a particularly rich vein of historiography. The galvanizing influence here has been the work of Judith Walkowitz, and it is in part because of her legacy that scholarly attention has focused, for the most part, on the figure of the prostitute and the feminist campaign which successfully forced the repeal of the Acts in 1886 (Walkowitz 1980). By contrast, there has been comparatively little written on the medical imperatives behind the Acts. Frank Mort's classic *Dangerous Sexualities: Medico-Moral Politics in England since 1830* (1987) provides the broader cultural context, while Peter Baldwin provides a synoptic political account (1999). Meanwhile, Phillipa Levine's *Prostitution, Race and Politics: Policing Venereal Disease in the British Empire* (2003) offers the suggestive idea that the CDAs were, in many ways, an imperial project reflected back onto the metropole. However, Catherine Lee's recent local study, *Policing Prostitution, 1856–1886: Deviance, Surveillance and Morality* (2013), has little to say about the role of the medical profession, while Anne Hanley's *Medicine, Knowledge and Venereal Diseases in England, 1886–1916* (2017) takes the date of repeal as its chronological starting point. Even Maria Isabel Romero Ruiz's work on the Lock Hospital in the nineteenth century, though it devotes space to a discussion of the Acts, does not take them as its primary focus (2014). Thus, somewhat surprisingly, we have no comprehensive study of such groups as the Association for Promoting the Extension of The Contagious Diseases Act of 1866 to the Civil Population of the United Kingdom, an organization which counted many medical practitioners among its members and which received support from pioneering female physician and suffragist Elizabeth Garrett Anderson. Nor do we have a particularly strong sense of the beliefs and motivations of those medical practitioners working under the Acts.

If medical authority was contested in the sphere of public health then other work has shown how it was also shaped by the broader social, political and economic forces of the period. In particular, medicine assumed an ambivalent position with regards to the market economy and to the liberal doctrines of free trade. In the early modern period, competition between 'orthodox' practitioners and 'unorthodox' quacks had taken place within a relatively unregulated but also less fully developed commercial economy. By the nineteenth century, however, medical practitioners were seeking greater protection and security from the state at a time of increasing commercialization and when the public were repeatedly told that only unrestrained competition could guarantee both quality and affordability. Historians have sought to tease out the intricacies of this ambivalence, demonstrating how medical practitioners might appeal (though not always successfully) to a language of the 'public good' in securing a protected place for 'orthodox' health care in the commercial marketplace (Searle 1998; Brown 2007). Moreover, as both Takahiro Ueyama and Claire Jones have demonstrated, medical practitioners were so enmeshed in a complex web of commercial relations that it was almost impossible to distinguish profit from principle in any case (Ueyama 2010; Jones 2013).

WAR, EMPIRE AND THE STATE

During the age of empire, advances in medicine and surgery meant that military medicine became an increasingly important aspect of any war effort. Throughout the period, Britain and most other nation states were engaged in combat, beginning with the French Revolutionary Wars in 1793 and culminating in the First World War in 1914. While some excellent studies consider cultural aspects of medicine and health during these wars, most focus on the experience of the patient, and gravitate toward the twentieth century – the topic of medical authority during war remains largely underexamined by the cultural historian.[6] This period has, however, provided fertile ground for social and military historians to explore the relationship between medicine and war (Harrison 1996; Cooter 1990; Curtin 1989). Social historians have recently begun to illuminate the interplay between professional and military authority in the medical context, and those studies necessarily touch on points of interest to the cultural history of this period. War created an environment in which the efforts of medical practitioners to cultivate legal and professional authority in broader society were brought into sharp focus. Where the medical care of soldiers was successful, medical participation in war strongly reinforced the growing authority of civilian medicine. For doctors, military service also provided avenues to advance socially and professionally (Ackroyd et al. 2006; Rosner 1999).

Throughout this period, the exigencies of war created opportunity for aspirant forms of medical knowledge to gain a foothold within the profession. Many British military surgeons who entered the service during the Napoleonic Wars had served an apprenticeship and received some formal education at a university. However, they were still disadvantaged compared to the Oxbridge educated physicians who dominated the military medical services. These new recruits fought for professional and military authority in the face of strong opposition. A key feature of this conflict was the military medical officers' push for recognition of an empirically-based approach to medicine over more traditional theoretical knowledge (Kelly 2011). Additionally, mirroring claims to status and authority in civilian life, military medical officers supported their pursuit of professional advancement with the exhibition of overt cultural signifiers associated with gentlemanly or officer classes, including both idealized masculine attributes and a refined education demonstrating 'knowledge of Edmund Burke's theory of the sublime[and] a properly developed understanding of the picturesque'.[7]

The military medical expertise Napoleonic practitioners promoted can be seen as one of the first examples of self-conscious professional medical specialization – a phenomenon that was to become a key medical development across this century. War often served as the crucible for these developments, arguably also crystallizing specialties such as orthopaedics and plastic surgery during the First World War.[8] War could also create opportunities for other medical professions, such as nursing and physiotherapy. The professionalization of nursing services was common to many armies during this period, and the context of the Crimean War is well known. Bertrand Taithe has demonstrated similar developments in France, identifying the emergence of lay (non-religious) nurses during the Franco-Prussian war, as French women embraced the opportunity to practice citizenship by volunteering with the Red Cross (Taithe 2001:111–12). One of the most significant cultural shifts in medicine can be seen coinciding with war at the end of this period when a new cohort of medical practitioners – female doctors – entered the medical services of the British and allied armies where they worked to prove their expertise and 'mettle' (Brock 2017; Murray 1920). Janet Watson's *Fighting Different Wars: Experience, Memory, and the First World War in Britain* (2004) notes that hospitals were not only sites for healing and death, but were also 'the locus for struggles for professional recognition, with women doctors seeking status equivalent to men and trained nurses seeking status as practitioners at all'. Women struggled on dual fronts to win over both military authorities and their professional colleagues. Clair Brock's recent study, *British Women Surgeons and their Patients* (2017), considers the social and cultural representation of female surgeons in the second half of the nineteenth century, and in her final two chapters on the Great War demonstrates how reporting of surgery by women in publications such as the suffragette *Common Causes* stressed the 'difficulty of procedures and feats of endurance' in order to preserve the financial, public and professional support female surgeons received from home.

Discrepancies between growing medical authority in civilian life and lower status within the army could precipitate change beyond the military context. In one of the most significant works to consider military medicine during this period, *The Medical War: British Military Medicine in the First World War* (2010), Mark Harrison surveys the wars of the age of empire and argues that two key aspects of medical authority – the respect given to medical advice by senior commanders, and the degree to which public scrutiny was exercised over medical arrangements – have always been crucial factors in the success of military medical arrangements. The frustrations of medical practitioners regarding their lack of military authority, and consequent inability to provide effective medical services, had been a feature of many wars throughout the century. In his essay, 'Before the World in Concealed Disgrace: Physicians, Professionalization and the 1898 Cuban Campaign of the Spanish American War' (1999), J. T. H. Connor shows that the failures of American doctors in the Spanish American war during the 1890s drew attention to the 'relative impotence' of military doctors in contrast to the increasing authority of their civilian counterparts and that this confusing disparity was seen as a reflection on the entire American profession. Connor argues that it was no coincidence that doctors began to mobilize through the American Medical Association in 1899, transforming the Association's journal into 'an especially aggressive and lobbyist organ'. At the same time, the organization established committees targeting legislative change which were first steps in the 'establishment of permanent machinery for the advancement of the AMA's political goals'. The political potency of national fitness and medical care for soldiers also continued to increase in Britain, reaching an apex during the South African War in 1899 and establishing strong links between military medicine and public morale. In the 1890s, the BMA and Royal Colleges supported army medical officers in a campaign seeking full commissioned officer and command status, resulting in The Royal Warrant of April 1898 granting them substantive rank and limited command (see Figure 8.3).[9]

In addition to fostering changing dynamics of authority within the medical profession, war could also have a profound effect on the public's perception of medicine. During the American Civil War, Shauna Devine (2014) shows that army doctors used the opportunities for learning, experiment and knowledge creation to establish medical authority and advance the professionalization of medicine. During the Crimean War, the failures of military medicine, and the claims of medical practitioners, were subjected to intense public and parliamentary scrutiny – the authority of doctors famously challenged by the

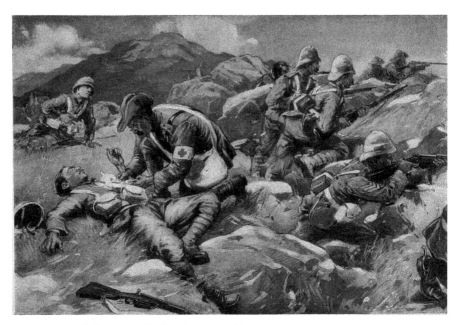

FIGURE 8.3: Military medical authority: 'A Non-combatant Hero – an Army Doctor at Work in the Firing Line' (*c.* 1900). Wellcome Collection.

nursing services and the claims of Florence Nightingale which posed both a professional and a gendered critique of medical authority (Shepherd 1991). Concerns about the health of soldiers, national fitness and the provision of medical care during war had been dominant themes in public discourse, even prior to the Crimea, and also following the Indian Rebellion in 1857. From the 1850s, the army came to occupy a central position in British public life and 'thereafter, militaristic and humanitarian sentiments were closely intertwined' in the defence of the empire (Harrison 2010: 3). By the time of the First World War, public interest in military medicine and the welfare of soldiers was very high, and was facilitated by extensive press reporting of the conflict. During the conflict, the images of military medicine offered to the public were intended to sustain public support for the war effort. Photographs depicted scenes of orderly tented hospital encampments, while postcards featured reassuring images of medical care. Reporters wrote, almost daily, stirring accounts of the heroism and self-sacrifice of doctors and nurses (Harrison 2010). Hospital gazettes such as *Happy Though Wounded* featured what Ana Carden-Coyne has labelled a 'compulsory cheerfulness', amplifying the propaganda of official photography and the press (2014). Along with the relative successes of military medicine, images reflecting medical competence and heroism significantly contributed to a wider medical authority within civilian society.

Perhaps the most intimate form of medical authority lies between practitioner and patient. A feature of military medicine has always been greater control over patient bodies and therapeutic choices than often exists in civilian life. Many historians have considered the implications of this as it relates to advances in medical treatment and the control of bodies both living and dead (Lawrence 1991; Devine 2014), but two recent studies explore the effects on the doctor–patient relationship in the final conflict of this period. Tracey Loughran, in *Shell-Shock and Medical Culture in First World War Britain* (2017), argues that this condition, so emblematic of the First World War, gave doctors an unusual degree of power over uniquely vulnerable patients. She shows how in applying diagnostic labels, choosing treatments and determining whether the soldier was fit to return to combat, the actions of doctors determined how patients suffered, and limited what potential the patient had for agency or resistance. This dynamic between doctor and patient, and the impact of war upon it, is examined closely in another of the most recent contributions to the history of the First World War. In her *The Politics of Wounds: Military Patients and Medical Power in the First World War* (2014), Ana Carden-Coyne illuminates the cultural life of military hospitals and the ways in which patients were subjected to medical authority in all its forms. She finds significance in the patient's experience of the triage system (who would be treated close to the front, who would be sent home for care, or who would be discharged), which often placed military priorities over the personal or medical needs of the patient. She shows that the consequent experience of disempowerment for patients led to a culture of resistance. Patients cultivated this resistance using humour, diaries and cartoons in hospital magazines mocking doctors as incompetent or as delighted torturers of the 'beleaguered wounded soldier'. However, she also draws out the alliances formed between civilian physicians and patients against the exercise of military power and military priorities in the provision of health care.

CONCLUSION

By the early twentieth century, then, medical authority was contested and complicated by a variety of factors. And yet at the same time, medical practitioners had probably never enjoyed greater esteem or public acclaim. The revolutions in surgery and bacteriology which characterized the later part of the nineteenth century served to make this what some have called the 'Golden Age' of medicine (Brandt and Gardner 2004). This paradox is perhaps most neatly encapsulated in George Bernard Shaw's *Doctor's Dilemma* (1906). Shaw's famous 'Preface' of 1909 is a scathing attack on the 'doubtful character of the medical profession', ranging from anti-vaccination and anti-vivisectionist sentiment though to the 'monstrous absurdity' of a commercial medical system in which the surgeon has 'a pecuniary interest in cutting off your leg' (1909/1987:

10). And yet the central protagonist of the play, Sir Colenso Ridgeon, is in many ways a conventional medical hero, proponent of precisely the kind of revolutionary new treatment that enhanced medicine's authority in this period. Shaw's solution to Ridgeon's personal dilemma of who to treat with limited resources is the same as his general solution to the problems of professional respectability. In both instances, the answer for Shaw lay in the development of a state-run system of health care that was in development in this period and which would come to fruition in the mid-twentieth century. However, as the experiences of the later twentieth and early twenty-first centuries have proved, the tensions between commerce and care, profit and public service, remain unresolved.

NOTES

1. For examples of the sociological literature, see Freidson 1970; Berlant 1975. For sociologically-inspired historical accounts, see Starr 1982; Waddington 1984.
2. On the cultural history of medicine, see Fissell 2004. For the 'compromise' of socio-cultural history, see Mandler 2004.
3. See also Shapin 1975.
4. On the Apothecaries Act, see Holloway 1966, Parts I– II; and Loudon 1992. On developments in other jurisdictions, see, for example, Ellis 1995; Frieden 1982; Rozenkrantz 1972; Johnson 2015.
5. For example, Rosen 1958; Porter 1998. Though Porter's account is much more contextualized and social historical and less inclined towards triumphalism, the approach is recognizably similar.
6. See, for example, Reznick 2011; Acton and Potter 2015; Linker 2011.
7. Colley 2005: 172–4; applied to the military context in Kelly 2011: 125. See also Kennedy 2013.
8. On orthopaedics, see Cooter 1993. For a recent treatment of plastic surgery informed by cultural history, see the essays collected in *Journal of War and Culture Studies* 10 (2017), 'Assessing the Legacy of the Gueules Cassées: from Surgery to Art'.
9. Note, however, that Harrison (2010: 5) argues that this change did not result in the hoped for military clout and the disputes of the 1890s 'blighted professional relationships for many years to come'.

BIBLIOGRAPHY

Abel, Emily K. (2007), *Tuberculosis and the Politics of Exclusion: A History of Public Health and Migration to Los Angeles*, New Brunswick, NJ: Rutgers University Press.

Abell, Mora (2009), *Doctor Thomas Monro: Physician, Patron and Painter*, Victoria, Canada: Trafford Publishing.

Abraham, Gerald (1945), *Rimsky-Korsakov: A Short Biography*, London: Duckworth.

Acevedo-Garcia, Dolores (2000), 'Residential Segregation and the Epidemiology of Infectious Diseases', *Social Science & Medicine* 51, no. 8: 1143–61.

Achebe, Chinua (1977), 'An image of Africa', *Massachusetts Review* 18, no. 4: 782–94.

Ackerknecht, Erwin (1948), 'Anticontagionism between 1821 and 1867', *Bulletin of the History of Medicine* 22: 562–93.

Ackerknecht, Erwin (1967), *Medicine at the Paris Hospital, 1794–1848*, Baltimore, MD: Johns Hopkins University Press.

Ackroyd, Marcus et al. (2006) *Advancing with the Army: Medicine, the Professions and Social Mobility in the British Isles 1790–1850*, Oxford: Oxford University Press.

Acton, Carol and Jane Potter (2015), *Working in a World of Hurt: Trauma and Resilience in the Narratives of Medical Personnel in Warzones*, Manchester: Manchester University Press.

Adams, Mark B. (ed.) (1990), *The Wellborn Science: Eugenics in Germany, France, Brazil, and Russia*. Oxford: Oxford University Press.

Addison, W. (1854), 'Notes on Epidemical Diseases', *Association Medical Journal* S3–2: 6–8.

Agland, Jamie (2009), 'Madness and Masculinity in the Caricatures of the Regency Crisis', in Richard Scully and Marian Quartly (eds), *Drawing the Line: Using Cartoons as Historical Evidence*, unpaginated, Clayton, Victoria, Australia: Monash Univ. ePress.

Aisenberg, Andrew R. (1999), *Contagion: Disease, Government, and the 'Social Question' in Nineteenth-Century France*, Stanford, CA: Stanford University Press.

Akehurst, Ann-Marie (2020), 'Quaker Architecture as an Agent of Cure at the York Friends' Retreat', *Quaker Studies* 25, no. 1: 45–76.

Albala, Ken (2014), 'Toward a Historical Dialectic of Culinary Styles', *Historical Research* 87, no. 238: 581–90.

Alberti, Samuel J. M. M. (2011), *Morbid Curiosities: Medical Museums in Nineteenth-Century Britain*, Oxford: Oxford University Press.

Alder, Ken (2007), 'Introduction', Focus section on 'Thick Things', *Isis* 98: 80–3.

Aldrete, J. A. (2004), 'Smallpox vaccination in the early 19th century using live carriers: the travels of Francisco Xavier de Balmis', *Southern Medical Journal* 97: 375–8.

Alexander, R. (1879), 'Practical Notes on the Treatment of Phthisis', *The Lancet* 114: 760–1.

Allen, Michelle (2008), *Cleansing the City: Sanitary Geographies in Victorian London*, Athens, OH: University of Ohio Press.

Anderson, Nancy (2012), 'Facing animals in the laboratory: lessons of nineteenth-century medical school microscopy manuals', in Nancy Anderson and Michael R. Dietrich (eds), *The Educated Eye: Visual Culture and Pedagogy in the Life Sciences*, 44–67, Hanover, NH: Dartmouth College Press.

Anderson, Stephanie (2008), '"Three Living Australians" and the Société d'Anthropologie de Paris, 1885', in Bronwen Douglas and Chris Ballard (eds), *Foreign Bodies: Oceania and the Science of Race 1750–1940*, 229–56, Canberra: ANU Press.

Anderson, Susan and Bruce H. Tabb (eds) (2002), *Water, Leisure and Culture: European Historical Perspectives*, New York: Berg.

Anderson, Warwick (1996a), 'Disease, Race and Empire', *Bulletin of the History of Medicine* 70, no. 1: 62–7.

Anderson, Warwick (1996b), 'Immunities of Empire: Race, Disease, and the New Tropical Medicine, 1900–1920', *Bulletin of the History of Medicine* 70, no. 1: 94–118

Anderson, Warwick (1997), 'The Trespass Speaks: White Masculinity and Colonial Breakdown', *American Historical Review* 102, no. 5:1343–70.

Anderson, Warwick (2003), *The Cultivation of Whiteness: Science, Health and Racial Destiny in Australia*, New York: Basic Books.

Anderson, Warwick (2006), *Colonial Pathologies: American Tropical Medicine, Race, and Hygiene in the Philippines*, Durham, NC: Duke University Press.

Anon. (1855), 'Association Intelligence', *Provincial Medical and Surgical Journal* 13, no. 138: 774–803.

Anon. (1872), 'The progress of medicine and surgery', *Edinburgh Review* 136: 252–65.

Anon. (1877), Editorial, *Nature* 16: 157–8.

Anon. (1883), 'The present state of medical science', *Edinburgh Review* 157: 481–508.

Anon. (1886), 'Review of *Compendium der Psychiatrie zum Gebrauche für Studierende und Aerzte*', *British Journal of Mental Science* 32, no. 138: 254–5.

Anon. (1893), 'The Traumatic Neuroses', *British Medical Journal* 2 (1716: 1115–16.

Anon. (1901), Editorial, *Jewish Chronicle*, 1 February.

Anon. (1906), 'Obituary Mary Putnam Jacobi', *British Medical Journal*, 30 June, 1568.

Anon. (1909), 'Obituary, David James Hamilton', *The Lancet*, 173: 730–1.

Anon. (n.d.), 'patent der Soja-Wurst', *Stiftung Bundeskanzler-Adenauer-Haus* http://adenauerhaus.de/downloads/ExpFeb12.pdf.

Appadurai, Arjun (1986), 'Introduction', in Arjun Appadurai (ed.), *The Social Life of Things: Commodities in Cultural Perspective*, Cambridge: Cambridge University Press.

Apple, Rima D. (1995), 'Science Gendered: Nutrition in the United States 1840–1940', in Harmke Kamminga and Andrew Cunningham (eds), *Science and Culture of Nutrition, 1840–1940*, 129–54, Amsterdam: Editions Rodopi B.V.

Arnold, D. (1993), *Colonizing the Body: State Medicine and Epidemic Disease in Nineteenth-Century India*, Berkeley: University of California Press.

Arnold, David (1999), '"An ancient race outworn": Malaria and Race in Colonial India', in Waltraud Ernst and Bernard Harris (eds), *Race, Society and Medicine, 1700–1960*, 123–43, London: Routledge.

Arnold, David (ed.) (1996), *Warm Climates and Western Medicine: The Emergence of Tropical Medicine, 1500–1900*, Amsterdam: Rodopi.

Arnott, Neil and J. P. Kay (1837–38), 'Report on the Prevalence of Certain Physical Causes of Fever in the Metropolis, Which Might be Removed by Proper Sanatory Measures', in *Fourth Annual Report of the Poor Law Commissioners, Supplement*, London: HMSO.

Arnup, K. (1992), '"Victims of Vaccination?" Opposition to Compulsory Immunization in Ontario, 1900–90', *Canadian Bulletin of Medical History* 9: 159–76.

Aronowitz, Robert (2008), 'Framing disease: an underappreciated mechanism for the social patterning of health', *Social Science & Medicine* 67, no. 1: 1–9.

Atkins, Peter (2012), 'Animal Wastes and Nuisances in Nineteenth-Century London', in Peter Atkins (ed.), *Animal Cities: Beastly Urban Histories*, 19–51, London: Routledge.

Atkins, Peter (ed.) (2012), *Animal Cities: Beastly Urban Histories*, London: Routledge.

Atwater, Wilbur Olin and C. F. Langworthy (1897), 'A Digest of Metabolism Experiments in Which the Balance of Income and Outgo Was Determined', *US Department of Agriculture. Office of Experiment Stations, Bulletin*. Washington, DC: Government Printing Office.

Bailey, Peter (1996), 'Breaking the Sound Barrier: A Historian Listens to Noise', *Body and Society* 2, no. 2: 49–66.

Bailin, Miriam (2007), *The Sickroom in Victorian Fiction: The Art of Being Ill*, Cambridge: Cambridge University Press.

Baldwin, Peter (1999), *Contagion and the State in Europe, 1830–1930*, Cambridge: Cambridge University Press.

[Banim, John and Michael Banim] (1831), *Chaunt of the Cholera: Songs for Ireland*, London: James Cochrane and Co.

Baratay, E. and E. Hardouin-Fugier (2002), *Zoo: A History of Zoological Gardens in the West*, London: Reaktion Books Ltd.

Barham, Peter (2004), *Forgotten Lunatics of the Great War*, London: Yale University Press.

Barker, Hannah (2009), 'Medical advertising and trust in late Georgian England', *Urban History* 36, no. 3: 379–98.

Barnes, David (2006), *The Great Stink of Paris and the Nineteenth-Century Struggle Against Filth and Germs*, Baltimore, MD: Johns Hopkins University Press.

Barnes, David S. (1995), *The Making of a Social Disease: Tuberculosis in Nineteenth-Century France*, Berkeley: University of California Press.

Barnett, L. Margaret (1995), '"Every Man His Own Physician": Dietetic Fads, 1890–1914', in Harmke Kamminga and Andrew Cunningham (eds), *Science and Culture of Nutrition, 1840–1940*, 155–78, Amsterdam: Editions Rodopi B.V.

Barnett, L. Margaret (1997), 'Fletcherism: The Chew-Chew Fad of the Edwardian Era', in David Smith (ed.), *Nutrition in Britain: Science, Scientists and Politics in the Twentieth Century*, 6–28. London: Routledge.

Bartrip, Peter W. J. and Sandra Burman (1983), *The Wounded Soldiers of Industry: Industrial Compensation Policy, 1833–1897*, Oxford: Oxford University Press.

Baschin, Marion (2016), '"Globules at Home": The History of Homeopathic Self-medication', *Social History of Medicine* 29, no. 4: 717–33.

Bashford, Alison (2003), 'Cultures of Confinement: Tuberculosis, Isolation and the Sanatorium', in Carolyn Strange and Alison Bashford (eds), *Isolation: Places and Practices of Exclusion*, 133–50, New York: Routledge.

Bashford, Alison (2004), *Imperial Hygiene: A Critical History of Colonialism, Nationalism and Public Health*, New York: Palgrave.

Bates, Christina (2012), *A Cultural History of the Nurse's Uniform*, Gatineau: Canadian Museum of Civilization.

Bates, Victoria (2016), '"Under cross-examination she fainted": sexual crime and swooning in the Victorian courtroom', *Journal of Victorian Culture* 21, no. 4: 456–70.

Baumgartner, Barbara (2016), 'Anatomy Lessons: Emily Dickinson's Brain Poems', *Legacy: A Journal of American Women Writers* 33, no. 1: 55–81.

Baxby, Derrick (1981), *Jenner's Smallpox Vaccine: The Riddle of Vaccinia Virus and its Origin*, London: Heinemann.

Bederman, Gail (2008), *Manliness and Civilization: A Cultural History of Gender and Race in the United States, 1880–1917*, Chicago: University of Chicago Press.

Beinart, William (2007), 'Transhumance, Animal Diseases and Environment in the Cape, South Africa', *South African Historical Journal* 58: 17–41.

Bell, Charles (1806), *Essays on the Anatomy of Expression in Painting*, London: Longman, Hurst, Rees, and Orme.

Bell, Charles (1824), *Essays on the Anatomy and Philosophy of Expression*, London: John Murray.

Bennett, Tony and Patrick Joyce (2010), 'Introduction', in Tony Bennett and Patrick Joyce (eds), *Material Powers: Cultural Studies, History and the Material Turn*, 1–21, Abingdon: Routledge.

Benson, E. (2011), 'Animal Writes: Historiography, Disciplinarity, and the Animal Trace', in L. Kalof and G. M. Montgomery (eds), *Making Animal Meaning*, 3–16, East Lansing: Michigan State University Press.

Bergen, Leo van (1999/2004), '"The Malingerers are to Blame": The Dutch Military Health Service before and during the First World War', in Roger Cooter, Mark Harrison and Steve Sturdy (eds), *Medicine and Modern Warfare*, 59–76, Amsterdam: Rodopi.

Berkowitz, Carin (2015), *Charles Bell and the Anatomy of Reform*, Chicago: University of. Chicago Press.

Berlant, Jeffrey (1975), *Profession and Monopoly*, Berkley: University of California Press.

Bernard, Claude (1865/2016), *Introduction à la médecine expérimentale*, Paris: BnF collection ebooks.

Berti, Ilaria (2016), '"Feeding the Sick upon Stewed Fish and Pork": Slave Health and Food in West Indies Sugar Plantation Hospitals', *Food & History* 14, no. 1: 81–106.

Bewell, Allan (1999), *Romanticism and Colonial Disease*, Baltimore, MD: Johns Hopkins University Press.

Bhattacharya, Sanjoy (1998), 'Re-devising Jennerian Vaccines? European Technologies, Indian Innovation and the Control of Smallpox in South Asia, 1850–1950', *Social Scientist* 26: 27–66.

Bhattacharya, Sanjoy, Mark Harrison and Michael Worboys (2005), *Fractured States: Smallpox, Public Health and Vaccination Policy in British India, 1800–1947*, Hyderabad: Orient Longman.

Bickham, T. (2008), 'Eating the Empire: Intersections of Food, Cookery and Imperialism in Eighteenth-Century Britain', *Past & Present* 198, no. 1: 71–109.

Binet, Alfred (1907), *The Mind and the Brain*, London: K. Paul, Trench, Trübner & Company Limited.

Bittel, Carla (2009), *Mary Putnam Jacobi and the Politics of Medicine in Nineteenth-Century America*, Chapel Hill: University of North Carolina Press.

Bivins, Roberta (2000), *Acupuncture, Expertise, and Cross-Cultural Medicine*, Basingstoke: Palgrave.

Blaine, Delabere (1802), *The Outlines of the Veterinary Art, or, The Principles of Medicine: As Applied to the Structure, Functions and Economy of the Horse, the Ox, the Sheep and the Dog*, London: T. N. Longman.

Bland Sutton, John (1885), 'On Hypertrophy and its Value in Evolution', *Proceedings of the Zoological Society of London*: 432–45.

Bland Sutton, John (1886), *An Introduction to General Pathology*, Philadelphia: Blakiston & Son.

Bland Sutton, John (1890), *Evolution and Disease*, London: Walter Scott.

Blatter, Jeremy (2014), 'The Psychotechnics of Everyday Life: Hugo Münsterberg and the Politics of Applied Psychology, 1887–1917', PhD thesis, Harvard University.

Blatter, Jeremy (2015), 'Screening the Psychological Laboratory: Hugo Münsterberg, Psychotechnics, and the Cinema, 1892–1916', *Science in Context* 28, no. 1: 53–76.

Block, Daniel (2005), 'Saving Milk Through Masculinity: Public Health Officers and Pure Milk, 1880–1930', *Food and Foodways* 13, no. 1–2: 115–34.

Blum, Nava and Elizabeth Fee (2008), 'The First Mental Hospital in China', *American Journal of Public Health* 98, no. 9: 1593.

Boddice, Rob (2011), 'Vivisecting Major: A Victorian Gentleman Scientist Defends Animal Experimentation', *Isis* 102: 215–37.

Boddice, Rob (2012), 'Species of Compassion: Aesthetics, Anaesthetics and Pain in the Physiological Laboratory', *19: Interdisciplinary Studies in the Long Nineteenth Century* 15, unpaginated.

Boddice, Rob (2014), 'German Methods, English Morals: Physiological Networks and the Question of Callousness, c.1870–1881', in Heather Ellis and Ulrike Kirchberger (eds), *Anglo-German Scholarly Relations in the Long Nineteenth Century*, 84–102, Leiden and Boston: Brill.

Boddice, Rob (2016), *The Science of Sympathy: Morality, Evolution and Victorian Civilization*, Urbana-Champaign: University of Illinois Press.

Boddice, Rob (2017), *Pain: A Very Short Introduction*, Oxford: Oxford University Press.

Boddice, Rob (2017a), 'Hysteria or Tetanus? Ambivalent Embodiments and the Authenticity of Pain', in Dolores Martin Moruno and Beatriz Pichel (eds), *Emotional Bodies: Studies on the Historical Performativity of Emotions*, 19–35, Urbana-Champaign: University of Illinois Press.

Boddice, Rob (2021), *Humane Professions: The Defence of Experimental Medicine, 1876–1914*, Cambridge: Cambridge University Press.

Boddice, Rob (ed.) (2014), *Pain and Emotion in Modern History*. Basingstoke: Palgrave.

Boddice, Rob and Daniel Lord Smail (2018), 'Neurohistory', in Peter Burke and Marek Tamm (eds), 301–25, *Debating New Approaches in History*, London: Bloomsbury.

Boddice, Rob and Mark Smith (2020), *Emotion, Sense, Experience*, Cambridge: Cambridge University Press.

Boissel, Jean (1993), *Gobineau, Biographie : Mythes et Réalité*, Paris: Berg International.

Boos, Florence (2013), 'Under Physical Siege: Early Victorian Autobiographies of Working-Class Women, *Philological Quarterly* 92, no. 2: 251–69.

Borden, Gail (1853), *The Meat Biscuit: Invented, Patented, and Manufactured*, New York: JH Brower & Co.

Borden, Gail and Ashbel Smith (1850), *Letter of Gail Borden Jr to Dr Ashbel Smith Setting Forth an Important Invention in the Preparation of A New Article of Food Termed Meatbiscuits; and the Reply of Dr Smith Thereto: Being a Letter Addressed to the American Association for the Promotion of Science*, Galveston, TX: Gibson & Cherry.

Bound Alberti, Fay (2010), *Matters of the Heart: History, Medicine, and Emotion*, Oxford: Oxford University Press.

Bourdieu, Pierre (1986), 'The forms of capital', in J. Richardson (ed.), *Handbook of Theory and Research for the Sociology of Education*, 46–58, New York: Greenwood.

Bourke, Joanna (1994), 'Housewifery in working-class England 1860–1914', *Past & Present* 143, no. 1: 167–97.

Bourke, Joanna (1996), *Dismembering the Male: Men's Bodies, Britain and the Great War*, London: Reaktion.

Bourke, Joanna (2014), 'Phantom Suffering: Amputees, Stump Pain and Phantom Sensations in Modern Britain', in Rob Boddice (ed.), *Pain and Emotion in Modern History*, 66–89, Houndmills: Palgrave.

Bourke, Joanna (2014), *The Story of Pain: From Prayer to Painkillers*, Oxford: Oxford University Press.

Boutin, Aimee (2015), *City of Noise: Sound and Nineteenth-Century Paris*, Chicago: University of Illinois Press.

Brandt, Allan M. (1987), *No Magic Bullet: A Social History of Venereal Disease in the United States since 1880*, Oxford: Oxford University Press.

Brandt Allan M. and Martha Gardner (2000), 'The Golden Age of Medicine?', in Roger Cooter and John Pickstone (eds), *Companion to Medicine in the Twentieth Century*, 21–37, London: Routledge.

Braun, Marta (1994), *Picturing Time: The Work of Etienne-Jules Marey (1830–1904)*, Chicago: University of Chicago Press.

Briggs, Asa (1961), 'Cholera and Society in the Nineteenth Century', *Past & Present* 19, no. 1: 76–96.

Brimnes, Niels (2004), 'Variolation, Vaccination and Popular Resistance in Early Colonial South India', *Medical History* 48: 199–228.

Brittan, Francesca (2006), 'Berlioz and the pathological fantastic: melancholy, monomania, and romantic autobiography', *19th-century Music* 29, no. 3: 211–39.

Broca, Paul (1863), 'Review of the Proceedings of the Anthropological Society of Paris, delivered June 4th, 1863', *Anthropological Review* 1, no. 2: 274–310.

Brock, Claire (2017), *British Women Surgeons and Their Patients, 1860–1918*, Cambridge: Cambridge University Press.

Brooks, Jane and Anne-Marie Rafferty (2007), 'Dress and distinction in nursing, 1860–1939: A corporate (as well as corporeal) armour of probity and purity', *Women's History Review* 16, no. 1: 41–57.

Brown, Michael (2007), 'Medicine, Quackery and the Free Market: The "War" Against Morison's Pills and the Construction of the Medical Profession, c.1830–c.1850', in Mark S. R. Jenner and Patrick Wallis (eds), *Medicine and the Market in England and its Colonies, c.1450– c.1850*, 238–61, Basingstoke: Palgrave.

Brown, Michael (2008), 'From foetid air to filth: the cultural transformation of British epidemiological thought, c. 1780–1848', *Bulletin for the History of Medicine* 82, no. 3: 515–44.

Brown, Michael (2010), '"Like a Devoted Army": Medicine, Heroic Masculinity and the Military Paradigm in Victorian Britain', *Journal of British Studies* 49, no. 3: 592–622.

Brown, Michael (2011), *Performing Medicine: Medical Culture and Identity in Provincial England, c.1760–1850*, Manchester: Manchester University Press.

Brown, Michael (2017), 'Surgery and Emotion: The Era Before Anaesthesia', in Thomas Schlich (ed.), *The Palgrave Handbook of the History of Surgery*, 327–47, Houdmills: Palgrave, 2017.

Brown, Prof. (1888), *Report on Eruptive Diseases of the Teats and Udders of Cows in Relation to Scarlet Fever in Man*, London: Agricultural Department, Privy Council Office.

Browne, Janet (1995), *Charles Darwin: Voyaging*, Princeton, NJ: Princeton University Press.

Brunton, Deborah (2008), *The Politics of Vaccination: Practice and Policy in England, Wales, Ireland, and Scotland, 1800–1874*, Rochester, NY: University of Rochester Press.

Bryder, Linda (1988), *Below the Magic Mountain: A Social History of Tuberculosis in Twentieth-Century Britain*, Oxford: Oxford University Press.

Buchanan, George (1857), *Report of the Medical Officer of Health for St. Giles District*, London: Board of Works.

Budd, Michael Anton (1997), *The Sculpture Machine: Physical Culture and Body Politics in the Age of Empire*, Basingstoke: Macmillan.

Bull, Michael and Les Black (eds) (2003), *The Auditory Culture Reader*, New York: Berg.

Budd, William (1863), 'Variola Ovina, Sheep's Small-Pox: Or the Laws of Contagious Epidemics Illustrated by an Experimental Type', *British Medical Journal* 2: 141–50.

Budd, William (1865), 'The Siberian Cattle Plague; or, the Typhoid Fever of the Ox', *British Medical Journal* 2: 169–79.

Bulloch, W. (1925), 'Emmanuel Klein', *Journal of Pathology and Bacteriology* 28: 684–99.

Burdett, B. (2011), 'Is Empathy the End of Sentimentality?', *Journal of Victorian Culture* 16, no. 2: 259–74.

Burdett, C. (2011a), '"The subjective inside us can turn into the objective outside": Vernon Lee's psychological aesthetics', *19: Interdisciplinary Studies in the Long Nineteenth Century*: 12.

Burkhardt, Richard (1999), 'Ethology, Natural History, the Life Sciences, and the Problem of Place', *Journal of the History of Biology* 32: 489–508.

Burnett, J. (1966), *Plenty and Want: A Social History of Diet in England from 1815 to the Present Day*, Edinburgh: Thomas Nelson.

Burnett, John, David Vincent and David Mayall (1984), *The Autobiography of the Working Class: An Annotated Critical Bibliography*, Brighton: Harvester.

Burney Frances (1812), letter to Esther Burney, 22 March, in Frances Burney, *Journals and Letters*, London: Penguin, 2001.

Busch, Jane Celia (1983), 'The Throwaway Ethic in America', PhD diss., University of Pennsylvania.

Bynum, W. F. (1990), '"C'est une Malade!" Animal Models and Concepts of Human Diseases', *Journal of the History of Medicine and Allied Sciences* 45: 397–413.

Bynum, W. F. (1994), *Science and the Practice of Medicine in the Nineteenth Century*, Cambridge: Cambridge University Press.

Bynum, W. F. (2000), 'Discarded diagnoses', *The Lancet*, 356, no. 9241: 1615.

Bynum, W. F. (2002), 'The Evolution of Germs and the Evolution of Disease: Some British Debates, 1870–1900', *History and Philosophy of the Life Sciences* 24: 53–68.

Cajal, Santiago Ramón y (1899), 'Comparative study of the sensory areas of the human cortex', in William Edward Story (ed.), *Clark University, 1889–1899: Decennial Celebration*, 311–82, Worcester, MA: Clark University Press.

Callen, Anthea (1995), *The Spectacular Body: Science, Method and Meaning in the Work of Degas*, London and New Haven, CT: Yale University Press.

Callen, Anthea (2018), *Looking at Men: Art, Anatomy, and the Modern Male Body*, London and New Haven, CT: Yale University Press.

Campbell, Margaret (1999), 'From Cure Chair to Chaise Longue: Medical Treatment and the Form of the Modern Recliner', *Journal of Design History* 12, no. 4: 327–43.

Campbell, Margaret (2005), 'What Tuberculosis did for Modernism: The Influence of a Curative Environment on Modernist Design and Architecture', *Medical History* 49, no. 4: 463–88.

Canghilhem, Georges (1965), *La Connaissance de la Vie*, Paris : J. Vrin.

Carden-Coyne, A. (2008), 'Painful bodies and brutal women: remedial massage, gender relations and cultural agency in military hospitals, 1914–1918', *Journal of War and Culture Studies* 1: 139–58.

Carden-Coyne, Ana (2009), *Reconstructing the Body: Classicism, Modernism, and the First World War*, Oxford: Oxford University Press.

Carden-Coyne, A. (2014), *The Politics of Wounds: Military Patients and Medical Power in the First World War*, Oxford: Oxford University Press.

Carlisle, Janice (2004), *Common Scents: Comparative Encounters in High-Victorian Fiction*, New York: Oxford University Press.

Carlyle, Thomas (1833–4/1918), *Sartor Resartus: The Life and Opinions of Herr Teufelsdröckh. In Three Books*, Oxford: Clarendon Press.

Carpenter, Kenneth J. (1994), *Protein and Energy: A Study of Changing Ideas in Nutrition*, Cambridge: Cambridge University Press.

Carpenter, Kenneth J. (2006) 'Nutritional Studies in Victorian Prisons', *Journal of Nutrition* 136, no. 1: 1–8.

Cartwright, Lisa (1995), *Screening the Body: Tracing Medicine's Visual Culture*, Minneapolis: University of Minnesota Press, 48–75.

Casper, Stephen T. (2014), *The Neurologists: A History of a Medical Speciality in Modern Britain, c. 1789–2000*, Manchester: Manchester University Press.

Cassidy, A., R. Dentinger, K. Schoefert and A. Woods (2017), 'Animal Roles and Traces in the History of Medicine, c.1880–1980', *BJHS Themes*: 1–23.

Cassier, Maurice (2005), 'Appropriation and Commercialization of the Pasteur Anthrax Vaccine', *Studies in History and Philosophy of Science Part C: Studies in History and Philosophy of Biological and Biomedical Sciences* 36: 722–42.

Cavallo, Sandra (2007), *Artisans of the Body in Early Modern Italy: Identities, Families, Masculinities*, Manchester: Manchester University Press.

Çelik, Zeynep (1993), *The Remaking of Istanbul: Portrait of an Ottoman City in the Nineteenth Century*, Berkeley: University of California Press.

Chambers, Thomas A. (2002), *Drinking the Waters: Creating an American Leisure Class at Nineteenth-Century Mineral Springs*, Washington, DC: Smithsonian Institution Press.

Chaplin, Simon (2009), 'John Hunter and the "Museum Oeconomy", 1750–1800', PhD diss., King's College London.

Chapman, Carleton B. (1967), 'Edward Smith (? 1818–1874), Physiologist, Human Ecologist, Reformer', *Journal of the History of Medicine and Allied Sciences* 22, no. 1: 1–26.

Charcot, J.-M. (1877) *Leçons sur les maladies du système nerveux faites a la Salpêtrière*, Paris: Adrien Delahaye.

Chartier, Roger (1988), *Cultural History*, Cambridge: Polity Press.

Cheadle, Dr. (1882), 'Introductory Address: A Discussion on Rickets', *British Medical Journal* 2: 1145–8.

Chevalier, Louis (1958), *Classes Laborieuses et Classes Dangereuses à Paris pendant la Première Moitié du XIXe siècle*, Paris : Plon.

Cheyne, George (1733), *The English malady: or, A treatise of nervous diseases of all kinds, as spleen, vapours, lowness of spirits, hypochondriacal, and hysterical distempers, etc.*, London: G. Strahan.

Churchill, Frederick (1976), 'Rudolf Virchow and the Pathologist's Criteria for the Inheritance of Acquired Characteristics', *Journal of the History of Medicine and Allied Sciences* 31: 117–48.

Churchill, Frederick (1997), 'Life Before Model Systems: General Zoology at August Weismann's Institute', *American Zoologist* 37: 260–8.

Claeys, Gregory and Lyman Tower Sargent (eds) (1999), *The Utopian Reader*, New York: New York University Press.

Clark, Emily (2015), 'Mad Literature: Insane Asylums in Nineteenth-Century America', *Arizona Journal of Interdisciplinary Studies* 4, no. 1: 42–64.

Clark, James (1829), *The Influence of Climate in the Prevention and Cure of Chronic Diseases, More Particularly of the Chest and Digestive Organs: Comprising an Account of the Principal Places Resorted to by Invalids in England and the South of Europe; A Comparative Estimate of their Respective Merits in Particular Diseases; and General Directions for Invalids while Travelling and Residing Abroad. With an appendix, containing a series of tables on climate*, London: Thomas and George Underwood.

Classen, Constance (1993), *Worlds of Sense: Exploring the Senses in History and Across Cultures*, London: Routledge.

Classen, Constance (ed.) (2014), *A Cultural History of the Senses*, 6 vols, London: Bloomsbury.

Cohen, William A. and Ryan Johnson (eds) (2004), *Filth: Dirt, Disgust and Modern Life*, Minneapolis: University of Minnesota Press.

Coleborne, Catharine (2010), *Madness in the Family: Insanity and Institutions in the Australasian Colonial World, 1860–1914*, London: Palgrave Macmillan.

Coleborne, Catharine (2015), *Insanity, Identity and Empire: Immigrants and institutional Confinement in Australia and New Zealand, 1873–1910*, Manchester: Manchester University Press.

Coleborne, Catharine and Dolly McKinnon (2011), *Exhibiting Madness in Museums: Remembering Psychiatry Through Collection and Display*, London: Routledge.

Coleman, William (1987), *Yellow Fever in the North: The Methods of Early Epidemiology*, Madison: University of Wisconsin Press.

Coleman, William and F. L. Holmes (eds) (1988), *The Investigative Enterprise: Experimental Physiology in Nineteenth-Century Medicine*, Berkeley: University of California Press.

Colley, Linda (2005) *Britons: Forging the Nation 1707–1837*, New Haven, CT: Yale University Press.

Collins, Joseph (1911), *The Way with the Nerves: Letters to a Neurologist on Various Modern Nervous Ailments, real and fancied, with replies thereto telling of their nature and treatment*, New York and London: G.P. Putnam's Sons.

Colomina, Beatriz (2007), *Domesticity at War*, Cambridge, MA: MIT Press.

Condrau, Flurin (2007), 'The Patient's View Meets the Clinical Gaze', *Social History of Medicine* 20: 525–40.

Condrau, Flurin (2010), 'Beyond the Total Institution: Towards a Reinterpretation of the Tuberculosis Sanatorium', in Flurin Condrau and Michael Worboys (eds), *Tuberculosis Then and Now: Perspectives on the History of an Infectious Disease*, 72–99, Montreal: McGill-Queen's University Press.

Cone, T. E. (1979), *History of American Pediatrics*, Boston: Little, Brown and Co.

Connor, J. T. H. (1999), '"Before the World in Concealed Disgrace": Physicians, Professionalization and the 1898 Cuban Campaign of the Spanish American War', in Roger Cooter, Mark Harrison and Steve Sturdy (eds). *Medicine and Modern Warfare*, 1–28. Amsterdam: Rodopi.

Cook, Noble David and William George Lovell (2001), *Secret Judgments of God: Old World Disease in Colonial Spanish America*, Norman: University of Oklahoma Press.

Cooter, Roger (1984), *The Cultural Meaning of Popular Science: Phrenology and the Organization of Consent in Nineteenth-Century Britain*, Cambridge: Cambridge University Press.

Cooter, Roger (1990) 'Medicine and the Goodness of War', *Canadian Bulletin of Medical History* 12: 147–59.

Cooter, Roger (1993), *Surgery and Society in Peace and War: Orthopaedics and the Organization of Modern Medicine, 1880–1948*, Basingstoke: Macmillan.

Cooter, Roger (1998), 'Malingering in modernity: psychological scripts and adversarial encounters during the First World War', in Roger Cooter, Mark Harrison and Steve Sturdy (eds), *War, Medicine and Modernity*, 125–48, Stroud: Sutton Press.

Cooter, Roger (2010), 'The Turn of the Body: History and the Politics of the Corporeal', *Arbor Ciencia, Pensamiento y Cultura*, 186: 393–405.

Cooter, R. (ed.) (1992), *In the Name of the Child: Health and Welfare, 1880–1940*, London: Routledge.

Cooter, Roger with Claudia Stein (2016), *Writing History in the Age of Biomedicine*, New Haven, CT: Yale University Press.

Copping, Matthew C. (2003), '"Honour Among Professionals": Medicine, Chemistry and Arsenic at the *Fin de Siècle*', PhD diss., University of Kent at Canterbury.

Corbin, Alain (1986), 'Commercial Sexuality in Nineteenth-Century France: A System of Images and Regulations', *Representations* 14: 209–19.

Corbin, Alain (1986), *The Foul and the Fragrant: Odor and the French Social Imagination*, Cambridge, MA: Harvard University Press.

Corbin, Alain (1995), *Time, Desire and Horror: Towards a History of the Senses*. Cambridge: Polity.

Corbin, Alain (1996), *Women for Hire: Prostitution and Sexuality in France after 1850*, Cambridge, MA: Harvard University Press.

Corbin, Alain (1998), *Village Bells: Sound and Meaning in the Nineteenth-Century French Countryside*, tran. Martin Thom, New York: Columbia University Press.

Cranefield, P. (1991), *Science and Empire: East Coast Fever in Rhodesia and the Transvaal*, Cambridge: Cambridge University Press.

Crary, Jonathan (1990), *Techniques of the Observer: On Vision and Modernity in the Nineteenth Century*, Cambridge, MA: MIT Press.

Crook, Tom (2007), 'Sanitary Inspection and the Public Sphere in Late Victorian and Edwardian Britain: A Case Study in Liberal Governance', *Social History* 32, no. 4: 369–93.

Crook, Tom (2016), *Governing Systems: Modernity and the Making of Public Health in England, 1830–1910*, Berkeley: University of California Press.

Crook, Tom and Mike Esbester (eds) (2016), *Governing Risks in Modern Britain: Danger, Safety and Accidents, c. 1800–2000*, Basingstoke: Palgrave.

Crook, Tom, Rebecca Gill and Bertrand Taithe (eds) (2011), *Evil, Barbarism and Empire: Britain and Abroad, c. 1830–2000*, Basingstoke: Palgrave.

Crook, T. and G. O'Hara (eds) (2011), *Statistics and the Public Sphere: Numbers and the People in Modern Britain, c. 1800–2000*, Abingdon: Routledge.

Crookshank, Edgar (1889), *History and Pathology of Vaccination: A Critical Inquiry*, London: HK Lewis.

Crozier, Anna (2007), 'Sensationalising Africa: British Medical Impressions of Sub-Saharan Africa, 1890–1939', *Journal of Imperial and Commonwealth History* 35, no. 3: 393–415.

Cryle, Peter and Elizabeth Stephens (2017), *Normality: A Critical Genealogy*, Chicago: University of Chicago Press.

Cunningham, Andrew and Perry Williams (eds) (1992), *The Laboratory Revolution in Medicine* Cambridge: Cambridge University Press.

Curtin, Philip D. (1961), 'The White Man's Grave: Image and Reality 1780–1850', *Journal of British Studies* 1, no. 1: 94–110.

Curtin, Philip D. (1989), *Death by Migration: Europe's Encounter with the Tropical World in the Nineteenth Century*, Cambridge: Cambridge University Press.

Curtin, Philip D. (1990), 'The End of the "White Man's Grave"? Nineteenth-century Mortality in West Africa', *Journal of Interdisciplinary History* 21, no. 1: 63–88.

Curtin, Philip D. (1998), *Disease and Empire: The Health of European Troops in the Conquest of Africa*, Cambridge: Cambridge University Press.

Curtis, Scott (2012), 'Photography and medical observation', in Nancy Anderson and Michael R. Dietrich (eds), *The Educated Eye: Visual Culture and Pedagogy in the Life Sciences*, 68–93, Hanover, NH: Dartmouth College Press.

Daston, Lorraine (ed.) (2008), *Things that Talk*, New York: Zone Books.

Daston, Lorraine and Peter Galison (1992), 'The Image of Objectivity', *Representations* 40, Special Issue: Seeing Science: 81–128.

Daston, Lorraine J. and Peter Galison (2010), *Objectivity*, Cambridge, MA: Zone Books, 133.

Daudet, Alphonse (2003), *In the Land of Pain*, trans. Julian Barnes, London: Jonathan Cape.

Davidoff, Leonore (1974), 'Mastered for Life: Servant and Wife in Victorian and Edwardian England', *Journal of Social History* 7, no. 4: 460–28.

Davidson, Luke (1996), '"Identities Ascertained": British ophthalmology in the first half of the nineteenth century', *Social History of Medicine* 9, no. 3: 313–33.

Davin, A. (1996), 'Loaves and Fishes: Food in Poor Households in Late Nineteenth-Century London', *History Workshop Journal* 41, no. 1: 167–92.

Davis, Audrey B. (1978), 'Historical Studies of Medical Instruments', *History of Science* 16: 107–33.

Davis, Audrey B. (1981), *Medicine and its Technology: An Introduction to the History of Medical Instrumentation*, Westport, CT: Greenwood Press.

Deacon, Harriet (1996), 'Racial Segregation and Medical Discourse in Nineteenth-Century Cape Town', *Journal of Southern African Studies* 22, no. 2: 287–308.

de Chadarevian, Soraya (1993), 'Graphical method and discipline: self-recording instruments in nineteenth-century physiology', *Studies in History and Philosophy of Science* 24, no. 2: 267–91.

Delaporte, François (1986), *Disease and Civilization: The Cholera in Paris, 1832*, Cambridge, MA: MIT Press.

de Rijcke, Sarah (2008), 'Light Tries the Expert Eye: The Introduction of Photography in Nineteenth-Century Macroscopic Neuroanatomy', *Journal of the History of the Neurosciences* 17: 349–66.

Derry, Margaret (2015), *Masterminding Nature: The Breeding of Animals, 1750–2010*, Toronto: University of Toronto Press.

Desmond, Adrian (1989), *The Politics of Evolution*, London: University of Chicago Press.

Devine, Shauna (2014), *Learning from the Wounded: The Civil War and the Rise of American Medical Science*, Chapel Hill: University of North Carolina Press.

Didi-Huberman, Georges (1982/2003), *Invention of Hysteria: Charcot and the Photographic Iconography of the Salpêtrière*, trans. Alisa Hartz, Cambridge, MA and London: MIT Press.

Dierig, Sven (2003), 'Engines for Experiment: Laboratory Revolution and Industrial Labor in the Nineteenth-Century City', *Osiris* 18, no. 1: 116–34.

Digby, Anne (1985), *Madness, Morality and Medicine: A Study of the York Retreat, 1796–1914*, Cambridge: Cambridge University Press.

Dixon, Thomas (2012), 'The Tears of Mr Justice Willes', *Journal of Victorian Culture* 17, no. 1: 1–23.

Dobson, Jessie (1962), 'John Hunter's Animals', *Journal of the History of Medicine and Allied Sciences* 27: 479–86.

Douglas, Mary (1966), *Purity and Danger: An Analysis of Concepts of Pollution and Taboo*, London: Routledge.

Dowbiggin, Ian (1991), *Inheriting Madness: Professionalization and Psychiatric Knowledge in Nineteenth-Century France*, Berkeley: University of California Press.

Dracobly, Alex (2003), 'Ethics and Experimentation on Human Subjects in Mid-Nineteenth-Century France: The Story of the 1859 Syphilis Experiments', *Bulletin of the History of Medicine* 77, no. 2: 332–66.

Drobnick, Jim (ed.) (2006), *The Smell Culture Reader*, New York: Berg.

Droin, Geneviève (2005), 'Endemic Goiter and Cretinism in the Alps', *International Journal of Anthropology* 20, no. 3–4: 307–24.

du Camp, Maxime (1878–80), *Les Convulsions de Paris*, Paris: Hachette.

Durbach, Nadja (2004), *Bodily Matters: The Anti-vaccination Movement in England, 1853–1907*, Durham NC: Duke University Press.

Dwork, D. (1987), 'The Milk Option: An Aspect of the History of the Infant Welfare Movement in England 1898–1908', *Medical History* 31, no. 1: 51–69.

Dwyer, Ellen (1987), *Homes for the Mad: Life Inside Two Nineteenth-Century Asylums*, New Brunswick, NJ: Rutgers University Press.

Dyck, Erika and Christopher Fletcher (eds) (2011), *Locating Health: Historical and Anthropological Investigations of Health and Place*, London: Pickering and Chatto.

Edgerton, David (2006), *The Shock of The Old: Technology and Global History since 1900*, London: Profile Books.

Editorial (1834), 'On Phthisis in Monkeys and Other Animals', *The Lancet* 22: 145–7.

Eigen, Joel (1995), *Witnessing Insanity: Madness and Mad-doctors in the English Court*, London: Yale University Press.

Eigen, Joel (2003), *Unconscious Crime, Mental Absence and Criminal Responsibility in Victorian London*, London: Johns Hopkins University Press.

Eigen, Joel (2016), *Mad Doctors in the Dock: Defending the Diagnosis, 1760–1913*, London: Johns Hopkins University Press.

Eisenberger, N. (2003), 'Does Rejection Hurt? An fMRI Study of Social Exclusion', *Science* 302: 290–2.

Ekirch, A. Roger (2001), 'Sleep we have lost: pre-industrial slumber in the British Isles', *American Historical Review* 106, no. 2: 343–86.

Ekirch, A. Roger (2006), *At Day's Close: Night in Times Past*, New York: WW Norton & Company.

Eliot, George (1871–2/2007), *Middlemarch*, London: CRW Publishing.

Elliot, Paul (1990), 'Vivisection and the Emergence of Experimental Physiology in Nineteenth Century France', in Nicolaas Rupke (ed.), *Vivisection in Historical Perspective*, 48–77, London: Routledge.

Ellis, J. D. (1995), *The Physician-Legislators of France: Medicine and Politics in the Early Third Republic, 1870–1914*, Cambridge: Cambridge University Press.

Ellis, Robert (2006), 'The Asylum, the Poor Law, and a Reassessment of the Four-Shilling Grant: Admissions to the County Asylums of Yorkshire in the Nineteenth Century', *Social History of Medicine* 19, no. 1: 55–71.

Engstrom, Eric J. (2003), *Clinical Psychiatry in Imperial Germany: A History of Psychiatric Practice*, Ithaca, NY: Cornell University Press.

Erichsen, John Eric (1867), *On Railway and Other Injuries of the Nervous System*, Philadelphia: Henry C. Lea.

Ernst, Waltraud (1991), *Mad Tales from the Raj: Colonial Psychiatry in South Asia, 1800–58*, London: Routledge.

Evans, R. J. (1987), *Death in Hamburg: State and Politics in the Cholera Years, 1830–1910*, Oxford: Clarendon Press.

Evans, Richard J. (1988), 'Epidemics and revolutions: cholera in nineteenth-century Europe', *Past & Present* 120: 123–46.

Eyler, J. (1986), 'The Epidemiology of Milk Borne Scarlet Fever', *American Journal of Public Health* 76: 573–84.

Farber, Paul Lawrence (2000), *Finding Order in Nature: The Naturalist Tradition from Linnaeus to E.O. Wilson*, Baltimore, MD: Johns Hopkins University Press.

Farley, John (1992), 'Parasites and the Germ Theory of Disease', in C. Rosenberg (ed.), *Framing Disease: Studies in Cultural History*, 33–49, New Brunswick, NJ: Rutgers University Press.

Feldman Barrett, Lisa (2006), 'Are emotions natural kinds?', *Perspectives on Psychological Science* 1: 28–58.

Feldman Barrett, Lisa (2006a), 'Solving the emotion paradox: categorization and the experience of emotion', *Personality and Social Psychology Review* 10: 20–46.

Fenton, T. (1865), Letter, *The American Phrenological Journal and Life Illustrated* 41, no. 6: 182.

Ferrières, Madeleine (2006), *Sacred Cow, Mad Cow: A History of Food Fears*, New York: Columbia University Press.

Fick, A. and J. Wislicenus (1866), 'On the Origin of Muscular Power', *London, Edinburgh and Dublin Philosophical Magazine and Journal of Science* 31, Supplement: 485–503.

Finlay, Mark R. (1992), 'Quackery and Cookery: Justus von Liebig's Extract of Meat and the Theory of Nutrition in the Victorian Age', *Bulletin of the History of Medicine* 66, no. 3: 404–18.

Finlay, Mark R. (1995), 'Early Marketing of the Theory of Nutrition: The Science and Culture of Liebig's Extract of Meat', in Harmke Kamminga and Andrew Cunningham (eds), *Science and Culture of Nutrition, 1840–1940*, 48–74, Amsterdam: Editions Rodopi B.V.

Finnegan, Diarmid (2008), '"An Aid to Mental Health": Natural History, Alienists and Therapeutics in Victorian Scotland', *Studies in History and Philosophy of Biological and Biomedical Sciences* 39: 326–37.

Fisher, John (1993), 'British Physicians, Medical Science, and the Cattle Plague, 1865–66', *Bulletin of the History of Medicine* 67: 61–9.

Fissell, Mary E. (2004), 'Making Meaning from the Margins: The New Cultural History of Medicine', in Frank Huisman and John Harley Warner (eds), *Locating Medical History: The Stories and their Meanings*, 364–89, Baltimore, MD: Johns Hopkins University Press.

Flaubert, Gustave (1881/2010), *Bouvard et Pecuchet*, Paris: Flammarion.

Flexner, S. (1925), 'Abraham Jacobi (1830–1919)', *Proceedings of the American Academy of Arts and Sciences* 60, no. 14: 626–9.

Flis, Nathan (2009), 'Images of the Toronto Provincial Asylum, 1846–1890', *Scientia Canadensis: Medical Sciences and Medical Buildings* 32, no. 1: 21–50.

Fogel, R. W. (2004), *The Escape from Hunger and Premature Death, 1700–2100*, Cambridge: Cambridge University Press.

Forrester, John (1994), 'Freud and collecting', in John Elsner (ed.), *The Cultures of Collecting*, 224–51, London: Reaktion.

Forth, Christopher E. (2008), *Masculinity in the Modern West: Gender, Civilization and the Body*, New York: Palgrave Macmillan.

Foucault, Michel (1961/1995), *Madness and Civilization: A History of Insanity in the Age of Reason*, trans. Richard Howard, London: Routledge.

Foucault, Michel (1963/2012), *The Birth of the Clinic*, London: Routledge.

Foucault, Michel (1969/1972), *The Archaeology of Knowledge*, trans. A. M. Sheridan Smith, London: Routledge.

Foucault, Michel (1975/2012), *Discipline & Punish: The Birth of the Prison*, New York: Vintage.

Foucault, Michel (1976/1990), *The History of Sexuality: An Introduction*, vol. 1, trans. Robert Hurley, New York: Vintage.

Foucault, Michel (1991), 'Governmentality', in G. Burchell, C. Gordon and P. Miller (eds), *The Foucault Effect: Studies in Governmentality*, 87–104, Chicago: University of Chicago Press.

Foucault, Michel (2007), *Security, Territory, Population: Lectures at the Collège de France, 1977–1978*, New York: Picador.

Franco, Nuno Henrique (2013), 'Animal Experiments in Biomedical Research: A Historical Perspective', *Animals* 3: 238–73.

Franco-Paredes, Carlos, Lorena Lammoglia and José Ignacio Santos-Preciado (2005), 'The Spanish Royal Philanthropic Expedition to Bring Smallpox Vaccination to the New World and Asia in the 19th Century', *Clinical Infectious Diseases* 41: 1285–9.

Frank, Johann Peter (1976), *A System of Complete Medical Police: Selections from Johann Peter Frank*, ed. Erna Lesky, Baltimore, MD: Johns Hopkins University Press.

Fraser, S. M. F. (1980), 'Leicester and Smallpox: The Leicester Method', *Medical History* 24: 315–32.

Freeman, W. T. (1900), 'Eczema and the Allied Diseases: An Outline of their Etiology, Pathology and Treatment', *The Lancet* 156, no. 4015: 398–401.

Freidson, Eliot (1970), *Profession of Medicine*, Chicago: University of Chicago Press.

French, Richard D. (1975), *Antivivisection and Medical Science in Victorian Society*, London and Princeton, NJ: Princeton University Press.

Freud, Sigmund (1921), *Massenpsychologie und Ich-analyse*, Vienna: Internationaler Psychoanalytischer Verlag.

Freud, Sigmund (1930/2002), *Civilization and Its Discontents*, London: Penguin.

Frieden, Nancy M. (1982), *Russian Physicians in an Era of Reform and Revolution 1856–1905*, Princeton, NJ: Princeton University Press.

Furst, Lilian R. (1998), *Between Doctors and Patients: The Changing Balance of Power*, Charlottesville: University Press of Virginia.

Furst, Lilian R. (2008), *Before Freud: Hysteria and Hypnosis in Later Nineteenth-Century Psychiatric Cases*, Lewisburg, PA: Bucknell University Press.

Galton, Francis (1855), *Hints to Travellers*, London: John Murray.

Gardner, L. I. (1959), 'Abraham Jacobi: Pediatric Pioneer', *Pediatrics* 24, no. 2: 282.

Garrison, F. H. (1919), 'Dr Abraham Jacobi (1830–1919), *Science* 50, no. 1283: 102.

Gatley, Katerina (2012), 'The Spouse, the Neurological Patient, and Doctors', in L. Stephen Jacyna and Stephen T. Casper (eds), *The Neurological Patient in History*, 81–108, Rochester, NY: Rochester University Press.

Gavin, Hector (1848), *Sanitary Ramblings: Being Sketches and Illustrations of Bethnal Green, A Type of the Condition of the Metropolis and Other Large Towns*, London: John Churchill.

Geertz, Clifford (1973), *The Interpretation of Cultures: Selected Essays*, New York: Basic Books.

Gere, Cathy (2017), *Pain, Pleasure, and the Greater Good: From the Panopticon to the Skinner Box and Beyond*, Chicago: University of Chicago Press.

Gesler, W. M. (1992), 'Therapeutic Landscapes: Medical Issues in Light of the New Cultural Geography', *Social Science and Medicine* 34: 735–46.

Gesler, W. M. (1998), 'Bath's Reputation as a Healing Place', in Robin A. Kearns and W. M. Gesler (eds), *Putting Health into Place: Landscape, Identity & Well-Being*, 17–35, Syracuse, NY: Syracuse University Press.

Gilbert, Pamela K. (2004), *Mapping the Victorian Social Body*, New York: SUNY Press

Gilbert, Pamela (2009), Cholera *and Nation: Doctoring the Social Body in Victorian England*, Albany, NY: SUNY Press, 2009.

Gilman, Sander (1982/1996), *Seeing the Insane: A Cultural History of Madness and Art in the Western World*, Lincoln: University of Nebraska Press.

Gilman, Sander (1991), *The Jew's Body*, London: Routledge.

Gilman, Sander L. (1993), 'The Image of the Hysteric', in Sander L. Gilman, Helen King, Roy Porter, G. S. Rousseau and Elaine Showalter (eds), *Hysteria Beyond Freud*, 345–452, Berkeley and Los Angeles: University of California Press.

Gilman, Sander L. (2008), *Fat: A Cultural History of Obesity*, Cambridge: Polity.

Gleadle, Kathryn (2003), 'The age of physiological reformers: rethinking gender and domesticity in the age of reform', in Arthur Burns and Joanna Innes (eds), *Rethinking the Age of Reform: Britain 1780–1850*, 200–19, Cambridge: Cambridge University Press.

Goldberg, Ann (1999), *Sex, Religion, and the Making of Modern Madness: The Eberbach Asylum and German Society, 1815–1849*, Oxford: Oxford University Press.

Goldberg, Daniel (2012), 'Pain Without Lesion: Debate Among American Neurologists, 1850–1900', *19: Interdisciplinary Studies in the Long Nineteenth Century* 15.

Goldberg, Daniel (2017), 'Pain, objectivity and history: understanding pain stigma', *Medical Humanities* 43, no. 4: 238–43.

Goldberg, Kevin D. (2011), 'Acidity and Power: The Politics of Natural Wine in Nineteenth-Century Germany', *Food and Foodways* 19, no. 4: 294–313.

Goldstein, Jan (1987), *Console and Classify: The French Psychiatric Profession in the Nineteenth Century*, Cambridge: Cambridge University Press.

Gooday, Graeme (2008), 'Placing or Replacing the Laboratory in the History of Science?', *Isis* 99, no. 4: 783–95.

Goodwin, Lorine Swainston (1999), *The Pure Food, Drink, and Drug Crusaders, 1879–1914*, Jefferson, NC: McFarland.

Gooldin, Sigal (2003), 'Fasting Women, Living Skeletons and Hunger Artists: Spectacles of Body and Miracles at the Turn of a Century', *Body & Society* 9, no. 2: 27–53.

Gordon, Bertram M. (2012), 'Reinventions of a Spa Town: the Unique Case of Vichy', *Journal of Tourism History* 4, no. 1: 35–55.

Gradmann, C. (2010), 'Robert Koch and the Invention of the Carrier State: Tropical Medicine, and Epidemiology Around 1900', *Studies in History and Philosophy of Biological and Biomedical Sciences* 41: 232–40.

Gray, Liz (2014), 'Body, Mind and Madness: Pain in Animals in Nineteenth-century Comparative Psychology', in Rob Boddice (ed.), *Pain and Emotion in Modern History*, 148–63, Basingstoke: Palgrave Macmillan

Green, Harvey (2012), 'Cultural History and the Material(s) Turn', *Cultural History* 1, no. 1: 61–82.

Greenberg, David F. (1988), *The Construction of Homosexuality*, Chicago: University of Chicago Press.

Grigsby, Darcy Grimaldo (1995), 'Rumor, Contagion, and Colonization in Gros's Plague-Stricken of Jaffa (1804)', *Representations* 51: 1–46.

Grob, Gerald (1994), *The Mad Among Us: A History of the Care of America's Mentally Ill*, New York: Free Press.

Guenther, Katja (2014), 'Exercises in therapy: neurological gymnastics between Kurort and hospital medicine, 1880–1945', *Bulletin of the History of Medicine* 88, no. 1: 102–31.

Guenther, Katja and Volker Hess (eds) (2016), 'Special Issue: Soul Catchers – A Material History of the Mind Sciences', *Medical History* 60, no. 3.

Guerrini, Anita (2003), *Experimenting with Humans and Animals: From Galen to Animal Rights*, Baltimore, MD: Johns Hopkins University Press.

Guillem-Llobat, Ximo (2014), 'The Search for International Food Safety Regulation. From the Commission Internationale Pour La Répression Des Falsifications to the Société Universelle de La Croix Blanche (1879–1909)', *Social History of Medicine* 27, no. 3: 419–39.

Guly, H. R. (2013), 'Medical Comforts during the Heroic Age of Antarctic Exploration', *Polar Record* 49, no. 2: 110–17.

Gunga, Hanns-Christian (2008), *Nathan Zuntz: His Life and Work in the Fields of High Altitude Physiology and Aviation Medicine*, San Diego: Academic Press.

Haalboom, A. F. (2017), 'Negotiating Zoonoses: Dealings with Infectious Diseases Shared by Humans and Livestock in The Netherlands (1898–2001)', PhD diss., Utrecht University.

Haggerty, R. J. (1997), 'Abraham Jacobi, MD, Respectable Rebel', *Pediatrics* 99, no. 3: 462–6.

Haig, Alexander and Kenneth G. Haig (1913), *Health through Diet: A Practical Guide to the Uric-Acid-Free Diet, Founded on Eighteen Years' Personal Experience*, London: Methuen & Co.

Hale, Piers J. (2014), *Political Descent: Malthus, Mutualism, and the Politics of Evolution in Victorian England*, Chicago: University of Chicago Press.

Hall, K. T., J. Loscalzo and T. J. Kaptchuk (2015), 'Genetics and the placebo effect: the placebome', *Trends in Molecular Medicine* 21: 285–94.

Haller, John S. (1971/1995), *Outcasts from Evolution: Scientific Attitudes of Racial Inferiority, 1859–1900*, Carbondale and Edwardsville: Southern Illinois University Press.

Halliday, Andrew (1828), *A General View of the Present State of Lunatics and Lunatic Asylums in Great Britain and Ireland*, London: Thomas and Paul Underwood.

Halpern, S. (1988), *American Pediatrics: The Social Dynamics of Professionalism, 1880–1980*, Berkeley: University of California Press.

Hamilton, Alice (1908), 'Industrial Diseases, with Special Reference to the Trades in which Women Are Employed', *Charities and the Commons* 20: 655–8.

Hamlin, Christopher (1996), *A Science of Impurity: Water Analysis in Nineteenth Century Britain*, Berkeley: University of California Press.

Hamlin, Christopher (1998), *Public Health and Social Justice in the Age of Chadwick: Britain, 1800–1854*, Cambridge: Cambridge University Press.

Hamlin, Christopher (2009), *Cholera: The Biography*, New York: Oxford University Press.

Hammonds, Evelyn (1999), *Childhood's Deadly Scourge: The Campaign to Control Diphtheria in New York City, 1880–1930*, Baltimore, MD: Johns Hopkins University Press.

Hanley, Anne (2017), *Medicine, Knowledge and Venereal Diseases in England, 1886–1916*, Basingstoke: Palgrave.

Hannaway, Caroline (1977), 'Veterinary Medicine and Rural Health Care in Pre-Revolutionary France', *Bulletin of the History of Medicine* 51: 431–47.

Hannaway, Caroline (1994), 'Vicq D'Azyr, Anatomy and a Vision of Medicine', in Ann La Berge and Mordechai Feingold (eds), *French Medical Culture in the Nineteenth Century*, 280–95, Amsterdam: Rodopi.

Hannaway, C. and A. La Berge (eds) (1998), *Constructing Paris Medicine*, Amsterdam: Rodopi.

Hardy, Anne (1992), 'Tracheotomy versus intubation: surgical intervention in diphtheria in Europe and the United States, 1825–1930', *Bulletin for the History of Medicine* 66: 536–59.

Hardy, Anne (1993), *Epidemic Streets: Infectious Disease and the Rise of Preventive Medicine, 1856–1900*, Oxford: Clarendon Press.

Hardy, Anne (1999), 'Food, Hygiene, and the Laboratory: A Short History of Food Poisoning in Britain, circa 1850–1950', *Social History of Medicine* 12, no. 1: 293–311.

Hardy, Anne (2003), 'Animals, Disease, and Man: Making Connections', *Perspectives in Biology and Medicine* 46: 200–15.

Hargrove, James L. (2006), 'History of the Calorie in Nutrition', *Journal of Nutrition* 136, no. 12: 2957–61.

Harpin, Anna and Jane Foster (eds) (2014), *Performance, Madness and Psychiatry: Isolated Acts*, London: Palgrave Macmillan.

Harrington, Anne (1989), *Medicine, Mind, and the Double Brain: A Study in Nineteenth-Century Thought*, Princeton, NJ: Princeton University Press.

Harrington, Ralph (2003), 'On the Tracks of Trauma: Railway Spine Reconsidered', *Social History of Medicine* 16, no. 2: 209–23.

Harris, Bernard (2004), 'Public Health, Nutrition, and the Decline of Mortality: The McKeown Thesis Revisited', *Social History of Medicine* 17, no. 3: 379–407.

Harrison, Barbara (1995), 'The Politics of Occupational Ill-health in Late Nineteenth Century Britain: The Case of the Match Making Industry', *Sociology of Health & Illness* 17, no. 1: 20–41.

Harrison, Brian (1973), 'Animals and the State in Nineteenth-Century England', *English Historical Review* 88: 786–820.

Harrison, Mark (1992), 'Quarantine, Pilgrimage, and Colonial Trade: India 1866–1900', *Indian Economic & Social History Review* 29, no. 2: 117–44.

Harrison, Mark (1996), 'The Medicalization of War: The Militarization of Medicine', *Social History of Medicine* 9, no. 2: 267–76.

Harrison, Mark (1996), '"The Tender Frame of Man": Disease, Climate and Racial Difference in India and the West Indies, 1760–1860', *Bulletin of the History of Medicine* 70, no. 1: 68–93.

Harrison, Mark (1999), *Climates and Constitutions: Health, Race, Environment and British Imperialism in India, 1600–1850*, New York: Oxford University Press.

Harrison, Mark (1999), 'Medicine and the Management of Modern Warfare: An Introduction', in Roger Cooter, Mark Harrison and Steve Sturdy (eds), *Medicine and Modern Warfare*, 1–28, Amsterdam: Rodopi.

Harrison, Mark (2006), 'Disease, Diplomacy and International Commerce: The Origins of International Sanitary Regulation in the Nineteenth Century', *Journal of Global History* 1, no. 2: 197–217.

Harrison, Mark (2010), *The Medical War: British Military Medicine in the First World War*, Oxford: Oxford University Press.

Harrison, Robert (1837), 'An Account of Tubercles in the Air-Cells of a Bird, and Some Observations on Tubercles in General', *Dublin Journal of Medical Science* 11: 227.

Harvey, David (1989), *The Condition of Postmodernity*, Oxford: Blackwell.

Harvey, David (2003), *Paris: Capital of Modernity*, New York: Routledge.

Harvey, J. (1990), 'Medicine and Politics: Dr Mary Putnam Jacobi and the Paris Commune', *Dialectical Anthropology* 15: 107–17.

Hashimoto, Akira (2010), 'Invention of a "Japanese Gheel": Psychiatric Family Care from a Historical and Transnational Perspective', in Waltraud Ernst and Thomas Mueller (eds), *Transnational Psychiatries: Social and Cultural Histories of Psychiatry in Comparative Perspective*, c.1800–2000, 142–71, Newcastle-upon-Tyne: Cambridge Scholars.

Hawkins, Sue and Andrea Tanner (2016) 'Food, glorious food: the functions of food in British children's hospitals, 1852–1914', *Food and History* 14, no. 1: 107–34.

Haynes, April (2003), 'The Trials of Frederick Hollick: Obscenity, Sex Education, and Medical Democracy in the Antebellum United States', *Journal of the History of Sexuality* 12, no. 4: 543–74.

Hayward, Rhodri (2004), 'Demonology, neurology, and medicine in Edwardian Britain', *Bulletin of the History of Medicine* 78, no. 1: 37–58.

Hegel, Georg (1931/2003), *The Phenomenology of Mind*, trans. J. B. Baillie, New York: Dover Publications.

Heggie, Vanessa (2005), 'Jewish Medical Charity in Manchester: Reforming Alien Bodies', *Bulletin of the John Rylands University Library of Manchester* 87, no. 1:111–32.

Heggie, Vanessa (2008) 'Lies, Damn Lies, and Manchester's Recruiting Statistics: Degeneration as an "Urban Legend" in Victorian and Edwardian Britain', *Journal of the History of Medicine and Allied Sciences* 63, no. 2: 178–216.

Heggie, Vanessa (2011), 'Domestic and domesticating education in the Victorian and Edwardian City', *History of Education* 40, no. 3: 273–90.

Heggie, Vanessa (2011), 'Health Visiting and District Nursing in Victorian Manchester: divergent and convergent vocations', *Women's History Review* 20, no. 3: 403–22.

Heggie, Vanessa (2016), 'Bodies, sport and science in the nineteenth century', *Past & Present* 231, no. 1: 169–200.

Heise, Ursula K., Jon Christensen and Michelle Niemann (2017), *The Routledge Companion to the Environmental Humanities*, New York: Routledge.

Herbert, Amanda E. (2009), 'Gender and the Spa: Space, Sociability and Self at British Health Spas, 1640–1714', *Journal of Social History* 43, no. 2: 361–83.

Hernández Brotons, Fanny (2017), 'The Experience of Cancer Illness: Spain and Beyond During the Second Half of the Nineteenth Century', PhD diss., Universidad Carlos III de Madrid.

Hickman, Clare (2013), *Therapeutic Landscapes: A History of English Hospital Gardens Since 1800*, Manchester: Manchester University Press.

Hicks, Dan (2010), 'The Material-Cultural Turn: Event and Effect', in Dan Hicks and Mary C. Beaudry (eds), *The Oxford Handbook of Material Culture Studies*, 25–98, Oxford: Oxford University Press.

Hierholzer, Vera (2007), 'The "War Against Food Adulteration": Municipal Food Monitoring and Citizen Self-Help Associations in Germany, 1870s–1880s', in Peter J. Atkins, Peter Lummel and Derek J. Oddy (eds), *Food and the City in Europe since 1800*, 117–30, Aldershot and Burlington, VT: Ashgate.

Higgs, E. (1991), 'Disease, Febrile Poisons and Statistics: The Census as a Medical Survey, 1841–1911', *Social History of Medicine* 4, no. 3: 465–78.

Hirshbein, Laura D. (2009), *American Melancholy: Constructions of Depression in the Twentieth Century*, New Brunswick, NJ: Rutgers University Press.

Hochadel, Oliver (n.d.), 'Science at the Nineteenth Century Zoological Garden: An Unfulfilled Promise?', unpublished manuscript.

Hoffman, Frederick L. (1909), 'Industrial Accidents and Industrial Diseases', *Publications of the American Statistical Association* 11, no. 88: 567–603.

Holloway, S. W. F. (1966), 'The Apothecaries' Act, 1815: a reinterpretation. Part I: the origins of the Act', *Medical History* 10: 107–29.

Holloway, S. W. F. (1966) 'Part II: the consequences of the Act', *Medical History* 10: 221–36.

Hollows, Joanne (2008), *Domestic Cultures*, Oxford: Oxford University Press.

Holt, Mack (2006), *Alcohol: A Social and Cultural History*, London: Berg.

Honigsbaum, Mark (2016), *Living with Enza: The Forgotten Story of Britain and the Great Flu Pandemic of 1918*, New York: Springer.

Hopwood, Nick (2004), 'Plastic Publishing in Embryology', in Nick Hopwood and Soraya de Chadarevian (eds), *Models: The Third Dimension of Science*, 170–206, Stanford, CA: Stanford University Press.

Horowitz, Roger, Jeffrey M. Pilcher and Sydney Watts (2004), 'Meat for the Multitudes: Market Culture in Paris, New York City, and Mexico City over the Long Nineteenth Century', *American Historical Review* 109, no. 4: 1055–83.

Horrocks, Sally M. (1994), 'Quality Control and Research: The Role of Scientists in the British Food Industry, 1870–1939', in J. Burnett and D. J. Oddy (eds), *The Origins and Development of Food Policies in Europe*, 130–45, Leicester: Leicester University Press.

House of Commons (1828), *Report from the Select Committee on Anatomy, 22 July 1828*, London: House of Commons.

Howse, Carrie (2006), 'From Lady Bountiful to Lady Administrator: Women and the Administration of Rural District Nursing in England, 1880–1925', *Women's History Review* 15, no. 3: 423–41.

Huber, M., M. van Vliet, M. Giezenberg et al. (2016), 'Towards a "Patient-Centred" Operationalisation of the New Dynamic Concept of Health: A Mixed Methods Study', *BMJ Open 2016*, 5:e010091. doi:10.1136/bmjopen-2015–010091.

Hubscher, Ronald (1999), *Les Maitres des Betes: Les Veterinaires dans la Societe Francaise (XVIIIe–XXe siecle)*, Paris: Edition Odile Jacob.

Hudson, John (1875), 'Epidemic of Hysterical Epilepsy and Tetanus', *The Lancet*, 9 October: 525–6.

Huisman, Frank and John Harley Warner (eds) (2004), *Locating Medical History: The Stories and Their Meanings*, Baltimore, MD: Johns Hopkins University Press.

Humphries, Margaret (2001), *Malaria: Poverty, Race, and Public Health in the United States*, Baltimore, MD: Johns Hopkins University Press.

Hunter, William (1784), *Introductory Lectures*, London: J. Johnson.

Hurst, Arthur F. (1918), 'War Contractures: Localized Tetanus, Reflex Disorder, or Hysteria', *British Journal of Surgery* 6: 579–605.

Hutchinson, Woods (1892), 'Darwinism and Disease', *Journal of the American Medical Association* 19: 147–51.

Huysmans, J-K. (1884), *A Rebours*, trans. Against the Grain or Against Nature, http://www.gutenberg.org/files/12341/12341–h/12341–h.htm.

Huzel, J. P. (2006), *The Popularization of Malthus in Early Nineteenth-Century England: Martineau, Cobbett and the Pauper Press*, Aldershot: Ashgate.

Hyman, Paula (1989), 'The Dreyfus Affair: The Visual and the Historical', *Journal of Modern History* 61, no. 6: 88–109.

Illich, Ivan (1974), 'Medical Nemesis', *The Lancet* 303, no. 7863: 918–21.

Jackson, Mark (ed.) (2011), *The Oxford Handbook of the History of Medicine*, Oxford: Oxford University Press.

Jackson, T. J. (1983), 'From Salvation to Self-Realization: Advertising and the Therapeutic Roots of the Consumer Culture, 1880–1930', in Richard Wightman Fox and T. J. Jackson Lears (eds), *The Culture of Consumption: Critical Essays in American History, 1880–1980*, 1–38, New York: Pantheon Books.

Jackson-Retondo, Elaine (2000), 'Manufacturing Moral Reform: Images and Realities of a Nineteenth-Century Prison', in Sally McMurry and Annmarie Adams (eds), *People, Power, Places: Perspectives in Vernacular Architecture*, vol. 8, 117–37, Knoxville: University of Tennessee Press.

Jacobi, A (1905), *The History of Paediatrics and its Relation to Others Sciences and Arts*, London: Royal College of Surgeons.

Jacyna, L. Stephen (1983), 'Images of John Hunter in the Nineteenth Century', *History of Science* 21: 85–108.

Jacyna, L. Stephen (1984), 'Principles of General Physiology: The Comparative Dimension to British Neuro-Science in the 1830s and 1840s', *Studies in the History of Biology* 7: 47–92.

Jacyna, L. Stephen (1984), 'The Romantic Programme and the Reception of Cell Theory in Britain', *Journal of the History of Biology* 17: 13–48.

Jacyna, L. Stephen (1994), *Philosophic Whigs: Medicine, Science, and Citizenship in Edinburgh, 1789–1848*, London: Routledge.

Jacyna, L. Stephen (2008), *Medicine and Modernism: A Biography of Henry Head*, Pittsburg: University of Pittsburg Press.

Jacyna, L. Stephen (2017), '"We Are Veritable Animals": The Nineteenth-Century Paris Menagerie as a Site for the Science of Intelligence', in Stephen T. Casper and Delia Gavrus (eds), *The History of the Mind and Brain Sciences: Technique, Technology, and Therapy*, 25–47, Rochester, NY: University of Rochester Press.

Jacyna, L. Stephen, and Stephen T. Casper (eds) (2012), *The Neurological Patient in History*, Rochester, NY: Rochester University Press.

James, F. A. J. L. (1989), 'Introduction', in F. James (ed.), *The Development of the Laboratory: Essays on the Place of Experiment in Industrial Civilization*, 184–217, New York: American Institute of Physics.

James, William (1902/1982), *The Varieties of Religious Experience*, Harmondsworth: Penguin Books.

Jardine, Nicholas (1992), 'The laboratory revolution in medicine as rhetorical and aesthetic accomplishment', in Andrew Cunningham and Perry Williams (eds), *The Laboratory Revolution in Medicine*, 304–23, Cambridge: Cambridge University Press.

Javelle, E. and D. Raoult (2020), 'COVID-19 pandemic more than a century after the Spanish flu', *The Lancet Infectious Diseases*, DOI:https://doi.org/10.1016/S1473-3099(20)30650-2.

Jenner, Edward (1807), letter to Phillips, 16 January, Royal College of Physicians, MS 735, f. 22.

Jennings, Eric T. (2006), *Curing the Colonizers: Hydrotherapy, Climatology, and French Colonial Spas*, Durham, NC: Duke University Press.

Jennings, Eric T. (2011), *Imperial Heights: Dalat and the Making and Undoing of French Indochina*, Berkeley: University of California Press.

Jewson, N. D. (1976), 'The Disappearance of the Sick-Man from Medical Cosmology, 1770–1870', *Sociology* 10, no. 2: 225–44.

Johnson, D. A. (2015), 'John Buchanan's Philadelphia Diploma Mill and the Rise of State Medical Boards', *Bulletin of the History of Medicine* 89, no. 1: 25–58.

Johnson, Steven (2007), *The Ghost Map: The Story of London's Most Terrifying Epidemic – and How it Changed Science, Cities, and the Modern World*, New York: Riverhead Books.

Jones, Claire L. (2013), *The Medical Trade Catalogue in Britain, 1870–1914*, London: Pickering & Chatto.

Jones, Claire L. (ed.) (2017), *Rethinking Modern Prostheses in Anglo-American Commodity Cultures, 1820–1939*, Manchester: Manchester University Press.

Jones, Colin and Roy Porter (eds) (2001), *Reassessing Foucault: Power, Medicine and the Body*, London: Routledge.

Jones, James H. (1993), *Bad Blood: The Tuskegee Syphilis Experiment*, New York: Free Press.

Jones, Kathleen (1972), *A History of the Mental Health Services*, London: Routledge and Kegan Paul.

Jones, Susan D. (2003), *Valuing Animals: Veterinarians and Their Patients in Modern America*, Baltimore, MD: Johns Hopkins University Press.

Jones, Susan D. (2010), *Death in a Small Package: A Short History of Anthrax*, Baltimore, MD: Johns Hopkins University Press.

Jordanova, Ludmilla (2000), *Defining Features: Medical and Scientific Portraits, 1600–2000*, London: Reaktion.

Jorland, G., A. Opinel and G. Weisz (eds) (2005), *Body Counts: Medical Quantification in Historical and Sociological Perspectives*, Montreal: McGill-Queens University Press.

Journal of Comparative Pathology and Therapeutics (1888–1900).

Joyce, Patrick (1994), *Democratic Subjects: The Self and the Social in Nineteenth-Century England*, Cambridge: Cambridge University Press.

Kaes, Anton (2010), *Shell Shock Cinema: Weimar Culture and the Wounds of War*, Princeton, NJ: Princeton University Press.

Keene, Melanie (2014), 'Familiar science in nineteenth-century Britain', *History of Science* 52: 53–71.

Keller, Richard C. (2001), 'Madness and Colonization: Psychiatry in the British and French Empires, 1800–1962', *Journal of Social History* 35, no. 2: 295–326.

Keller, Richard C. (2007), *Colonial Madness: Psychiatry in French North Africa*, Chicago: University of Chicago Press.

Kelley, Victoria (2010), *Soap and Water: Cleanliness, Dirt and the Working Classes in Victorian and Edwardian Britain*, London: I.B. Taurus.

Kelly, Catherine (2010), 'Medicine and the Egyptian Campaign: The Development of the Military Medical Officer during the Napoleonic Wars c. 1798–1801', *Canadian Bulletin of Medical History* 27, no. 2: 321–42.

Kelly, Catherine (2011), *War and the Militarization of British Army Medicine, 1793–1830*, London: Pickering & Chatto.

Kelly, Dorothy (2011), 'Balzac's Disorienting Orientalism: "Une Passion dans le desert"', *Nineteenth-Century French Studies* 40, no. 1: 1–17.

Kelly, Laura (2013), *Irish Women in Medicine, c.1880s–1920s: Origins, Education and Careers*, Manchester: Manchester University Press.

Kelly, Laura (2017), *Irish Medical Education and Student Culture, c.1850–1950*, Liverpool: Liverpool University Press.

Kennaway, James (2012), *Bad Vibrations: The History of the Idea of Music as a Cause of Disease*, London: Ashgate.

Kennedy, Catriona (2013), *Narratives of the Revolutionary and Napoleonic Wars: Military and Civilian Experience in Britain and Ireland*, Basingstoke: Palgrave Macmillan.

Kenny, Nicholas (2014), *The Feel of the City: Experiences of Urban Transformation*, Toronto: University of Toronto Press.

Kenny, Nicolas (2015), 'City Glow: Streetlights, Emotions, and Nocturnal Life, 1880s–1910s', *Journal of Urban History* 43, no. 1: 91–114.

Kern, Stephen (2003), *The Culture of Time and Space, 1880–1918*, Cambridge, MA: Harvard University Press.

Kete, Katherine (ed.) (2007), *A Cultural History of Animals*, vol. 5: *The Age of Empire (1800–1920)*, London: Bloomsbury.

Kiechle, Melanie A. (2017), *Smell Detectives: An Olfactory History of Nineteenth-Century Urban America*, Seattle: University of Washington Press.

Killen, Andreas (2006), *Berlin Electropolis: Shock, Nerves, and German Modernity*, Berkeley: University of California Press.

Kim, Hoi-Eun (2014), *Doctors of Empire: Medical and Cultural Encounters between Imperial Germany and Meiji Japan*, Toronto: University of Toronto Press.

Kirk, Robert G. W. (2016), 'The Birth of the Laboratory Animal: Biopolitics, Animal Experimentation, and Animal Wellbeing', in Matthew Chrulew and Dinesh Joseph Wadiwel (eds), *Foucault and Animals*, 193–221, Leiden and Boston: Brill.

Kirk, R. G. W. and N. Pemberton (2013), *Leech*, London: Reaktion Books Ltd.

Kirk, R. G. W. and M. Worboys, M. (2011), 'Medicine and Species: One Medicine, One History?' in Mark Jackson (ed.), *The Oxford Handbook of the History of Medicine*, 561–77, Oxford: Oxford University Press.

Kitta, A. (2011), *Vaccinations and Public Concern in History: Legend, Rumour, and Risk Perception*, New York: Routledge.

Klein, Ursula and E. C. Spary (eds) (2010), *Materials and Expertise in Early Modern Europe: Between Market and Laboratory*, Chicago: University of Chicago Press.

Klestinec, Cynthia (2010), 'Practical Experience in Anatomy', in Charles T. Wolfe and Ofer Gal (eds), *The Body as Object and Instrument of Knowledge: Embodied Empiricism in Early Modern Science*, 33–57, Dordrecht: Springer.

Kline, Ronald and Trevor Pinch (1996), 'Users as Agents of Technological Change: The Social Construction of the Automobile in the Rural United States', *Technology and Culture* 37, no. 4: 763–95.

Knox, Frederick John (1836), *The Anatomist's Instructor, and Museum Companion; being practical directions for the formation and subsequent management of anatomical museums*, Edinburgh: Adam and Charles Black.

Koch, Tom (2005), *Cartographies of Disease: Maps, Mapping, and Medicine*, Redlands, CA: ESRI Press.

Koven, Seth (2006), *Slumming: Sexual and Social Politics in Victorian England*, Princeton, NJ: Princeton University Press.

Kraut, Alan M. (1995), *Silent Travelers: Germs, Genes, and the Immigrant Menace*, Baltimore, MD: Johns Hopkins University Press.

Krementsov, Nikolai (2008), 'Hormones and the Bolsheviks: From Organotherapy to Experimental Endocrinology, 1918–1929', *Isis* 99, no. 3: 486–518.

Kudlick, Catherine J. (1996), *Cholera in Post-Revolutionary Paris: A Cultural History*, Berkeley: University of California Press.

Kurlansky, Mark (1997), *Cod: A Biography of the Fish That Changed the World*, London: Vintage.

La Berge, A. (2005), 'Medical Statistics at the Paris School: What was at stake', in Gérard Jorland, Annick Opinel and George Weisz (eds), *Body Counts: Medical Quantification in Historical and Sociological Perspectives*, 89–108, Montreal: McGill-Queens University Press.

La Berge, Ann and Elizabeth Fowler (2002), *Mission and Method: The Early Nineteenth-Century French Public Health Movement*, Cambridge: Cambridge University Press.

Laberge, M.-P. (1987), 'Les Instituts Pasteur du Maghreb: La recherche scientifique dans le cadre de la politique coloniale', *Revue Française d'Histoire d'Outre-Mer* 74: 27–42.

Laderman, Gary (2003), *Rest in Peace: A Cultural History of Death and the Funeral Home in Twentieth-Century America*, Oxford: Oxford University Press.

Laennec, R. T. H. (1829), *A Treatise on the Diseases of the Chest and on Mediate Auscultation*, trans. John Forbes, London: Underwood.

Lambert, R. J. (1962), 'A Victorian National Health Service: State Vaccination 1855–71', *Historical Journal* 5: 1–18

Langdon Down, J. (1866), 'Observations on an Ethnic Classification of Idiots', *London Hospital Report* 3: 259–60.

Lansbury, Carol (1985), *The Old Brown Dog: Women, Workers and Vivisection in Edwardian England*, Madison, WI: Madison University Press.

Latour, Bruno (1983), 'Give Me a Laboratory and I will Raise the World', in K. Knorr-Cetina and M. Mulkay (eds), *Science Observed: Perspectives on the Social Study of Science*, 141–70, London: Sage.

Latour, Bruno (1988), *The Pasteurization of France*, trans. A. Sheridan and J. Law, Cambridge, MA: Harvard University Press.

Latour, Bruno (1992), 'The Costly Ghastly Kitchen', in Andrew Cunningham and Perry Williams (eds), *The Laboratory Revolution in Medicine*, 295–303, Cambridge: Cambridge University Press.

Lawlor, Clark (2006), *Consumption and Literature: The Making of the Romantic Disease*, New York: Palgrave MacMillan.

Lawrence, Christopher (1979), 'The nervous system and society in the Scottish Enlightenment', in Barry Barnes and Steven Shapin (eds), *Natural Order: Historical Studies of Scientific Culture*, 19–40, London: Sage.

Lawrence, Christopher (1985), 'Incommunicable knowledge: science, technology and the clinical art in Britain 1850–1914', *Journal of Contemporary History* 20, no. 4: 503–20.

Lawrence, Christopher (1985), 'Ornate Physicians and Learned Artisans: Edinburgh medical men 1726–1776', in William F. Bynum and Roy Porter (eds), *William Hunter and the Eighteenth-Century Medical World*, 153–76, Cambridge: Cambridge University Press.

Lawrence, Christopher (1996), 'Disciplining Disease: Scurvy, the Navy and Imperial Expansion, 1750–1825', in D. Miller and P. Reill (eds), *Visions of Empire*, 80–106, Cambridge: Cambridge University Press.

Lawrence, Christopher (1998), 'Medical minds, surgical bodies: corporeality and the doctors', in Christopher Lawrence and Steven Shapin (eds), *Science Incarnate: Historical Embodiments of Natural Knowledge*, 156–201, Chicago: University of Chicago Press.

Lawrence, Christopher and Michael Brown (2016), 'Quintessentially Modern Heroes: Surgeons, Explorers, and Empire, c.1840–1914', *Journal of Social History* 50, no. 1: 148–78.

Lawrence, Ghislaine (1992), 'The ambiguous artifact: surgical instruments and the surgical past', in Christopher Lawrence (ed.), *Medical Theory, Surgical Practice*, 295–314, London and New York: Routledge.

Leavitt, Judith Walzer and Whitney Walton (1984), '"Down to Death's Door": Women's Perceptions of Childbirth in America', in Judith Walzer Leavitt (ed.), *Women and Health in America: Historical Readings*, 155–65, Madison: University of Wisconsin Press.

Leavitt, Sarah (2002), *From Catherine Beecher to Martha Stewart: A Cultural History of Domestic Advice*, Chapel Hill: University of North Carolina Press.

Lederer, Susan E. (1995), *Subjected to Science: Human Experimentation in America Before the Second World War*, Baltimore, MD: Johns Hopkins University Press.

Lee, Catherine (2013), *Policing Prostitution, 1856–1886: Deviance, Surveillance and Morality*, London: Pickering and Chatto.

Lee, Paula Young (2008), *Meat, Modernity, and the Rise of the Slaughterhouse*, London: University of New Hampshire Press.

Lefebvre, Henri (1992), *The Production of Space*, trans. Donald Nicholson-Smith, Hoboken, NJ: Wiley-Blackwell.

Le Goff, Jacques and Jean-Charles Sournia (1985), *Les Maladies ont une Histoire*, Paris: Le Seuil.

Legrand du Saule (1896), 'L'État Mental des Parisiens pendant le siège de Paris', *Chronique Médicale*: 77–80, 119–21, 147–51.

Léonard, Jacques (1978), *Les Médecins de l'Ouest au 19ème siècle*, Paris: Librairie Champion.

Levine, Philippa (2003), *Prostitution, Race, and Politics: Policing Venereal Disease in the British Empire*, London: Routledge.

Lewenson, Sandra B. and Eleanor Krohn Herrmann (eds) (2007), *Capturing Nursing History*, New York: Springer.

Li, Shang-Jen (2002), 'Natural History of Parasitic Disease: Patrick Manson's Philosophical Method', *Isis* 93: 206–28.

Li Chiu, Martha (1991), 'Mind, Body, and Illness in a Chinese Medical Tradition', PhD diss., Harvard University.

Lidsky, Paul (1982), *Les Écrivains contre la Commune*, Paris: François Maspéro.

Lieffers, C. (2012), '"The Present Time Is Eminently Scientific": The Science of Cookery in Nineteenth-Century Britain', *Journal of Social History* 45, no. 4: 936–59.

Lindsay, W. L. (1854), 'Clinical Notes on Cholera', *Association Medical Journal* S3–2: 834–41.

Linker, Beth (2011), 'Shooting Disabled Soldiers: Medicine and Photography in World War I America', *Journal of the History of Medicine and Allied Sciences* 66, no. 3: 313–46.

Linton, D. S. (2005), *Emil von Behring: Infectious Disease, Immunology, Serum Therapy*, Philadelphia: American Philosophical Society.

Livingstone, David (1999), 'Tropical Climate and Moral Hygiene: The Anatomy of a Victorian Debate', *British Journal for the History of Science* 32, no. 1: 93–110.

Livingstone, David (2003), *Putting Science in its Place: Geographies of Scientific Knowledge*, Chicago: University of Chicago Press.

Local Government Board (1887), 'Supplement to Sixteenth Annual Report, containing Report of Medical Officer, 1886', *Parliamentary Papers*, C.5171.

Local Government Board (1889), 'Supplement to Eighteenth Annual Report, containing Report of Medical Officer, 1888', *Parliamentary Papers*, C.5813

Logan, Cheryl (2002), 'Before There Were Standards: The Role of Test Animals in the Production of Empirical Generality in Physiology', *Journal of the History of Biology* 35: 329–63.

Logan, Melville (1997), *Nerves and Narratives: A Cultural History of Hysteria in 19th-Century British Prose*, Berkeley: University of California Press.

Lomax, E. M. R. (1996), *Small and Special: The Development of Hospitals for Children in Victorian Britain*, London: Wellcome Institute for the History of Medicine.

Lombroso, Cesare and William Ferrero (1895), *The Female Offender*, New York: Appleton and Company.

Long, James (1841), 'Introductory Lecture Delivered at the Liverpool Medical Institution', *Provincial Medical and Surgical Journal* 3: 23–9.

Loudon, Irvine (1992), 'Medical Practitioners 1750–1850 and the Period of Medical Reform in Britain', in Andrew Wear (ed.), *Medicine in Society: Historical Essays*, 219–47, Cambridge: Cambridge University Press.

Loughran, Tracey (2017), *Shell-Shock and Medical Culture in First World War Britain*, Cambridge: Cambridge University Press.

Low, Michael Christopher (2008), 'Empire and the Hajj: Pilgrims, plagues, and pan-Islam under British surveillance, 1865–1908', *International Journal of Middle East Studies* 40, no. 2: 269–90.

Löwy, Ilana (1992), 'From Guinea Pigs to Man: The Development of Haffkine's Anticholera Vaccine', *Journal of the History of Medicine and Allied Sciences* 47: 270–309.

Löwy, Ilana (2007), 'The Social History of Medicine: Beyond the Local', *Social History of Medicine* 20, no. 3: 465–82.

Lummel, Peter, Peter Atkins and Derek Oddy (eds), *Food and the City in Europe since 1800*, Aldershot and Burlington, VT: Ashgate.

Lupton, Deborah (2012), *Medicine as Culture: Illness, Disease and the Body*, New York: Sage.

Lutz, Tom (1991), *American Nervousness, 1903: An Anecdotal History*, Ithaca, NY: Cornell University Press.

Lynch, Michael E. (1988), 'Sacrifice and the transformation of the animal body into a scientific object: laboratory culture and ritual practice in the neurosciences', *Social Studies of Science* 18, no. 2: 265–89.

Lyons, Maryinez (2002), *The Colonial Disease: A Social History of Sleeping Sickness in Northern Zaire, 1900–1940*, Cambridge: Cambridge University Press.

Macalpine, Ida and Richard Hunter (1969), *George III and the Mad Business*, London: Allen Lane/Penguin Press.

MacDonald, Helen (2006), *Human Remains: Dissection and its Histories*, New Haven, CT: Yale University Press.

Macilwaine, S. W. (1900), 'What is a Disease?', *British Medical Journal* 2, no. 2085: 1703–4.

Macilwaine, S. W. (1911), *Medical Revolution: A Plea for National Preservation of Health Based upon the Natural Interpretation of Disease*, London: P.S. King.

Mack, Adam (2015), *Sensing Chicago: Noisemakers, Strikebreakers and Muckrakers*, Chicago: University of Chicago Press.

Mackaman, Douglas Peter (1998), *Leisure Settings: Bourgeois Culture, Medicine and the Spa in Modern France*, Chicago: University of Chicago Press.

MacKay, Michael (2009), 'The Rise of a Medical Speciality: The Medicalization of Elite Equine Medical Care, 1680–1800', PhD diss., University of York.

MacKenzie, John (1988), *The Empire of Nature: Hunting, Conservation and British Imperialism*, Manchester: Manchester University Press.

MacMichael, William (1827/1915), *The Gold-Headed Cane*, New York: Hoeber.

Macpherson, John (1866), *Cholera in its Home: With a Sketch of the Pathology and Treatment of the Disease*, London: John Churchill & Sons.

Maehle, Andreas-Holger (2009), *Doctors, Honour and the Law: Medical Ethics in Imperial Germany*, Basingstoke: Palgrave.

Maerker, Anna (2013), 'Anatomizing the Trade: Designing and Marketing Anatomical Models as Medical Technologies, c.1700–1900', *Technology and Culture* 54, no. 3: 531–62.

Maglen, Krista (2005), 'Importing trachoma: The introduction into Britain of American ideas of an "immigrant disease", 1892–1906', *Immigrants & Minorities* 23, no. 1: 80–99.

Mahone, Sloan (2006), 'The psychology of rebellion: colonial medical responses to dissent in British East Africa', *Journal of African History* 47: 241–58.

Malpas, C. (2004), 'Jules Guerin Makes his Market: The Social Economy of Orthopaedic Medicine in Paris, c. 1825–1845', in W. de Blecourt and C. Usborne (eds), *Cultural Approaches to the History of Medicine*, London: Palgrave.

Mandler, Peter (2004), 'The Problem with Cultural History', *Social and Cultural History* 1, no. 1: 94–117.

Manthorpe, Catherine (1986), 'Science or Domestic Science? The Struggle to Define an Appropriate Science Education for Girls in Early Twentieth-century England', *History of Education* 15, no. 3: 195–213.

Marcellus, Jane (2008), 'Nervous Women and Noble Savages: The Romanticized "Other" in Nineteenth-Century US Patent Medicine Advertising', *Journal of Popular Culture* 41, no. 5: 784–808.

Mariani-Costantini, Renato and Aldo Mariani-Costantini (2007), 'An Outline of the History of Pellagra in Italy', *Journal of Anthropological Science* 85: 163–71.

Markus, Thomas A. (1993), *Buildings & Power: Freedom and Control in the Origin of Modern Building Types*, London and New York: Routledge.

Marland, Hilary (2004), *Dangerous Motherhood: Insanity and Childbirth in Victorian Britain*, London: Palgrave Macmillan.

Marland, Hilary (2006), 'Languages and Landscapes of Emotion: Motherhood and Puerperal Insanity in the Nineteenth Century', in Fay Bound Alberti (ed.), *Medicine, Emotion, and Disease, 1700–1950*, 53–78, Basingstoke: Palgrave.

Marriott, John (2003), *The Other Empire: Metropolis, India and Progress in the Colonial Imagination*, Manchester: Manchester University Press.

Martin, James Ranald (1856), *The Influence of Tropical Climates on European Constitutions, including Practical Observations on the Nature and Treatment of the Diseases of Europeans on their Return from Tropical Climates, new edition*, London: John Churchill.

Martineau, Harriet (1845), *Life in the Sickroom*, Boston: William Crosby.

[Martineau, Harriet] (1852), 'What there is in a button', *Household Words*, 17 April, vol. 5: 106–12.

Marx, Leo and Merritt Roe Smith (eds) (1995), *Does Technology Drive History? The Dilemma of Technological Determinism*, Cambridge, MA, and London: MIT Press.

Maudsley, Henry (1871), *Body and Mind: An Inquiry into their Connection and Mutual Influence, specially in Reference to Mental Disorders*, New York: D. Appleton and Company.

Mayhew, Henry (1849), 'A Visit to the Cholera Districts of Bermondsey', *Morning Chronicle*, 24 September.

Mayo, Elizabeth (1863), *Lessons on Objects, Graduated Series; Designed for Children Between the Ages of Six and Fourteen Years*, New York: Scribner.

McCarthy, Angela (2016), *Migration, Ethnicity, and Madness: New Zealand, 1860–1910*, Liverpool: Liverpool University Press.

McClelland, Charles E. (2002), *The German Experience of Professionalization: Modern Learned Professions and their Organizations from the Early Nineteenth Century to the Hitler Era*, Cambridge: Cambridge University Press.

McDonough, Patrick (2008), *Idiocy: A Cultural History*, Liverpool: Liverpool University Press.

McGregor, Neil (2010), *A History of the World in 100 Objects*, London: Penguin.

McHugh, P. (1980), *Prostitution and Victorian Social Reform*, London: Croom Helm.

McIntosh, James et al. (1913), 'Parasyphilis of the Nervous System', *Brain* 36, no. 1: 1–30.

McShane, C. and J. Tarr (2007), *The Horse and the City: Living Machines in the Nineteenth Century*, Baltimore, MD: Johns Hopkins University Press.

Mental Deficiency Sub-Committee Minutes (1914–17), 'Mental Deficiency Act, 1913: Memorandum of the Town Clerk for the Information of the Asylums Committee for the Care of the Mentally Defective' (BCC1/AF/7/1/1), 7–9, Birmingham Archives, Library of Birmingham.

Mepham, T. B. (1993), '"Humanizing" Milk: The Formulation of Artificial Feeds for Infants (1850–1910)', *Medical History* 37, no. 3: 225–49.

Mercer, Philip (1972), *Sympathy and Ethics: A Study of the Relationship between Sympathy and Morality with Special Reference to Hume's Treatise*, Oxford: Clarendon Press.

Messner, Algelika C. (2009), 'Translations and TransFormations: Toward Creating New Men in Early Twentieth-Century China', in Poonam Bala (ed.), *Biomedicine as a Contested Site: Some Revelations in Imperial Contexts*, 99–114, Lanham, MD: Lexington Books.

Méthot, Pierre-Olivier (2012), 'Why Do Parasites Harm Their Host? On the Origin and Legacy of Theobald Smith's "Law of Declining Virulence", 1900–1980', *History and Philosophy of the Life Sciences* 34: 561–601.

Micale, Mark (1995), *Approaching Hysteria: Disease and Its Interpretations*, Princeton, NJ: Princeton University Press.

Micale, Mark S. (2008) *Hysterical Men: The Hidden History of Male Nervous Illness*, Cambridge, MA: Harvard University Press.

Micale, S. and Roy Porter (1995), *Approaching Hysteria: Disease and its Interpretations*, Princeton, NJ: Princeton University Press.

Miller, Daniel (2005), 'Introduction', in Daniel Miller (ed.), *Materiality*, 1–50, Durham, NC: Duke University Press.

Miller, Ian (2009), 'Necessary torture? Vivisection, suffragette force-feeding, and responses to scientific medicine in Britain c. 1870–1920', *Journal of the History of Medicine and Allied Sciences* 64, no. 3: 333–72.

Milles, Dietrich (1995), 'Working Capacity and Calorie Consumption: The History of Rational Physical Economy', in Harmke Kamminga and Andrew Cunningham (eds), *Science and Culture of Nutrition, 1840–1940*, 75–96, Amsterdam: Editions Rodopi B.V.

Mishra, Saurabh (2011), 'Beasts, Murrains, and the British Raj: Reassessing Colonial Medicine in India from the Veterinary Perspective, 1860–1900', *Bulletin of the History of Medicine* 85, no. 4 (Winter): 587–619.

Mitsuda, Tatsuya (2017), 'Entangled Histories: German Veterinary Medicine, 1770–1900', *Medical History* 61: 25–47.

Mogil, Jeffrey, Alexander Tuttle, Sarasa Tohyama, Tim Ramsay, Jonathan Kimmelman, Petra Schweinhardt and Gary Bennett (2015), 'Increasing placebo responses over time in U.S. clinical trials of neuropathic pain', *Pain* 156, no. 12: 2616–26.

Mood, Jonathan (2009), '"If We're Petticoat Clothed, We're Major Minded": Working-class Women and the Meat Boycott of 1872', *Women's History Review* 18, no. 3: 409–26.

Mooney, Graham (1999), 'Public Health Versus Private Practice: the Contested Development of Compulsory Infectious Disease Notification in Late-Nineteenth Century Britain', *Bulletin of the History of Medicine* 73, no. 2: 238–67.

Mooney, Graham (2013), 'The Material Consumptive: Domesticating the Tuberculosis Patient in Edwardian England', *Journal of Historical Geography* 42: 152–66.

Mooney, Graham (2015), *Intrusive Interventions: Public Health, Domestic Space, and Infectious Disease Surveillance in England, 1840–1914*, Rochester, NY: University of Rochester Press.

Moore, Wendy (2005), *The Knife Man: Blood, Body-snatching and the Birth of Modern Surgery*, London: Bantam.

Moran, James E. (2000), *Committed to a State Asylum: Insanity and Society in Nineteenth-Century Quebec and Ontario*, Montreal: McGill-Queen's University Press.

Moran, James (2019), *Madness on Trial: A Transatlantic History of English Civil Law and Lunacy*, Manchester: University of Manchester Press.

Moran, James, Leslie Topp and Jonathan Andrews (eds) (2011), *Madness, Architecture and the Built Environment: Psychiatric Spaces in Historical Context*, New York: Routledge.

[Morley, Henry] (1858), 'Use and abuse of the dead', *Household Words* 17, no. 3 (April): 361–5.

Morris, R. J. (1976), *Cholera 1832: The Social Response to an Epidemic*, London: Croom Helm.

Mort, Frank (1987), *Dangerous Sexualities: Medico-Moral Politics in England since 1830*, London: Routledge.

Moscoso, Javier (2012), *Pain: A Cultural History*, Basingstoke: Palgrave.

Moscoso, Javier (2016), 'From the History of Emotions to the History of Experience: The Multiple Layers of Material Expressions', in Elena Delgado, Pura Fernández and Jo Labanyi (eds), *Engaging the Emotions in Spanish Culture and History*, 176–91, Nashville, TN: Vanderbilt Press.

Moscoso, Javier and Juan Manuel Zaragoza (2014), 'Historias del Bienestar. Desde la historia de las emociones a las políticas de la experiencia', *Cuadernos de Historia Contemporánea* 36: 73–89.

Moscucci, Ornella (2005), 'Gender and Cancer in Britain, 1860–1910: The Emergence of Cancer as a Public Health Concern', *American Journal of Public Health* 95, no. 8: 1312–21.

Moseley, Benjamin (1800), *A Treatise on Sugar, with Miscellaneous Medical Observations*, 2nd edn, London: John Nichols.

Müller-Wille, Staffan and Hans-Jörg Rheinberger (2012), *A Cultural History of Heredity*, Chicago: University of Chicago Press.

Murchison, Charles (1865), 'On the Points of Resemblance between Cattle-Plague and Small-Pox', *The Lancet* 86: 724–6.

Murchison, Charles (1866), 'On the Points of Resemblance between Cattle-Plague and Small-Pox', *The Lancet* 87: 58–61, 119–20.

Murdoch, Lydia (2015), 'Anti-Vaccination and the Politics of Grief in Late-Victorian England', in S. Olsen (ed.), *Childhood, Youth and Emotions in Modern History: National, Colonial and Global Perspectives*, 242–60, Basingstoke: Palgrave.

Murdoch, Lydia (2015), 'Carrying the Pox: The Use of Children and Ideals of Childhood in Early British and Imperial Campaigns Against Smallpox', *Journal of Social History* 48: 511–35.

Murray, Caitlin (2007), 'The "Colouring of the Psychosis": Interpreting Insanity in the Primitive Mind', *Health and History* 9, no. 2: 7–21.

Murray, Flora (1920), *Women as Army Surgeons: Being the History of the Women's Hospital Corps in Paris, Wimereux and Endell Street; September 1914–October 1919*, London: Hodder & Stoughton.

Murray, Jamieson (1909), *A History of the Reading Pathological Society*, London: John Bale, Sons & Co.

Murray, Narisara (2000), 'From Birds of Paradise to Drosophila: The Changing Roles of Scientific Specimens in Europe and America to 1920', in L. Kalof and B. Resl (eds), *A Cultural History of Animals*, vol. 6: *The Modern Age (1920–2000)*, 119–37, London: Bloomsbury.

Musselman, Elizabeth Green (2012), *Nervous Conditions: Science and the Body Politic in Early Industrial Britain*, Albany, NY: State University of New York Press.

Narter, Meltem (2006), 'The Change in the Daily Knowledge of Madness in Turkey', *Journal for the Theory of Social Behaviour* 36, no. 4: 409–24.

Nead, Lynda (2005), *Victorian Babylon: People, Streets, and Images in Victorian London*, New Haven, CT: Yale University Press.

Neill, Deborah (2009), 'Finding the "Ideal Diet": Nutrition, Culture, and Dietary Practices in France and French Equatorial Africa, c. 1890s to 1920s', *Food and Foodways* 17, no. 1: 1–28.

Newman, Laura (2017), 'Making germs real: germ theories of disease and occupational knowledge in Britain, c.1880–1930', PhD diss., King's College London.

Newsom Kerr, Matthew L. (2018), *Contagion, Isolation and Biopolitics in Victorian London*, New York: Palgrave.

Niall, P. A. S. and Juergen Mueller (2002), 'Updating the Accounts: Global Mortality of the 1918–1920 "Spanish" Influenza Pandemic', *Bulletin of the History of Medicine* 76, no. 1: 105–15.

Nieto-Galan, A. (2015), 'Mr Giovanni Succi Meets Dr Luigi Luciani in Florence: Hunger Artists and Experimental Physiology in the Late Nineteenth Century', *Social History of Medicine* 28, no. 1: 64–81.

Nightingale, Florence (1990), *Ever yours, Florence Nightingale: Selected Letters*, ed. Martha Vicinus and Bea Nergaard, Cambridge, MA: Harvard University Press.

Nitrini, Ricardo (2000), 'The History of Tabes Dorsalis and the Impact of Observational Studies in Neurology', *Archives of Neurology* 57, no. 4: 605–6.

Njoh, Ambe J. (2008), 'Colonial philosophies, urban space, and racial segregation in British and French colonial Africa', *Journal of Black Studies* 38, no. 4: 579–99.

Novak, Daniel A. (2008), *Realism, Photography and Nineteenth-Century Fiction*, vol. 60, Cambridge: Cambridge University Press.

Noyes Brothers and Cutler (1888), *Illustrated Catalogue of Surgical, Dental and Veterinary Instruments*, St Paul, MN: Pioneer Press Company.

Nyhart, Lynn (1995), *Biology takes Form: Animal Morphology and the German Universities, 1800–1900*, Chicago: University of Chicago Press.

Nyhart, Lynn (2009), *Modern Nature: The Rise of the Biological Perspective in Germany*, London: University of Chicago Press.

O'Brien, Patricia (1983), 'The Kleptomania Diagnosis: Bourgeois Women and Theft in Late Nineteenth-Century France', *Journal of Social History* 17, no. 1: 65–77.

O'Connor, Erin (2000), *Raw Material: Producing Pathology in Victorian Culture*, Chapel Hill, NC: Duke University Press.

Oddy, Derek (1983), 'Urban Famine in Nineteenth-Century Britain: The Effect of the Lancashire Cotton Famine on Working-Class Diet and Health', *Economic History Review* 36, no. 1: 68–86.

Oddy, Derek, (2007), 'Food Quality in London and the Rise of the Public Analyst, 1870–1939', in Peter J. Atkins, Peter Lummel and Derek J. Oddy (eds), *Food and the City in Europe since 1800*, 91–104, Aldershot and Burlington, VT: Ashgate.

Oddy, Derek (2008), 'Hunger: A History', *Reviews in History* 695 (October), http://www.history.ac.uk/reviews/review/695.

Oppenheim, Janet (1988), *The Other World: Spiritualism and Psychical Research in England, 1850–1914*, Cambridge: Cambridge University Press.

Oppenheim, Janet (1991), *Shattered Nerves: Doctors, Patients and Depression in Victorian England*, Oxford: Oxford University Press.

Orwell, George (2001), *The Road to Wigan Pier*, New York: Penguin Classics.

Osborn, Emily Lynn (2004), '"Rubber Fever", Commerce and French Colonial Rule in Upper Guinée, 1890–1913', *Journal of African History* 45, no. 3: 445–65.

Osborne, Michael A. (2014), *The Emergence of Tropical Medicine in France*, Chicago: University of Chicago Press.

Osborne, Thomas (1996), 'Security and Vitality: Drains, Liberalism and Power in the Nineteenth Century', in Andrew Barry, Thomas Osborne and Nikolas Rose (eds), *Foucault and Political Reason: Liberalism, Neo-Liberalism and the Rationalities of Government*, 99–121, Chicago: University of Chicago Press.

Osler, William (1925), *Aequanimitas, with other Addresses to Medical Students and Practitioners of Medicine*, 2nd edn, Philadelphia: P. Blakiston's Son.

Otis, Laura (2000), *Membranes: Metaphors of Invasion in Nineteenth-Century Literature, Science, and Politics*, Baltimore, MD: Johns Hopkins University Press.

Otis, Laura (2002), 'The metaphoric circuit: organic and technological communication in the nineteenth century', *Journal of the History of Ideas* 63, no. 1: 105–28.

Otis, Laura (2007), *Müller's Lab: The Story of Jakob Henle, Theodor Schwann, Emil duBois-Reymond, Hermann von Helmholtz, Rudolf Virchow, Robert Remak, Ernst Haeckel, and Their Brilliant, Tormented Advisor*, Oxford: Oxford University Press.

Ott, Katherine (1996), *Fevered Lives: Tuberculosis in American Culture since 1870*, Cambridge, MA: Harvard University Press.

Otter, Chris (2008), *The Victorian Eye: A Political History of Light and Vision in Britain, 1800–1910*, Chicago: University of Chicago Press.

Otter, Chris (2011), 'Hippophagy in the UK: A Failed Dietary Revolution', *Endeavour* 35, no. 2–3: 80–90.

Oudshoorn, Nelly and Trevor Pinch (eds) (2003), *How Users Matter: The Co-Construction of Users and Technology*, Cambridge, MA: MIT Press.

Outram, Dorinda (1988), *The Body and the French Revolution*, New Haven, CT: Yale University Press.

Packard, Randall M. and Peter J. Brown (1997), 'Rethinking Health, Development, and Malaria: Historicizing a Cultural Model in International Health', *Medical Anthropology* 17, no. 3: 181–94.

Parascandola, John (2008), *Sex, Sin, and Science: A History of Syphilis in America*, Westport, CT: Praeger.

Parker, Joan E. (2001), 'Lydia Becker's "School for Science": A Challenge to Domesticity', *Women's History Review* 10, no. 4: 629–50.

Parle, Julie (2003), 'Witchcraft or Madness? The Amandiki of Zululand, 1894–1914', *Journal of Southern African Studies* 29, no. 1: 105–32.

Parry-Jones, William Ll. (1972), *The Trade in Lunacy: A Study of Private Madhouses in England in the Eighteenth and Nineteenth Centuries*, London: Routledge and Kegan Paul.

Parry-Jones, William Ll. (1981), 'The Model of Geel Lunatic Colony and Its Influence on the Nineteenth-Century Asylum System in Britain', in Andrew Scull (ed.), *Madhouses, Mad-Doctors and Madmen: The Social History of Psychiatry in the Victorian Era*, 201–17, London: Athlone Press.

Paul, Harry W. (2011), *Henri de Rothschild, 1872–1947: Medicine and Theater*, London: Routledge.

Pauly, Phillip (1984), 'The Appearance of Academic Biology in Late Nineteenth Century America,' *Journal of the History of Biology* 17: 369–97.

Payer, Peter (2007), 'The Age of Noise: Early Reactions in Vienna, 1870–1914', *Journal of Urban History* 33: 773–93.

Pelling, Margaret (1978), *Cholera, Fever and English Medicine 1825–1865*, Oxford: Oxford University Press

Percivall, W. (1823), *Elementary Lectures in the Veterinary Art*, London: Longman.

Perkins, Linda M. (1983), 'The Impact of the "Cult of True Womanhood" on the Education of Black Women', *Journal of Social Issues* 39, no. 3: 17–28

Petitjean, P., C. Jami and A. M. Moulin (eds) (1992), *Science and Empires: Historical Studies about Scientific Development and European Expansion*, Amsterdam: Rodopi.

Philippon, Jacques and Jacques Poirier (2008), *Joseph Babinski: A Biography*, Oxford: Oxford University Press.

Phillips, Howard (2014), 'The Recent Wave of "Spanish" Flu Historiography', *Social History of Medicine* 27, no. 4: 789–808.

Pick, Daniel (1986), 'The faces of anarchy: Lombroso and the politics of criminal science in post-unification Italy', *History Workshop Journal* 21, no. 1: 60–86.

Pick, D. (1989), *Faces of Degeneration: A European Disorder, c.1848–1918*, Cambridge: Cambridge University Press.

Picker, John M. (2003), *Victorian Soundscapes*, New York: Oxford University Press.

Pickstone, John V. (1981), 'Bureaucracy, Liberalism and the Body in post-Revolutionary France: Bichat's Physiology and the Paris School of Medicine', *History of Science* 19, no. 2: 115–42.

Pickstone, John V. (1992), 'Dearth, dirt and fever epidemics: rewriting the history of British "public health", 1780–1850', in T. Ranger and P. Slack (eds), *Epidemics and Ideas: Essays on the Historical Perception of Pestilence*, 125–48, Cambridge: Cambridge University Press.

Pickstone, John V. (1999), 'How Might We Map the Cultural Fields of Science? Politics and Organisms in Restoration France', *History of Science* 37, no. 3: 347–64.

Pickstone, John (2000), *Ways of Knowing: A New History of Science, Technology and Medicine*, Manchester: Manchester University Press.

Pinel, Patrice (1992), *Naissance d'un Fléau. Histoire de la Lutte contre le Cancer en France 1890–1940*, Paris: Métaillé,

Pinel, Philippe (1801), *Traité medico-philosophique sur l'aliénation mentale, ou la manie*, Paris: Richard.

Pitzner, Donald E. (ed.) (1997), *America's Communal Utopias*, Chapel Hill: University of North Carolina Press.

Pols, Hans (2012), 'Notes from Batavia, the Europeans' Graveyard: The Nineteenth-Century Debate on Acclimatization in the Dutch East Indies', *Journal of the History of Medicine and Allied Sciences* 67, no. 1: 120–48.

Poovey, Mary (1995), *Making a Social Body: British Cultural Formation, 1830–1864*, Chicago: University of Chicago Press.

Porter, Dorothy (1998), *Health, Civilization and the State*, London: Routledge.

Porter, Dorothy and Roy Porter (1988), 'The Politics of Prevention: Anti-Vaccinationism and Public Health in Nineteenth-Century England', *Medical History* 32: 231–52.

Porter, Roy (1985), 'The Patient's View: Doing Medical History from Below', *Theory and Society* 14, no. 2: 175–98.

Porter, Roy (1985), 'William Hunter: a surgeon and a gentleman', in William F. Bynum and Roy Porter (eds), *William Hunter and the Eighteenth-Century Medical World*, 7–34, Cambridge: Cambridge University Press.

Porter, Roy (1987/1990), *Mind Forg'd Manacles: A History of Madness in England from the Restoration to the Regency*, London: Penguin.

Porter, Roy (1987/1996), *A Social History of Madness: Stories of the Insane*, London: Phoenix.

Porter, Roy (1989), *Health for Sale: Quackery in England 1660–1850*, Manchester: Manchester University Press.

Porter, Roy (1993), 'Man, Animals and Medicine at the Time of the Founding of the Royal Veterinary College', in A. R. Michell (ed.), *History of the Healing Professions*, vol. 3, 19–30, Wallingford: CABI.

Porter, Roy (1997), *Rewriting the Self: Histories from the Renaissance to the Present*, London: Psychology Press.

Porter, Roy (2001), *Bodies Politic: Disease, Death and the Doctors in Britain, 1650–1900*, London: Reaktion.

Porter, Roy (ed.) (1990), *The Medical History of Waters and Spas, Medical History Supplement no. 10*, London: Wellcome Institute.

Porter, Roy and G. S. Rousseau (2000), *Gout: The Patrician Malady*, New Haven, CT: Yale University Press.

Porter, Theodore M. (1986), *The Rise of Statistical Thinking, 1820–1900*, Princeton, NJ: Princeton University Press.

Porter, TheodoreM. (1996), *Trust in Numbers: The Pursuit of Objectivity in Science and Public life*, Princeton, NJ: Princeton University Press.

Poskett, James (2017), 'Phrenology, Correspondence, and the Global Politics of Reform, 1815–1848', *History Journal*, 60, no. 2: 409–42.

Powell, Anne (2009), *Women in the War Zone: Hospital Service in the First World War*, Stroud: History Press.

Putnam, R. (1925), *The Life and Letters of Mary Putnam Jacobi*, New York: G. P. Putnam's Sons.

Qureshi, Sadiah (2011), *Peoples on Parade: Exhibitions, Empire, and Anthropology in Nineteenth Century Britain*, Chicago and London: University of Chicago Press.

Rabinbach, Anson (1990/1992), *The Human Motor: Energy, Fatigue and the Origins of Modernity*, Berkeley: University of California Press.

Ramsden, E. and D. Wilson (2013), 'The Suicidal Animal: Science and the Nature of Self-Destruction', *Past & Present* 224: 201–42.

Ray, Arthur J. (1984), 'The Northern Great Plains: Pantry of the Northwestern Fur Trade, 1774–1885', *Prairie Forum* 9, no. 2: 263–80.

Reader, John (2008), *The Untold History of the Potato*, London: Vintage.

Reddy, William (2001), *The Navigation of Feeling: A Framework for the History of Emotions*, Cambridge: Cambridge University Press.

Rees, Danny (2014), 'Down in the Mouth: Faces of Pain', in Rob Boddice (ed.), *Pain and Emotion in Modern History*, 164–86, Basingstoke: Palgrave Macmillan.

Reid, Donald (1991), *Paris Sewers and Sewermen: Realities and Representations*, Cambridge, MA: Harvard University Press.

Reinarz, Jonathan (2014), *Past Scents: Historical Perspectives on Smell*, Chicago: University of Illinois Press.

Reinarz, Jonathan and Rebecca Wynter (2015), 'Introduction: Towards a history of complaining about medicine', in Jonathan Reinarz and Rebecca Wynter (eds), *Complaints, Controversies and Grievances in Medicine: Historical and Social Science Perspectives*, 1–33, London: Routledge.

Reiser, Stanley Joel (2009), *Technological Medicine*, Cambridge: Cambridge University Press.

Reiss, Benjamin (2008), *Theaters of Madness: Insane Asylums and Nineteenth-Century American Culture*, Chicago: University of Chicago Press.

Reuter, Shelley Z. (2006) 'The Genuine Jewish Type: Racial Ideology and Anti-Immigrationism in Early Medical Writing about Tay-Sachs Disease', *Canadian Journal of Sociology /Cahiers Canadiens de sociologie* 31, no. 3: 291–323.

Reznick, Jeffrey (2011), *Healing the Nation: Soldiers and the Culture of Caregiving in Britain during the Great War*, Manchester: Manchester University Press

Richardson, Ruth (1988/2001), *Death, Dissection, and the Destitute*, 2nd edn, London, Phoenix Press.

Risse, Guenter (1999), *Mending Bodies, Saving Souls: A History of Hospitals*, Oxford: Oxford University Press.

Ritvo, Harriet (1987), *The Animal Estate: The English and Other Creatures in the Victorian Age*, Cambridge, MA: Harvard University Press.

Ritvo, Harriet (1995), 'Border Trouble: Shifting the Line between People and Other Animals', *Social Research* 62: 481–500.

Roberts, M. J. D. (2009), 'The Politics of Professionalization: MPs, Medical Men, and the 1858 Medical Act', *Medical History* 53, no. 1: 37–56.

Romano, T. M. (1997), 'The Cattle Plague of 1865 and the Reception of "The Germ Theory" in Mid-Victorian Britain', *Journal of the History of Medicine and Allied Sciences* 52: 51–80.

Romano, Terrie (2002), *Making Medicine Scientific: John Burdon Sanderson and the Culture of Victorian Science*, London: Johns Hopkins University Press.

Roper, M. (2009), *The Secret Battle: Emotional Survival in the Great War*, Manchester: Manchester University Press.

Rose, F. Clifford (ed.) (2004), *Neurology of the Arts: Painting, Music, Literature*, London: Imperial College Press.

Rose, Nikolas (1999), *Powers of Freedom: Reframing Political Thought*, Cambridge: Cambridge University Press.

Rosen, G. (1942), 'Changing Attitudes of the Medical Profession to Specialisation', *Bulletin of the History of Medicine* 12: 343–54.

Rosen, George (1944), *The Specialization of Medicine with Particular Reference to Ophthalmology*, New York: Froben Press.

Rosen, George (1958), *A History of Public Health*, New York: M.D. Publications.

Rosenberg, Charles (1962), *The Cholera Years: The United States, 1832, 1849 and 1866*, Chicago: University of Chicago Press.

Rosenberg, Charles (1966), 'Cholera in Nineteenth-Century Europe: A Tool for Social and Economic Analysis', *Comparative Studies in Society and History* 8, no. 4: 452–63.

Rosenberg, Charles (1995), *The Trial of the Assassin Guiteau: Psychiatry and the Law in the Gilded Age*, Chicago: University of Chicago Press.

Rosenberg, Charles E., Janet Golden and Steven J. Peitzman (1992), 'Framing Disease', *Hospital Practice* 27, no. 7: 179–221.

Rosner, Lisa (1999), *The Most Beautiful Man in Existence: The Scandalous Life of Alexander Lessassier*, Philadelphia: University of Pennsylvania Press.

Rothfels, Nigel (2002), *Savages and Beasts: The Birth of the Modern Zoo*, Baltimore, MD: Johns Hopkins University Press.

Rothman, Sheila (1994), *Living in the Shadow of Death: Tuberculosis and the Social Experience of Illness in American History*, New York: Basic Books.

Rousseau, G., M. Gill, D. Haycock and M. Herwig (eds) (2003), *Framing and Imagining Disease in Cultural History*, New York: Springer.

Rowley, W. (1805), *Cow-Pox Inoculation, No Security Against Small-Pox Infection*. London: J. Harris.

Rozenkrantz, Barbara G. (1972), *Public Health and the State: Changing Views in Massachusetts 1842–1936*, Cambridge, MA: Harvard University Press.

Ruiz, Maria Isabel Romero (2014), *The London Lock Hospital in the Nineteenth Century: Gender, Sexuality and Social Reform*, Oxford: Peter Lang.

Ruiz-Gómez, Natasha (2013), 'The "scientific artworks" of Doctor Paul Richer', *Medical Humanities* 39: 4–10.

Rupke, Nicolaas (ed.) (1990), *Vivisection in Historical Perspective*, London: Routledge.

Rupke, Nicolaas A. (ed.) (2000), *Medical Geography in Historical Perspective*, *Medical History Supplement No. 20*, London: Wellcome Trust Centre for the History of Medicine at UCL.

Rylance, Rick (2000), *Victorian Psychology and British Culture, 1850–1880*, Oxford: Oxford University Press.

Sakula, Alex (1982), 'Baroness Burdett-Coutts' Garden Party: The International Medical Congress. London, 1881', *Medical History* 26, no. 2: 183–90.

Salisbury, Laura and Andrew Shail (eds) (2010), *Neurology and Modernity: A Cultural History of Nervous Systems, 1800–1950*, London: Palgrave Macmillan.

Sappol, Michael (2004), *A Traffic of Dead Bodies: Anatomy and Embodied Social Identity in Nineteenth-Century America*, Princeton, NJ: Princeton University Press.

Schiebinger, Londa (2004), *Plants and Empire: Colonial Bioprospecting in the Atlantic World*, Cambridge, MA: Harvard University Press.

Schiller, Francis (1992), *Paul Broca: Founder of French Anthropology, Explorer of the Brain*, Oxford: Oxford University Press.

Schivelbusch, Wolfgang (1995), *Disenchanted Night: The Industrialization of Light in the Nineteenth Century*, trans. Angela Davies, Berkeley: University of California Press.

Schivelbusch, Wolfgang (2014), *The Railway Journey: The Industrialization of Time and Space in the Nineteenth Century*, Berkeley: University of California Press.

Schlich, Thomas (2007), 'Surgery, Science and Modernity: Operating Rooms and Laboratories as Spaces of Control', *History of Science* 45: 231–56.

Schlich, Thomas (2015), '"The Days of Brilliancy are Past": Skill, Styles and the Changing Rules of Surgical Performance, ca. 1820–1920', *Medical History* 59, no. 3: 379–403.

Scholliers, Peter (2007), 'Food Fraud and the Big City: Brussels' Responses to Food Anxieties in the Nineteenth Century', in Peter Atkins, Peter Lummel and Derek Oddy (eds), *Food and the City in Europe Since 1800*, 77–90, Aldershot: Ashgate.

Scholliers, Peter (2012), 'The Many Rooms in the House: Research on Past Foodways in Modern Europe', in Kyri W. Clafin and Peter Scholiers (eds), *Writing Food History: A Global Perspective*, 59–71, London: Bloomsbury.

Schweber, L. (2006), *Disciplining Statistics: Demography and Vital Statistics in France and England, 1830–1885*, Durham, NC: Duke University Press.

Scott, Ann, Mervyn Eadie and Andrew Lees (eds) (2012), *William Richard Gowers 1845–1915: Exploring the Victorian Brain*, Oxford: Oxford University Press.

Scull, Andrew (1979), *Museums of Madness: The Social Organization of Insanity in 19th Century England*, London: Allen Lane.

Scull, Andrew (2005), *The Most Solitary of Afflictions: Madness and Society in Britain, 1700–1900*, New Haven, CT: Yale University Press.

Scull, Andrew (2009), *Hysteria: The Biography*, Oxford: Oxford University Press.

Scull, Andrew (2015), 'A culture of complaint', in Jonathan Reinarz and Rebecca Wynter (eds), *Complaints, Controversies and Grievances in Medicine: Historical and Social Science Perspectives*, 37–55, London: Routledge.

Scull, Andrew (2015), *Madness in Civilization: A Cultural History of Insanity, from the Bible to Freud, from the Madhouse to Modern Medicine*, Princeton, NJ: Princeton University Press.

Scully, Richard and Marian Quartly (eds) (2009), *Drawing the Line: Using Cartoons as Historical Evidence*, Victoria: Monash University ePress.

Searle, Geoffrey (1998), *Morality and the Market in Victorian Britain*, Oxford: Clarendon.

Sevcenko, Nicolau (2010), *A Revolta da Vacina*, São Paulo: Cosac Naify.

Shah, Nayan (2001), *Contagious Divides: Epidemics and Race in San Francisco's Chinatown*, Berkeley: University of California Press.

Shapin, Steven (1975), 'Phrenological Knowledge and the Social Structure of Early Nineteenth-Century Edinburgh', *Annals of Science* 32, no. 3: 219–24.

Shaw, George Bernard (1909/1987), *The Doctor's Dilemma: A Tragedy*, Harmondsworth: Penguin.

Shepherd, John (1991), *The Crimean Doctors: A History of the British Medical Services in the Crimean War*, 2 vols, Liverpool: Liverpool University Press.

Showalter, Elaine (1985/1987), *The Female Malady: Women, Madness and English Culture, 1830–1980*, Harmondsworth: Penguin.

Sielke, Sabine (2008), 'The Brain – is wider than the Sky – or: Re-Cognizing Emily Dickinson', *Emily Dickinson Journal* 17, no. 1: 68–85.

Sigerist, Henry (1951), *A History of Medicine: Primitive and Archaic Medicine*, New York: Oxford University Press.

Silberman, Steve (2015), *NeuroTribes: The Legacy of Autism and the Future of Neurodiversity*, New York: Avery.

Sillitoe, Helen (1933), *A History of the Teaching of Domestic Subjects*, London: Metheun & Co Ltd.

Simon, John (1850), 'A Course of Lectures in General Pathology', *The Lancet* 56: 138.

Simon, Rita J. and Heather Ahn-Redding (2006), *The Insanity Defence the World Over*, New York: Rowman and Littlefield.

Simonds, J. B. (1848), *A Practical Treatise on Variola Ovina, or Smallpox in Sheep*, London: n.p.

Simpson, J. Y. (1868), *Proposal to Stamp out Small-Pox and Other Contagious Diseases*, Edinburgh: Edmonston and Douglas.

Sinha, Mrinalini (1995), *Colonial Masculinity: The 'Manly Englishman' and the 'Effeminate Bengali' in the Late Nineteenth Century*, Manchester: Manchester University Press.

Sirotkina, Irina (2002), *Diagnosing Literary Genius: A Cultural History of Psychiatry in Russia, 1880–1930*, London: Johns Hopkins University Press.

Sirotkina, Irina (2007), 'The Politics of Etiology: Shell Shock in the Russian Army, 1914–1918', in Angela Brintlinger and Ilya Vinitsky (eds), *Madness and the Mad in Russian Culture*, 117–29, Toronto: University of Toronto Press.

Skinner, C. (2016), 'Medical Discovery as Suffrage Justification in Mary Putnam Jacobi's 1894 New York campaign rhetoric', *Advances in the History of Rhetoric* 19, no. 3: 251–75.

Smail, Daniel Lord (2008), *On Deep History and the Brain*, Berkeley and Los Angeles: University of California Press.

Smith, Adam (1759/2009), *The Theory of Moral Sentiments*, London: Penguin.

Smith, F. B. (2006), 'The Contagious Diseases Acts Reconsidered', *Social History of Medicine* 19, no. 3: 197–215.

Smith, Leonard (1999), *'Cure, Comfort and Safe Custody': Public Lunatic Asylums in Early Nineteenth-Century England*, London: Leicester University Press.

Smith, Leonard (2007), *Lunatic Hospitals in Georgian England, 1750–1830*, London: Routledge.

Smith, Leonard (2014), *Insanity, Race and Colonialism: Managing Mental Disorder in the Post-Emancipation British Caribbean, 1838–1914*, London: Palgrave Macmillan.

Smith, Mark M. (2001), *Listening to Nineteenth-Century America*, Chapel Hill: University of North Carolina Press.

Smith, Roger (1992), *Inhibition: History and Meaning in the Sciences of Mind and Brain*, Berkeley: University of California Press.

Smith, S. D. (2001), 'Coffee, Microscopy, and the Lancet's Analytical Sanitary Commission', *Social History of Medicine* 14, no. 2: 171–97.

Smithcors, J. (1959), 'Medical Men and the Beginnings of Veterinary Medicine in America', *Bulletin of the History of Medicine* 33: 330–41.

Sontag, Susan (1978), *Illness as Metaphor*, New York: Farrar, Strauss and Giroux.

Sournia, Charles (1990), *A History of Alcoholism*, Oxford: Blackwell.

Spencer, Herbert (1876), 'The Comparative Psychology of Man', *Mind* 1, no. 1: 16–17.

Spencer, Herbert (1878), 'Consciousness under chloroform', *Missouri Dental Journal* 10: 575–80.

Spiering, Menno (2006), 'Food, Phagophobia and English National Identity', in Thomas M. Wilson (ed.), *Food, Drink and Identity in Europe*, 31–48, Amsterdam: Rodolphi.

Stadler, Peter (1988/1993), *Pestalozzi. Geschichtliche Biographie*, 2 vols, Zurich: Verlag NZZ.

Stallybrass, Peter and Allon White (1986), *The Politics and Poetics of Transgression*, Ithaca, NY: Cornell University Press.

Stanziani, Alessandro (2007), 'Municipal Laboratories and the Analysis of Foodstuffs in France under the Third Republic: A Case Study of the Paris Municipal Laboratory, 1878–1907', in Peter J. Atkins, Peter Lummel and Derek J. Oddy (eds), *Food and the City in Europe since 1800*, 105–16, Aldershot and Burlington, VT: Ashgate.

Starr, Paul (1982), *The Social Transformation of American Medicine*, New York: Basic Books.

Steere-Williams, J. (2010), 'The Perfect Food and the Filth Disease: Milk-Borne Typhoid and Epidemiological Practice in Late Victorian Britain', *Journal of the History of Medicine and Allied Sciences* 65: 514–45.

Steinitz, Lesley (2017), 'The Language of Advertising: Fashioning Health Consumers at the *Fin de Siècle*', in Mary Addyman, Laura Wood and Christopher Yiannitsaros (eds), *Food, Drink, and the Written Word in Britain, 1820–1945*, 135–63, London: Routledge.

Stepan, Nancy Leys (2001), *Picturing Tropical Nature*, Ithaca, NY: Cornell University Press.

Stern, Alexandra Minna (2006), 'Yellow Fever Crusade: US Colonialism, Tropical Medicine, and the International Politics of Mosquito Control, 1900–1920', in Alison Bashford (ed.), *Medicine at the Border: Disease, Globalization and Security, 1850 to the Present*, 41–59, New York: Palgrave.

Stiles, Anne (2012), *Popular Fiction and Brain Science*, Cambridge: Cambridge University Press.

Stiles, Anne, Stanley Finger and Francois Boller (eds) (2013), *Literature, Neurology and Neuroscience: Historical and Literary Connections*, Oxford: Elsevier.

Stirling, Jeannette (2010), 'Hystericity and hauntings: the female and the feminised', in *Representing Epilepsy: Myth and Matter*, Liverpool: Liverpool University Press.

Stocking, George (1991), *Victorian Anthropology*, New York: Simon and Schuster.

Stoddard, Charles William (1912), 'A Bit of Old China', in *In the Footsteps of the Padres*, new edn, 123–43, San Francisco: A.M. Robertson.

Storie, Elizabeth (1859), *Autobiography of Elizabeth Storie, a narrative of Glasgow, who was subjected to much injustice at the hands of some members of the medical, legal and clerical professions*, Reel 12, Working Class Autobiographies, British Library microfilm.

Stowe, Steven (2004), *Doctoring the South: Southern Physicians and Everyday Medicine in the Mid-Nineteenth Century*, Chapel Hill: University of North Carolina Press.

Strange, Julie-Marie (2005), *Death, Grief and Poverty in Britain, 1870–1914*, Cambridge: Cambridge University Press.

Sturdy, Harriet and William Parry-Jones (1999), 'Boarding-out insane patients: the significance of the Scottish system 1857–1913', in Peter Bartlett and David Wright (eds), *Outside the Walls of the Asylum: The History of Care in the Community, 1750–2000*, 86–114, London: Athlone.

Sturdy, S. (2007), 'Scientific Method for Medical Practitioners: The Case Method of Teaching Pathology in Early Twentieth-Century Edinburgh', *Bulletin for the History of Medicine* 81, no. 4: 760–92.

Sturdy, S. (2011), 'Looking for Trouble: Medical Science and Clinical Practice in the Historiography of Modern Medicine', *Social History of Medicine* 24, no. 3: 739–57.

Sugaya, Norioki (2010), *Flaubert Épistémologue: Autour du Dossier Médical de Bouvard et Pécuchet*, Amsterdam: Rodopi.

Suzuki, Akihito (2003), 'The state, the family, and the insane in Japan, 1900–1945', in Roy Porter and David Wright (eds), *The Confinement of the Insane: International Perspectives, 1800–1965*, 193–225, Cambridge: Cambridge University Press.

Suzuki, Akihito (2006), *Madness at Home: The Psychiatrist, the Patient and the Family in England, 1820–1860*, Oakland: University of California Press.

Swartz, Sally (1995), 'The Black Insane in the Cape, 1891–1920', *Journal of Southern African Studies* 21, no. 3: 399–415.

Sweet, Ryan (2017), '"Get the best article in the market": prostheses for women in nineteenth-century literature and commerce", in Claire L. Jones (ed.), *Rethinking Modern Prostheses in Anglo-American Commodity Cultures, 1820–1939*, 114–36, Manchester: Manchester University Press.

Szreter, Simon (2014), 'The prevalence of syphilis in England and Wales on the eve of the Great War: re-visiting the estimates of the Royal Commission on Venereal Diseases 1913–1916', *Social History of Medicine* 27, no. 3: 508–29.

Taithe, Bertrand (1999), 'The Rise and Fall of European Syphilisation: The Debates on Human Experimentation and Vaccination of Syphilis', in F. X. Eder, L. Hall and G. Hekma, *Sexual Cultures in Europe: Themes in Sexuality*, 2, 34–77, Manchester: Manchester University Press, 1999.

Taithe, Bertrand (2001), *Citizenship and Wars: France in Turmoil 1870–1871*, London: Routledge.

Taylor, Jesse Oak (2016), *The Sky of Our Manufacture: The London Fog in British Fiction from Dickens to Woolf*, Charlottesville: University of Virginia Press.

Teigen, P. (1984), 'William Osler and Comparative Medicine', *Canadian Veterinary Journal* 25: 400–5.

Teuteberg, H. J. (2007), 'The Birth of the Modern Consumer Age: Food Innovations from 1800', in Paul Freedman (ed.), *Food: The History of Taste*, 232–61, Berkeley and Los Angeles: University of California Press.

Thibert, Félix (1844), *Musée d'anatomie pathologique: bibliothèque de médecine et de chirurgie pratiques représentant en relief les altérations morbides du corps humain*, Paris: C.H. Lambert.

Thompson, E. P. (1966), *The Making of the English Working Class*, New York: Vintage Books.

Thompson, Emily (2004), *The Soundscape of Modernity: Architectural Acoustics and the Culture of Listening in America*, Cambridge, MA: MIT Press.

Thomson, Mathew (2006), *Psychological Subjects: Identity, Culture and Health in Twentieth Century Britain*, Oxford: Oxford University Press.

Thorsheim, Peter (2006), *Inventing Pollution: Coal, Smoke, and Culture in Britain since 1800*, Athens, OH: Ohio University Press.

The Times (1849), 22 October: 4.

Timmermann, Carsten and Julie Anderson (eds) (2006), *Devices and Designs: Medical Technologies in Historical Perspective*, London: Palgrave Macmillan.

Tomes, Nancy (1984), *The Art of Asylum-Keeping: Thomas Story Kilbride and the Origins of American Psychiatry*, Cambridge: Cambridge University Press.

Tomes, N. (1998), *The Gospel of Germs: Men, Women and the Microbe in American Life*, Cambridge, MA: Harvard University Press.

Tooley, Henry (1823), *History of the Yellow Fever: As it Appeared in the City of Natchez, in the Months of August, September & October, 1823, second edition*, Washington, MS: Andrew Marschalk; National Library of Medicine, http://resource.nlm.nih.gov/2575026R.

Trachtenberg, Alan (1982), *The Incorporation of American Culture and Society in the Gilded Age*, New York: Hill and Wang.

Transactions of the Odontological Society (1856–89).

Transactions of the Pathological Society of London (1846–81).

Treitel, Corinna (2007) 'Food Science/Food Politics: Max Rubner and "Rational Nutrition" in Fin-de-Siecle', in Peter Lummel, Peter J. Atkins and Derek J. Oddy (eds), *Food and the City in Europe since 1800*, 51–62, Aldershot and Burlington, VT: Ashgate.

Trentman, Frank (2004), 'Beyond Consumerism: New Historical Perspectives on Consumption', *Journal of Contemporary History* 39, no. 3: 373–401.

Tristan, Flora, 'London Prostitutes, 1839', in John Carey (ed.), *Eyewitness to History*, 310–13, New York: Avon Books.

Truax, R. (1952), *The Doctors Jacobi*, Boston: Little, Brown and Company.

Tuells, J. (2002), 'Francisco Xavier Balmis (1753–1819), a pioneer of international vaccination', *Journal of Epidemiology and Community Health* 56: 802.

Tuells, J. and S. M. R. Martin (2011), 'Francisco Xavier Balmis y las Juntas de Vacuna, un ejemplo pionero para implementar la vacunación', *Salud pública de México* 53: 172–7.

Tuke, Samuel (1813), *Description of the Retreat, an institution near York, for insane persons of the Society of Friends*, Philadelphia: Isaac Peirce.

Tuke, Samuel (1815), *Practical Hints on the Construction and Economy of Pauper Lunatic Asylums*, York: William Alexander.

Turner, James (1980), *Reckoning with the Beast*, Baltimore, MD: Johns Hopkins University Press.

Twohig, Peter (2005), *Labour in the Laboratory: Medical Laboratory Workers in the Maritimes*, Montreal: McGill-Queens University Press.

Ueyama, Takahiro (2010), *Health in the Marketplace: Professionalism, Therapeutic Desires, and Medical Commodification in Late-Victorian London*, California: Society for the Promotion of Science and Scholarship.

United Kingdom, Parliament (1866a), *First Report of the Commissioners Appointed to Inquire into the Origin and Nature, &c. of the Cattle Plague, Cd. 3591*, London: Stationary Office.

United Kingdom, Parliament (1866b), *Second Report of the Commissioners Appointed to Inquire into the Origin and Nature, &c. of the Cattle Plague, Cd. 6000*, London: Stationary Office.

United Kingdom, Parliament (1866c), *Third Report of the Commissioners Appointed to Inquire into the Origin and Nature, &c. of the Cattle Plague, Cd. 3656*, London: Stationary Office.

United Kingdom Parliament (1876), *Report of the Royal Commission on the Practice of Subjecting Live Animals to Experiments for Scientific Purposes, C. 1397*, London: Stationary Office.

United States Patent and Trademark Office (1912), *U.S. Patent no. 1021146*, http://pdfpiw.uspto.gov.

Valentine, Gill and Ruth Butler (1999), 'The Alternative Fairy Story: Diana and the Sexual Dissidents', *Journal of Gender Studies* 8, no. 3: 295–302.

Valenze, Deborah M. (2011), *Milk: A Local and Global History*, New Haven, CT: Yale University Press.

van Bergen, Leo (1999/2004), '"The Malingerers are to Blame": The Dutch Military Health Service before and during the First World War', in Roger Cooter, Mark Harrison and Steve Sturdy (eds), *Medicine and Modern Warfare, 59–76*, Amsterdam: Rodopi.

van Bergen, L. (2009), *Before My Helpless Sight: Suffering, Dying and Military Medicine on the Western Front, 1914–1918*, Amsterdam: Rodopi.

Vaughan, Megan (1991), *Curing their Ills: Colonial Power and African Illness*, Stanford: CA: Stanford University Press.

Veale, Lucy (2010), 'An Historical Geography of the Nilgiri Cinchona Plantations, 1860–1900', PhD diss., University of Nottingham.

Vernon, James (2007), *Hunger: A Modern History*, Cambridge, MA: Belknap.

Virdi, Jaipreet (2020) , *Hearing Happiness: Deafness Cures in History*, Chicago and London: University of Chicago Press.

Waddington, Ivan (1984), *The Medical Profession in the Industrial Revolution*, Dublin: Gill and Macmillan.

Waddington, Keir (2003), '"Unfit for Human Consumption": Tuberculosis and the Problem of Infected Meat in Late Victorian Britain', *Bulletin of the History of Medicine* 77, no. 3: 636–61.

Waddington, Keir (2012), '"We Don't Want Any German Sausages Here!" Food, Fear, and the German Nation in Victorian and Edwardian Britain', *Journal of British Studies* 52, no. 4: 1017–42.

Walkowitz, J. R. (1980), *Prostitution and Victorian Society: Women, Class and the State*, Cambridge: Cambridge University Press.

Wall, L. L. (2006), 'The medical ethics of Dr J Marion Sims: a fresh look at the historical record', *Journal of Medical Ethics* 32: 346–50.

Wallace, Alfred Russel (1898), *Vaccination A Delusion, Its Penal Enforcement A Crime*, London: Swan Sonnenschein.

Wallis, Jennifer (2017), *Investigating the Body in the Victorian Asylum: Madness in the Flesh*, London: Palgrave Macmillan.

Walsh, Stephen (2003), *Stravinsky: A Creative Spring: Russia and France, 1882–1934*, Berkeley: University of California Press.

Walshe, Walter Hayle (1846), *The Nature and Treatment of Cancer*, London: Taylor and Walton.

Warner, John Harley (1986), *The Therapeutic Perspective: Medical Practice, Knowledge and Identity in America, 1820–1885*, Princeton, NJ: Princeton University Press.

Warner, John Harley (1998), 'Orthodoxy and Otherness: Homeopathy and Regular Medicine in Nineteenth-Century America', in Robert Jütte, Guether B. Risse and

John Woodward (eds), *Culture, Knowledge, and Healing: Historical Perspectives of Homeopathic Medicine in Europe and North America*, 5–29, Amsterdam: Rodopi.

Warner, John Harley (2003), *Against the Spirit of System: The French Impulse in Nineteenth-Century American Medicine*, Baltimore, MD: Johns Hopkins University Press.

Warner, John Harley (2014), 'The Fielding H. Garrison Lecture: The Aesthetic Grounding of Modern Medicine', *Bulletin of the History of Medicine* 88, no. 1: 1–47.

Warner, John Harley and James M. Edmondson (2009), *Dissection: Photographs of a Rite of Passage in American Medicine 1880–1930*, New York: Blast Books.

Warner Osborn, Matthew (2014), *Rum Maniacs: Alcoholic Insanity in the Early American Republic*, Chicago: University of Chicago Press.

Waters, Catherine (2008), *Commodity Culture in Dickens's Household Words: The Social Life of Goods*, Aldershot: Ashgate.

Watson, A. (2008), *Enduring the Great War: Combat, Morale, and Collapse in the German and British Armies, 1914–1918*, Cambridge: Cambridge University Press.

Watson, Janet (2004), *Fighting Different Wars: Experience, Memory, and the First World War in Britain*, Cambridge: Cambridge University Press.

Weaver, Lawrence T. (2010), '"Growing Babies": Defining the Milk Requirements of Infants 1890–1910', *Social History of Medicine* 2, no. 2: 320–37.

Weindling, Paul (1991), 'Bourgeois Values, Doctors and the State: The Professionalization of Medicine in Germany, 1848–1933', in David Blackbourn and Richard J. Evans (eds), *The German Bourgeoisie: Essays on the Social History of the German Middle Classes from the Late Eighteenth to the Early Twentieth Century*, 198–223, New York and London: Routledge.

Weiner, Dora B. (1994), 'Le geste de Pinel: The History of a Psychiatric Myth', in Mark S. Micale and Roy Porter (eds), *Discovering the History of Psychiatry*, 232–47, Oxford: Oxford University Press.

Weisz, George (1995), *The Medical Mandarins: The French Academy of Medicine in the Nineteenth and Early Twentieth Centuries*, Oxford: Oxford University Press.

Weisz, George (2003), 'The Emergence of Medical Specialization in the Nineteenth Century', *Bulletin of the History of Medicine* 77, no. 3: 536–74.

Weisz, George (2006), *Divide and Conquer: A Comparative History of Medical Specialization*, Oxford: Oxford University Press.

Weitzman, Ronald (1971), 'An introduction to Adorno's music and social criticism', *Music & Letters* 52, no. 3: 287–98.

Wells, Susan (2001), *Out of the Dead House: Nineteenth-Century Women Physicians and the Writing of Medicine*, Madison: University of Wisconsin Press.

Werrett, Simon (2013), 'Recycling in Early Modern Science', *British Journal for the History of Science* 46, part 4, no. 161: 627–46.

Werrett, Simon (2014), 'Matter and Facts: Material Culture in the History of Science', in Robert Chapman and Alison Wylie (eds), *Material Evidence: Learning from Archaeological Practice*, 339–52, New York: Routledge.

Werrett, Simon (2019), *Thrifty Science: Making the Most of Materials in the History of Experiment*, Chicago: University of Chicago Press.

Wessely, Simon (2003), 'Malingering: historical perspectives', in Peter W. Halligan, Christopher Bass and David A. Oakley (eds), *Malingering and Illness Deception*, 31–41, Oxford: Oxford University Press.

White, Anthony and Edzard Ernst (2004), 'A Brief History of Acupuncture', *Rheumatology* 43, no. 5: 662–3.

White, Paul (2006), 'Sympathy under the Knife: Experimentation and Emotion in Late Victorian Medicine', in Fay Bound Alberti (ed.), *Medicine, Emotion and Disease, 1700–1950*, 100–24, Basingstoke: Palgrave.

White, Paul (2009), 'Darwin's Emotions: The Scientific Self and the Sentiment of Objectivity', *Isis* 100: 811–26.

Whorton, James (2011), *The Arsenic Century: How Victorian Britain was Poisoned at Home, Work & Play*, Oxford: Oxford University Press.

Wilkinson, Lise (1992), *Animals and Disease: An Introduction to the History of Comparative Medicine*, Cambridge: Cambridge University Press.

Willenfelt, Johanna (2014), 'Documenting Bodies: Pain Surfaces', in Rob Boddice (ed.), *Pain and Emotion in Modern History*, 260–76, Basingstoke and New York: Palgrave Macmillan.

Williams, D. E (1976), 'Were "hunger" rioters really hungry', *Past & Present* 71, no. 1: 70–5.

Williams, W. Roger (1888), *The Principles of Cancer and Tumour Formation*, London: John Bale & Sons.

Willis, Martin (2006), 'Unmasking Immorality: Popular Opposition to Laboratory Science in Late Victorian Britain', in David Clifford et al. (eds), *Repositioning Victorian Sciences: Shifting Centres in Nineteenth-Century Scientific Thinking*, 207–18, London: Anthem Press.

Wilson, Elizabeth (1985), *Adorned in Dreams: Fashion and Modernity*, Los Angeles: University of California Press.

Wilson, Fiona (2004), 'Indian Citizenship and the Discourse of Hygiene/Disease in Nineteenth-Century Peru', *Bulletin of Latin American Research* 23, no. 2: 165–80.

Winter, Jay (2014), *Sites of Memory, Sites of Mourning: The Great War in European Cultural History*, Cambridge: Cambridge University Press.

Wise, M. Norton and Crosbie Smith (1990) 'Work and Waste: Political Economy and Natural Philosophy in Nineteenth-Century Britain (III)', *History of Science* 27, no. 3: 221–61.

Wolf, Jacqueline (2009), *Deliver Me from Pain: Anesthesia and Birth in America*, Baltimore, MD: Johns Hopkins University Press.

Woloshyn, Tania (2013), 'Le Pays du Soleil: The Art of Heliotherapy on the Côte d'Azur', *Social History of Medicine* 26, no. 1: 74–93.

Wood, Whitney (2014), '"When I Think of What is Before Me, I Feel Afraid": Narratives of Fear, Pain and Childbirth in Late Victorian Canada', in Rob Boddice (ed.), *Pain and Emotion in Modern History*, 187–203, Basingstoke and New York: Palgrave Macmillan.

Woods, Abigail (2013), 'From Practical Men to Scientific Experts: British Veterinary Surgeons and the Development of Government Scientific Expertise, c.1878–1919', *History of Science* 51: 457–80.

Woods, Abigail (2016), 'Animals and Disease', in Mark Jackson (ed.), *Routledge History of Disease*, 147–64, London: Routledge.

Woods, Abigail (2017), 'Animals in the History of Human and Veterinary Medicine', in H. Kean and P. Howell (eds), *Routledge Companion to Animal–Human History*, 147–70, London: Routledge.

Woods, Abigail (2017), 'Animals in Surgery', in Thomas Schlich (ed.), *Handbook of the History of Surgery*, 115–31, Basingstoke: Palgrave Macmillan.

Woods, Abigail (2017), 'Doctors in the Zoo: Connecting Human and Animal Health in British Zoological Gardens, c1828–1890', in Abigail Woods, Michael Bresalier, Angela Cassidy and Rachel Mason Dentinger (eds), *One Health and its Histories:*

Animals and the Shaping of Modern Medicine, 27–69, Basingstoke: Palgrave Macmillan.

Woods, Abigail (2017), 'From Co-ordinated Campaigns to Water-Tight Compartments: Diseased Sheep and their Investigation in Britain, c.1880–1920', in Abigail Woods, Michael Bresalier, Angela Cassidy and Rachel Mason Dentinger (eds), *One Health and its Histories: Animals and the Shaping of Modern Medicine*, 71–117, Basingstoke: Palgrave Macmillan.

Woods, Abigail (2017), 'From One medicine to Two: The Evolving Relationship between Human and Veterinary Medicine in England, 1791–1835', *Bulletin of the History of Medicine* 91, no. 3: 494–523.

Woods, Abigail, Michael Bresalier, Angela Cassidy and Rachel Mason Dentinger (eds) (2017), *One Health and its Histories: Animals and the Shaping of Modern Medicine*, Basingstoke: Palgrave Macmillan.

Woodworth, John M. (1875), *The Cholera Epidemic of 1873 in the United States*, Washington, DC: Government Printing Office; National Library of Medicine, http://resource.nlm.nih.gov/64760840R.

Worboys, Michael (1991), 'Germ Theories of Disease and British Veterinary Medicine, 1860–1890', *Medical History* 35: 308–27.

Worboys, Michael (2000), *Spreading Germs: Disease Theories and Medical Practice in Britain 1865–1900*, Cambridge: Cambridge University Press.

Worth Estes, J. (1996), 'The Medical Properties of Food in the Eighteenth Century', *Journal of the History of Medicine and Allied Sciences* 51, no. 1: 127–54.

Wynter, Rebecca (2011), '"Good in all respects": appearance and dress at Staffordshire County Lunatic Asylum, 1818–1854', *History of Psychiatry* 22, no. 1: 40–57.

Wynter, Rebecca (2015), 'Horrible dens of deception: Thomas Bakewell, Thomas Mulock, and anti-asylum sentiments, c.1815–58', in Thomas Knowles and Serena Trowbridge (eds), *Insanity and the Lunatic Asylum in the Nineteenth Century*, 11–27, London: Pickering & Chatto.

Wynter, Rebecca (2015), 'Pictures of Peter Pan: Institutions, Local definitions of "Mental Deficiency", and the Filtering of Children in Early Twentieth-Century England', *Family and Community History* 18, no. 2: 122–38.

Youatt, William (1836), 'Comparative Pathology', *Veterinarian* 9: passim.

Young, Linda (2003), *Middle-Class Culture in the Nineteenth Century: America, Australia and Britain*, London: Palgrave.

Zimmerman, Andrew (2001), *Anthropology and Antihumanism in Imperial Germany*, Chicago and London: University of Chicago Press.

Zola, Émile (1880/1964), *The Naturalist Novel*, New York: Harvest House.

CONTRIBUTORS

Rob Boddice is Senior Research Fellow at the Academy of Finland Centre of Excellence in the History of Experiences. His recent books include *The History of Emotions* (2018), *A History of Feelings* (2019) and (with Mark Smith) *Emotion, Sense, Experience* (2020).

Michael Brown is Reader in History in the Department of Humanities at the University of Roehampton (UK). He works on the cultural history of medicine and surgery in the long nineteenth century as well as the histories of gender and war. He is the author of *Performing Medicine: Medical Culture and Identity in Provincial England, c.1760–1850* (2011), as well as a number of journal articles and book chapters. He is currently a Wellcome Trust Investigator in Medical Humanities and Social Sciences, leading a team investigating the relationships between surgery and emotion in Britain from 1800 to the present.

Stephen T. Casper is Associate Professor of History (Clarkson University, NY) and Associate Director of the Clarkson Honors Program. He is an historian of the mind and brain sciences and has published extensively on the history of neurology, psychiatry, neuroscience and critical neuroscience. His latest volume (co-edited with Delia Gavrus) is *The History of the Brain and Mind Sciences: Technique, Technology, Therapy* (2017). He is current writing a monograph, tentatively entitled *Punch Drunk and Dementia: A Modern History of Concussion, 1870 to 2012.*

Vanessa Heggie is a lecturer in the History of Science and Medicine at the University of Birmingham (UK). She has published widely on a range of topics relating to nineteenth- and twentieth-century history of medicine and science, from district visiting in Victorian Britain to sex testing in modern sporting events. Her most recent book is *Higher and Colder: A History of Extreme Physiology and Exploration* (forthcoming).

Catherine Kelly is a Reader in Law at the University of Bristol. She holds degrees in Law (ANU) and History (Oxford). Her research focuses on the law's interaction with science and medicine in both historical and contemporary contexts. Catherine has previously been awarded a Harold White Fellowship at the National Library of Australia, a Caird Short-Term Research Fellowship at the National Maritime Museum, and from 2005 to 2008 held the Clifford Norton Studentship in the History of Science at The Queen's College, Oxford. She is the author of *War and the Militarization of British Army Medicine, 1793–1830* (2011), as well as a number of journal articles and book chapters.

Anna Maerker is Senior Lecturer in the History of Medicine at King's College London. Her work on the material culture of science and medicine, and on public history, includes the monograph *Model Experts: Wax Anatomies and Enlightenment in Florence and Vienna, 1775–1815* (2011) and the co-edited work *History, Memory and Public Life: The Past in the Present* (2018), with Adam Sutcliffe and Simon Sleight.

Matthew Newsom Kerr is Associate Professor of History at Santa Clara University, California. He is author of *Contagion, Isolation, and Biopolitics in Victorian London* (2018), as well as a number of articles that examine the politics and culture of nineteenth-century public health.

Jonathan Reinarz is Professor of the History of Medicine at the University of Birmingham (UK), and past-President of the European Association for the History of Medicine and Health (2017–19). He has published widely on the history of medicine, including hospitals, medical education and the senses over the period covered by this volume. His current research, funded by the AHRC (UK), examines the history of burns injuries in Britain, 1800–2000.

Bertrand Taithe is Professor of Cultural History at the University of Manchester. He is a founding member and executive director of the Humanitarian and Conflict Response Institute at Manchester and has been editor of the *European Review of History – Revue européenne d'histoire* since 1994. He has published extensively on the history of poverty, medicine and war, and the history of humanitarianism.

Abigail Woods is Professor of the History of Human and Animal Health and Head of the Department of History at King's College London. She recently completed a five-year Wellcome Trust-funded programme of research on the interlinked histories of human and animal health in modern Britain. This gave rise to the volume (co-authored with Michael Bresalier, Angela Cassidy and Rachel Mason Dentinger) *One Health and its Histories: Animals and the Shaping of Modern Medicine* (2017).

Rebecca Wynter is Postdoctoral Research Fellow on 'Forged by Fire: Burns Injury and Identity in Britain, *c.*1800–2000', funded by the AHRC, and Lecturer in History at the Centre for Research in Quaker Studies (University of Birmingham and Woodbrooke, Birmingham). She is Roy Porter Prize Chair for the Society for the Social History of Medicine, and Reviews Editor for *Quaker Studies*. Rebecca has published on the histories of psychiatry, mental health, neurology, ambulance and First World War medicine. Her latest book, co-edited with Pink Dandelion, is *A Quaker Conscientious Objector: The Prison Letters of Wilfrid Littleboy, 1917–1919* (2020).

INDEX